www.harcourt-international.com

Bringing you products from all Harcourt Health Sciences companies including Baillière Tindall, Churchill Livingstone, Mosby and W.B. Saunders

- ▶ **Browse** for latest information on books, journals and electronic products

- ▶ **Search** for information on over 20 000 published titles with full product information including tables of contents and sample chapters

- ▶ **Keep up to date** with our extensive publishing programme in your field by registering with eAlert or requesting postal updates

- ▶ **Secure online ordering** with prompt delivery, as well as full contact details to order by phone, fax or post

- ▶ **News** of special features and promotions

If you are based in the following countries, please visit the country-specific site to receive full details of product availability and local ordering information

USA: www.harcourthealth.com

Canada: www.harcourtcanada.com

Australia: www.harcourt.com.au

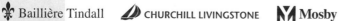 Baillière Tindall   CHURCHILL LIVINGSTONE   Mosby   W.B. SAUNDERS

Kohai Educational Centre
41 Roehampton Avenue,
Toronto, Ontario, M4P 1P9

Psychiatric Drugs Explained

For Churchill Livingstone:

Senior Commissioning Editor: Jacqueline Curthoys
Project Manager: Jane Dingwall
Design Direction: Judith Wright

Psychiatric Drugs Explained

THIRD EDITION

David Healy MD FRCPsych

Director
North Wales Department of Psychological Medicine
University of Wales
College of Medicine
Bangor
UK

Foreword by

Cedric Knight

Independent Newham Users' Forum
London
UK

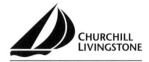

CHURCHILL
LIVINGSTONE

EDINBURGH LONDON NEW YORK PHILADELPHIA ST LOUIS SYDNEY TORONTO 2002

Second edition 1997
Third edition 2002

ISBN 0 443 07018 0

British Library Cataloguing in Publication Data
A catalogue record for this book is available from the British Library

Library of Congress Cataloging in Publication Data
A catalog record for this book is available from the Library of
Congress

Note
Medical knowledge is constantly changing. As new information
becomes available, changes in treatment, procedures, equipment and
the use of drugs become necessary. The author and the publishers
have, as far as it is possible, taken care to ensure that the information
given in this text is accurate and up to date. However, readers are
strongly advised to confirm that the information, especially with
regard to drug usage, complies with the latest legislation and
standards of practice.

The
publisher's
policy is to use
**paper manufactured
from sustainable forests**

Printed in China

Contents

Foreword

About the closest I have ever been to a medical qualification was recently playing the role of psychiatrist on stage, performing with a group of other survivors and users of mental health services. It was a short scene, designed to illustrate the gulf in understanding between doctor and patient, and the dominance of medication issues in mental health.

The portrayal was meant to be an over-the-top caricature based on a few bad encounters but, alarmingly, many people later commented how realistic it was. As it was an *avant garde* kind of play, I was to ask the audience as to what I as the psychiatrist should do with my 'difficult' patient. Suggestions included 'Change the medication', 'Take the medication yourself', 'Give him a hug', and most simply, 'Listen to him'. It was surprisingly easy to justify the doctor's appalling behaviour, and I realised that he was a product of his circumstances as much as the patient was.

A major factor preventing transparency and proper listening (besides the regular invalidation of anyone with a mental health diagnosis) must be the frequency of corporately-sponsored campaigns to increase 'compliance' with medication. These mention various strategies, including, apparently benignly, providing information leaflets. However, that such information is given to the end of changing behaviour, rather than as a natural right, may cause one to be suspicious of the information. The prescribing and taking of medication appears to a detached observer almost to be an end in itself. Letters in journals even admonish that the effect of publishing certain research will be that 'misinformation, fear, and apathy may result in the avoidance of effective treatment', which is hardly scientific and certainly patronising to those who ostensibly benefit.

Fortunately, with the help of a good library (and to a lesser extent the internet), it is possible for determined users to read the primary sources. In my own recovery from mental distress, I would go as far as to say that understanding the 'treatments' was far more helpful than the treatments themselves. Not everyone has the time to do this, so it is a useful part of 'self-management' for users and carers to be pointed (by professionals or self-help groups) to relevant sections of an established reference like *Psychiatric Drugs Explained.*

The author, David Healy, is unusual in psychiatry in that he retains a sociological and historical view of the subject. Having hindsight is important not only in understanding the roots of current practice and the serendipitous discovery of many drugs, but also in recognising the failure of medical institutions in the past to respond appropriately to, say, tardive dyskinesia or benzodiazepine dependence. Wariness of probable new abuses is one of many reasons that public policy makers increasingly look to the user movement for guidance.

I find it significant that when the philosopher Michel Foucault was investigating the historical relationship between knowledge and power, he first chose to critique, of all the possible areas of human endeavour, psychiatry. *Histoire de la folie* was an influence on the 'antipsychiatry' movement, but more importantly gave rise to some of the ideas now called 'postmodernism'. Postmodernists often argue against the very possibility of scientific impartiality and regard public health as no less subjective and politically charged than policing. It is true there are problems in attempting to objectify human mental states, in deciding whose objectification you go with. For example, saying someone is suicidal and melancholic may be less helpful than saying she is bullied and belittled by her husband and has no one to talk to. But to me, a postmodern view ultimately makes it hard to distinguish between helping someone and abusing them, as everything could be seen simultaneously as help and abuse.

Most of us, including those forced into scepticism by experience, are not going to give up on the possibility of scientific objectivity, of eventual convergence of our beliefs with the truth. Here we have all kinds of substances, from herbs and spices to phenylpiperazines and phenethylamines, that can have profound effects on mental states and bodily processes. The exact response may be highly individual and is often learned, but it clearly is a legitimate area for scientific investigation. Furthermore, in what area is it more important to eliminate external biases and ensure an impartial two-way flow of information, than in the overcoming of one's mental distress, which is difficult enough as it is?

This book attempts to encapsulate a range of common psychiatric viewpoints. Besides its lucidity and (relative) accessibility, many will find it useful because it restricts itself to what is actually known about psychiatric drugs. Conjectures are indicated as such. For example, there is little mention of the much-popularised theories that, because most neuroleptics and antidepressants lower dopamine activity or increase serotonin (5HT) activity respectively (among many other effects), psychosis and depression must therefore involve abnormally high dopamine or low serotonin. Combining experience with many hours poring over journals, I personally concluded such theories were fallacious.

Dr Healy is also well known for his involvement in psychopharmacological controversies. One is in emphasising the continued association, first publicised by Martin Teicher of Harvard and others, between the 'SSRI antidepressants' and suicide, when compared to older drugs. In short, one view suggests that someone on an SSRI for a year has a one in a thousand excess risk of suicide compared to someone with untreated depression. This would add up to a bigger, if less visible, drug tragedy than thalidomide. The point that this effect is independent of any pre-existing depression (just like the point that the dependence issues with the same drugs are physical, not psychological) is percolating through the psychiatric and regulatory institutions only with agonising slowness. The way to resolve a controversy like this is obviously through further research, yet, astonishingly, there have been no studies to test the association with fluoxetine explicitly.

The second controversy is to suggest that despite these increased risks, the same drugs should be available without prescription. I am not yet convinced, although over-the-counter status would target those who *themselves* judge the benefits outweigh any adverse reactions. Further, by obviating disabling psychiatric labels, such moves might help break down the subjective barriers between 'normal' (I understand this, so it is not a problem) and 'abnormal' (I do not understand this, so it should be treated), without invalidating the decades of research into psychoactive drugs summarised here.

2001   Cedric Knight

Preface

The first edition of this book started from a set of consensus statements that I helped to draw up in 1990, along with other members of the Aberconwy mental health team. This team includes community nurses, social workers, a clinical psychologist and doctors. Our interest was to produce consensus statements about how both antipsychotics and antidepressants work, so that an individual encountering different members of the team would not get contradictory views on these drugs. Our hunch at the time was that most people can assimilate and handle far more information about their condition and its treatment than they are ordinarily given credit for. Nothing I have seen in the 10 years since has persuaded me to the contrary.

Since 1990, events would appear to be moving in this direction. All medicines now include information inserts, which, although commonly constructed with one eye on protecting the legal position of the company making the medicine, are nevertheless a step forward. In America, pharmaceutical companies have begun to advertise directly to consumers – this is less clearly a step forward but can be seen as part of a general trend that will pull the consumers of medication into the process of managing their own conditions. A number of other medicines that were formerly available only on prescription are now on sale over the counter. If H_2-blocking agents can be sold in this way, there seems little reason why the selective serotonin reuptake inhibitors (SSRIs) could not be made similarly available. The consequences for the 'mental health marketplace' of such a switch might be quite dramatic. Only recently, a change of this nature would have been inconceivable, but now it may be only a matter of a few years away. Should it happen, the role of therapists will be much more clearly to advise rather than to prescribe (i.e. to order).

The larger picture in which the prescription and consumption of medicines takes place is therefore changing. The fine print of available drugs is also changing. The SSRIs had appeared when the first edition of this book was published, but Prozac had not yet become the media phenomenon it subsequently became. There is now a post-SSRI generation of antidepressants and a post-clozapine generation of antipsychotics. In other areas there has been the increasing use of sodium valproate and other anticonvulsants for bipolar disorders and the appearance of new agents for dementias and sexual dysfunction. There have been other developments as well. Dependence on psychotropic drugs, for instance, has been more clearly mapped than before.

In revising this book – as in writing it in the first place – I have accumulated a growing list of people to whom I owe a debt, including Ian Rickard, Ian Murray, Robin Holden, Colin Peters, Jane Hollywood, Jeanne Hughes,

Rebecca Sykes, John Harlow, Adrian Pugh, Anne Hall, Hilary Yeadon, Pat Corns, Ruth Allerhand, Barry Broadmeadow, Bill White, Louise Doughty, Julia Pook, Gwyneth Jones, Tony Roberts, Kate Fitzgerald, Brian Williams, Phil Thomas, David King, Brian Leonard and many others.

I also owe a great deal to colleagues from the pharmaceutical industry, including Brian Tiplady, Roger Pindar, George Beaumont, Peter Waldmeier and others. Many of the ideas that I put forward in the various chapters of this book have been very heavily influenced by these contacts. These colleagues, rather than I, have provided many of the criticisms of the industry and many of the examples that I use to illustrate potential problems associated with the commercialisation of psychotropic compounds. There are two points to take out of this. One is that, while it is relatively easy to paint a dark picture of the pharmaceutical industry where psychotropic medication is concerned, many of those who work within the industry are aware of the problems and take a responsible attitude towards them. It would be a mistake to think that the psychopharmaceutical industry is somehow the repository of all problems to do with mental health and that the prescribers and takers of drugs are innocent parties to what is done to them.

The truth is more complex. The medical profession cannot escape blame for many of the problems produced by psychotropic prescribing. But, equally, as Sir William Osler at the end of the 19th century remarked before the modern pharmaceutical industry had been established, one of the most characteristic features of human beings, compared with other animals, lies in their propensity to self-medicate. We are inveterate takers of compounds aimed at adjusting our internal equilibrium or balance – first this way and then that way. This is a process we've been at for millennia with various herbs, potions, compresses, purgatives and emetics – a process from which health food stores now profit. The significance of the contemporary position is that this process has become much more regulated and structured than it ever was before, and our automatic access to available compounds has been curtailed. An increasingly large industrial enterprise has geared itself up to supply our needs and, in the process, this enterprise has commandeered the science that can be extracted from our attempts to regulate our internal balance.

Herein lies a potential problem. It is one thing to restrict the use of drugs. It is quite another thing to restrict information about drugs. While, clearly, there is no censor of drug information, in practice the 'system' operates at almost every turn to frustrate an individual's access to the information they need to make the decisions that they – and no one else – should be making about their life. I see the information in this book as the bare minimum that people taking psychotropic drugs need to inform their choices; it should not be seen as an effort to push at the boundaries of what information people should have access to.

This edition of this book includes a set of User Issue boxes throughout. These represent something of a return to the original inspiration for the book, which was heavily oriented towards users.

David Healy

Abbreviations

AAMI	age-associated memory impairment
ACE	angiotensin-converting enzyme
ACh	acetylcholine
ADH	antidiuretic hormone
ADHD	attention-deficit hyperactivity disorder
BZ	benzodiazepine (receptor)
cGMP	cyclic guanosine monophosphate
CPAP	continuous positive airways pressure
D	dopamine (receptor)
DNA	deoxyribonucleic acid
DSM-III	Diagnostic and Statistical Manual for Mental Disorders, 3rd edition
ECT	electroconvulsive therapy
FDA	Food and Drug Administration
GABA	γ-aminobutyric acid
GAD	generalised anxiety disorder
GTN	glyceryl trinitrate
5HT	5-hydroxytryptamine
LSD	lysergic acid diethylamide
MAOI	monoamine oxidase inhibitor
MID	multi-infarct dementia
MRC	Medical Research Council
NMD	N-methyl-D-aspartate
NMS	neuroleptic malignant syndrome
OCD	obsessive–compulsive disorder
OTC	over the counter
PDE	phosphodiesterase
PTSD	post-traumatic stress disorder
RCT	randomised clinical trial
REM	rapid eye movement
RTA	road traffic accident
S	serotonin (receptor)
SAQ	self-assessment questionnaire
SDAT	senile dementia of the Alzheimer type
SDLT	senile dementia of the Lewy body type
SSRI	selective serotonin reuptake inhibitor
THA	tetrahydroaminoacridine
tPA	tissue plasminogen activator

Introduction

There are typically three parties to the act of taking any psychotropic drug: the taker, the prescriber and the company that produces and markets the drug. All three are bound up by the history of our attitudes to psychological problems, to psychotropic drug taking and to the processes of industrialization taking place both within the pharmaceutical industry and within medicine. All three are also shaped by changing attitudes in society at large, one of which involves an increasing awareness of the rights of the individual, included in which is a right to information about treatments they may be given.

These forces have conspired in recent years to bring about the production of handbooks about drugs, which cover their mode of action, their potential benefits and their possible side effects. However, such handbooks have consisted mostly of lists of drugs with bold statements of reputed modes of action and comprehensive lists of side effects. These give little flavour of how the drugs concerned may interfere with individual functioning or impinge on individual well-being.

One of the aims of this book, in contrast to these others, is to produce a text that will make the issues live. To this end, there is a lot of detail about the history of different drugs. On the question of what the various drugs do, both current thinking and current confusions are outlined. Too much certainty is, I believe, the enemy of both progress and science. And apparent academic certainty tends to invalidate the perceptions of a drug taker – who is actually one of the individuals best placed to contribute to the further development of psychopharmacology.

I have also included an attempt to assess the influence of the pharmaceutical industry on the perceptions of both clinicians and patients.

More importantly, rather than simply give a list of benefits and side effects, I have attempted to give a fuller description of what the experience of the side effects may be like and how these impinge on normal living. Trying to put some flesh on the bare bones of a list of side effects means that I have had to compromise between being comprehensive and being significant. Readers should be aware that this book does not include every known side effect. It does not include precise figures as to the frequency of each side effect. It does not include all known interactions with other compounds. What it does include are the reactions and interactions that occur regularly, and the book attempts to give some feel for how important or otherwise these are.

What emerges, nevertheless, is a list of side effects that in many respects is rather fearsome – to add to a set of motives on the part of both prescribers and the pharmaceutical industry that are often venal. Many of my colleagues will wonder whether taking this course of action is advisable. I have a number of reasons for thinking it is.

CONSUMERS AND COMPLIANCE

The final arbiter of whether psychotropic medication is useful or not is the taker. The taking of any psychiatric drug involves a trade-off between the benefits the drug confers and the risks it entails. Until recently, prescribers have been accustomed to making this trade-off for those for whom they prescribe. In general medicine, where respiratory or cardiac function is concerned, this is often the only possible course of action. But where psychotropic drugs are concerned, this is not the only option and – arguably – is not the best option.

In psychiatry, prescribers often moan about non-compliance with the regimens they prescribe. In the absence of any systematic work on why the takers of the drugs we prescribe are non-compliant, the vacuum tends to be filled with a vague view that patient recalcitrance amounts almost to a culpable or moral failing. It seems that we rarely stop to appreciate that anyone worth their salt is going to think seriously about continuing treatments with medications that may obliterate their sex life, make them suicidal or generally make them feel worse than they were before they began treatment. There have always been prescribers sensitive to issues like this. But there have also been far too many of us who, when faced with complaints about the medications we have prescribed, have tended almost reflexly to increase the dose of what has been prescribed or to add some antidote to counteract the side effects of the first prescription, rather than to listen carefully to the substance of the complaint.

We are taking a tremendous burden on ourselves in proceeding this way. But, more importantly, in doing so we neglect the services of a group of potential mental health workers whose services come for free – our patients. Fully informing the client of the nature of the compounds, of their potential benefits and equally of their limitations and side effects, and of the available alternatives, at the very least would have the merit of deflecting legal criticism. More importantly, however, it has the potential benefit of enlisting the takers of psychotropic drugs in the enterprise of handling their own condition, regarding which they may often be uniquely sensitive.

INDIVIDUAL END-POINTS

The reason for this latter claim is that, where drugs are concerned, one person's cure may be another's poison. My first awareness of this came from a very simple practical exercise, almost 30 years ago in medical school. A group of 10 of us were given a beta-blocker to take. This should slow the heart rate, and it did – for nine of us – but one of the group had a marked increase in heart rate. This suggested that she was 'wired up' differently to the rest of us.

A few years later the lesson was brought home again in a study giving clonidine to some colleagues. Clonidine lowers the concentration of noradrenaline in the bloodstream, and in the group as a whole it clearly did so, but in 20% of those investigated it produced an increase.

In the central nervous system, where there is a multiplicity of receptors for each drug to act on, and where all of us have different proportions of each of these, the likelihood of a uniform response to any one drug is rather low. A diversity of responses, rather than uniformity, should be expected. Nevertheless, in practice prescribers tend to operate as though uniform responses were the norm. It is emerging that in some cases this inflexibility may be fatal. Where psychological problems are concerned, however, we traditionally have had the escape route of blaming the undesirable behaviour of our patients – such as their killing themselves because the drugs we prescribe make them feel worse – on the neurosis or irrationality that brought them for treatment in the first instance. This avenue of escape – blaming the patient – is one we should be reluctant to adopt.

PHARMACOPSYCHOLOGY

There is another reason for taking this approach, which is that the takers of psychotropic drugs are potentially engaged in a scientific experiment every time they consume a prescribed medication. By treating psychotropic drugs just like any other group of drugs, most books manage to obscure the scientific drama involved.

At the end of the 19th century, when the first psychoactive agents became available, Emil Kraepelin coined a name for the study of the effects of these drugs on psychological functioning: pharmacopsychology. The current term is psychopharmacology. The difference between these two terms indicates a major shift in the thinking that has taken place over the course of the last 100 years, a shift that to some extent needs to be reversed today to restore balance to the field.

Psychopharmacology today is science concerned with discovering the receptors that psychoactive drugs bind to, the levels they achieve in the brain and the benefits that these drugs offer to hospital services or general practitioners in reducing the disruption caused by psychological problems, or the frequency of attendance of individuals with mental health problems.

Pharmacopsychology, in contrast, as conceived by Kraepelin, was a discipline that would concern itself with exploring the construction of the psyche by means of the use of drugs. Every taking of a psychoactive drug, from tea and coffee to alcohol or barbiturates, Kraepelin believed, could potentially reveal something about the way psychological operations function or about how the constituent parts of the psyche are put together.

This remains a legitimate scientific programme today. It has been suspended over the past 50 years, largely because of our reluctance to take at face value the verbal reports of individuals who take the drugs we prescribe. This reluctance has been engendered in part by behaviourist theories of psychology, which have in general ignored any so-called 'internal mental events'. It has been reinforced by the psychoanalytical approaches to psychological disorder, which have broadly proposed that there is no point in paying much heed to the obvious or face-value meanings of what individuals with psychological problems may say, as there would be no problem if their statements could be taken at face value. Finally, this reluctance has been supplemented by psychopharmacologists who, in trying to unravel the mysteries of the mechanisms of action of psychoactive compounds and of brain functioning, have in general paid little heed to the statements of the takers of these drugs, and have focused instead on the drugs as probes of physiological status.

However, even a biologically reductionist programme could have benefited significantly from paying more heed to the statements of psychotropic drug takers. For example, I believe, there could never have been a dopamine hypothesis of schizophrenia if the statements of individuals taking neuroleptics had been taken into account (see Ch. 1).

What seems to be needed today is the re-creation of a science of pharmacopsychology. Such a science would work closely with the takers of psychotropic drugs to determine what changes they experience on the compounds they take, in an effort to work back from those experiences to an understanding of how the mind works.

To this end, any readers of this book who themselves are taking psychotropic medication are encouraged to write to the author, if they have had experiences not covered by the present book, or if they can put into graphic or concrete terms what effect some drug has had on their lives – for better or for worse. Far from being simply material to add to a catalogue of side effects, such reports will contain valuable clues for future experimental investigation.

Management of the psychoses

SECTION CONTENTS

The antipsychotics

INTRODUCTION

Traditionally, three major categories of psychiatric illness have been described. These are schizophrenia, manic–depressive psychosis and a third group of disorders variously termed the paranoid, reactive or sensitive psychoses, which more recently have been called the delusional disorders.

Any appearances of diagnostic precision are misleading, however. Since the Second World War, there has been a tendency to label all serious psychiatric conditions as schizophrenia and the pharmacological management of serious conditions, in practice, reduces to the management of what is called schizophrenia (Healy 2001). In recent years, the concept of schizophrenia has been fragmenting. Disorders, such as borderline personality disorder and delusional disorder, have been distinguished from schizophrenia. This process is likely to continue with developments in pharmacogenetics and neuroimaging.

The management of schizophrenia has also reduced in the past 30 years to the clinical employment of a group of drugs once called the neuroleptics, now more often called antipsychotics, which have been supposed to be in some way specifically therapeutic for schizophrenia. The antipsychotics are a group of drugs of which chlorpromazine and haloperidol were among the original compounds, and clozapine and a number of what are called 'atypical antipsychotics' are now perhaps the most commonly prescribed. These drugs were once also called major tranquillisers, although they are certainly not tranquillisers, in the sense that diazepam (Valium) or chlordiazepoxide (Librium) are.

In practice, however, the antipsychotics are used for conditions such as mania and obsessive–compulsive disorder, as well as a range of severe anxiety states and even as hypnotics. Accordingly, there will also be references to the use of antipsychotics in the chapters on the management of both the affective disorders and anxiety. There is, furthermore, a place for the use of both benzodiazepines and psychostimulants in the management of schizophrenia or severe psychotic disturbances, which will be outlined in their respective sections.

One further point needs to be borne in mind. There has been considerable controversy over whether the antipsychotic drugs led to the emptying of the mental hospitals or whether this was happening before their introduction. This is not an issue that can be answered easily. There were, and almost certainly are, people whose lives have been transformed for the better by these drugs, but the availability of the drugs does something else: it engenders confidence and a willingness to take risks. The existence of this group of drugs provides a safety net, which has meant that some people have been talked to or discharged home who previously would have been left to vegetate in back wards. It is often not possible to tease apart contributions made by the drugs, the interaction or the discharge. The point is that no drug is ever given in isolation. The talking that goes with drug administration and the context in which it is given may be of critical importance (Healy 2001).

An example drawn from psychotherapy may highlight the issues. In the 1960s and 1970s, there was a vogue for token economy programmes in many

Table 1.1 The antipsychotics

Generic drug name	UK trade name	US trade name
First generation		
chlorpromazine	Largactil	Thorazine
flupentixol	Fluanxol/Depixol	–
zuclopenthixol	Clopixol	–
perphenazine	Fentazin	Trilafon
trifluoperazine	Stelazine	Stelazine
pericyazine	Neulactil	Neulactil
promazine	Sparine	–
loxapine	Loxitan/Loxapac	Loxitane
sulpiride	Sulpitil/Dolmatil/Sulparex	–
haloperidol	Serenace/Haldol/Dozic	Haldol
pimozide	Orap	Orap
fluphenazine	Moditen/Modecate	Moditen
molindone	–	Moban/Lidone
Second generation		
clozapine	Clozaril	Clozaril
risperidone	Risperdal	Risperdal
olanzapine	Zyprexa	Zyprexa
sertindole	Serdolect	–
quetiapine	Seroquel	Seroquel
ziprasidone	Zeldox	Zeldox
amisulpride	Solian	–
zotepine	Zoleptil	–

hospitals. Schemes were put in place whereby in return for 'good' behaviours patients would receive tokens, which they could then use to buy cigarettes or other benefits. It seemed to work. But did it do so because of the principles of learning theory involved, or because it forced patients and nursing staff to spend more time talking to one another, or because it offered patients some more control of their lives in wards that were heavily regulated? Today, there is interest in cognitive approaches for hallucinations and delusions – but do these work because of something new or because, hoping that they may work, we are encouraged to spend more time with patients?

The interaction between two human beings may be incredibly potent. The giving and taking of psychotropic drugs should be part of and should facilitate such interactions, rather than substitute for them.

Table 1.1 lists first- and second-generation antipsychotic drugs.

HISTORY OF THE ANTIPSYCHOTICS

Chlorpromazine, the first of the antipsychotics, was discovered in 1952. Its use for nervous disorders led on to the synthesis of the antidepressants, the anxiolytics and all other drugs now used for nervous problems. Despite this enormous effect on all our lives, no Nobel Prize was ever given for its discovery – owing to a bitter controversy over who discovered it. This controversy is relevant to the question of what these drugs do.

Chlorpromazine was first synthesised in 1950 with the intention of producing a centrally acting antihistamine for the control of cardiorespiratory shock and related conditions. In the course of its use as part of an anaesthetic cocktail in 1952, Henri Laborit, a surgeon, described a striking change in subjects who had taken it: they were not sedated in the usual way with anaesthetic agents, but rather appeared to become indifferent to what was going on around them. Laborit described this as an ataractic effect. It was visible within minutes of having had the drug and it came on in normal subjects.

In 1952, Jean Delay and Pierre Deniker reported that chlorpromazine was of benefit in controlling states of manic and psychotic agitation. There was no suggestion initially that chlorpromazine was likely in any way to be specific to schizophrenia. That came later. In the mid-1950s, chlorpromazine was being reported as being useful for almost every psychiatric condition (hence its European trade name Largactil – Large Action).

Laborit on the one side, and Delay and Deniker on the other, have contested the priority in the discovery of chlorpromazine. Taking sides in this dispute depends on whether you see the antipsychotics as being in some way curative of psychotic illness or as producing a more general anti-agitation effect in anyone who takes it, whether or not they have a psychological problem.

Within a few years of their use, it became clear that the new group of drugs produced extrapyramidal side effects, most notably parkinsonism. As further compounds came on stream, it seemed that only those that produced extrapyramidal effects brought about benefits in the psychoses. This led to two things. One was that the drugs as a group came to be called neuroleptics by Delay, a term that literally means 'nerve seizing'. This insight in turn led on to the dopamine hypothesis of schizophrenia. The second effect was that for 30 years little effort was put into finding antipsychotics that would not produce extrapyramidal effects – atypical antipsychotics, as such agents are now called. It is only in recent years with the rediscovery of clozapine, a drug almost devoid of extrapyramidal effects, that the picture is changing.

ARE ANTIPSYCHOTICS ANTISCHIZOPHRENIC?

The evidence that the antipsychotics are antischizophrenic comes from a series of studies showing that subjects who take them after discharge from hospital are much less likely to be readmitted than those who do not (Johnstone et al 1988). The dopamine hypothesis of schizophrenia was based on this kind of evidence. Briefly, this hypothesis states that as all antipsychotics block the dopamine system in the brain, and as they are beneficial in schizophrenia, there must be something wrong with the dopamine system in the brains of individuals with schizophrenia.

A major research enterprise then developed around attempts to test the dopamine hypothesis and to develop new drugs active on the dopamine system. From a sociological point of view, there have been two consequences of this. One has been that many researchers have had a vested interest in believing that antipsychotics are antischizophrenic. In addition, given the 'known' abnormalities in the dopamine system in schizophrenia, the fact that the drugs work on the dopamine system seems to mean that they are antischizophrenic.

For those who take the approach that antipsychotics do reverse the core disturbance in schizophrenia, the usual response to patients not getting better has been to give more of the drugs, and the idea that an individual might not take their drugs is viewed very seriously. In addition, the idea of paying much heed to what the takers of the drugs have to say about whether they are helpful or not has seemed irrelevant: after all, these drugs cure an illness, a cardinal manifestation of which is supposedly a lack of judgement.

The view taken throughout this chapter is that the antipsychotics are not specifically antischizophrenic. In daily practice, many people who are agitated will be prescribed an antipsychotic, whether or not they have schizophrenia. And, whether or not the person has schizophrenia, it makes sense to pay heed to whether they say the drug they are on is suiting them or not.

There is also evidence from a number of studies that patients who use these drugs 'cleverly', that is who take the drugs when they feel themselves 'slipping' but discontinue when they feel better again, are no more likely to be readmitted to hospital than patients who take the drugs continuously (Healy 1990). The evidence from these trials, however, is compromised by the fact that antipsychotics can cause dependence, and this may produce relapses on discontinuation.

Further evidence in favour of the notion that antipsychotics are anti-agitation rather than antischizophrenic agents comes from three sources. First, while antipsychotics may help patients get out of hospital, they self-evidently do not cure schizophrenia. Second, brain imaging studies have revealed that the dopamine system in the brain of individuals with schizophrenia is normal (Healy 1991). Finally, the reports from individuals who take these drugs point to anti-agitation effects rather than cure.

But what of the evidence that these drugs work on the dopamine system? The fact that the drugs are useful and work through the dopamine system can also be taken to indicate that, whatever is wrong in schizophrenia, it cannot be wrong with the dopamine system. A good analogy would be with the use of aspirin in rheumatoid arthritis. Aspirin works on the prostaglandin system. The fact that it is helpful (not curative) in arthritis indicates that, whatever is wrong in this condition, there is nothing wrong with the prostaglandin system.

HOW ANTIPSYCHOTICS WORK

During the 1960s it was shown that brain cells work by releasing neurotransmitters. There are now known to be up to 100 different neurotransmitters, with millions of them released every second. Neurotransmitters act by binding to a receptor protein on their target cell. Most drugs that act on the brain do so by attaching themselves to these receptors, either blocking or enhancing the action of the neurotransmitter that naturally binds there.

Most neurotransmitters have at least six or seven different receptors to which they bind. Ordinarily the drugs in current clinical use will bind to one or two of these but not all, so that some, but not all, actions of that particular neurotransmitter are enhanced or blocked. However, the same medications will also bind to the receptors of other neurotransmitter systems. Thus, while antipsychotics primarily act on the dopamine system, they also act on the noradrenaline, serotonin (5-hydroxytryptamine; 5HT), acetylcholine and other systems. These are Cocktail Compounds rather than Magic Bullets, which only hit one target.

Dopamine

Dopamine was one of the first brain neurotransmitters discovered. Arvid Carlsson discovered it in the late 1950s. It was subsequently shown that Parkinson disease involves a loss of dopamine-containing nerve cells and that disease could be treated with the dopamine precursor, L-dopa, or with dopamine agonists. The antipsychotics all bind to and block the dopamine 2 receptor – they are D_2 antagonists.

What does blocking D_2 receptors do? In very low doses, it will reduce stereotypies. This lays the basis for the use of these drugs in Tourette syndrome, where sufferers have stereotyped utterances and gestures, which interrupt normal speech and behaviour. Many individuals in the throes of a psychosis display repetitive thinking and actions, which seem almost stereotyped, and, indeed, agitation may make us all stereotyped to some extent.

Blocking the dopamine system also produces a feeling of indifference, a sense of being shielded from stress – a 'who cares' feeling that many people under stress find immensely useful. It is for this reason that the antipsychotics have also been called major tranquillisers. But the tranquillisation they produce is not like the wave of calm relaxation that Librium, Valium or alcohol produces. Subjectively, it is much more a case of finding oneself not getting worked up rather than finding oneself tranquillised down. Objectively, it can look more like immobilisation than sedation.

Serotonin and the atypical antipsychotics

In addition to binding to D_2 receptors, almost all antipsychotics act on the serotonin (5HT) system, binding in particular to serotonin S_2 receptors (see Ch. 12). Despite the fact that LSD (lysergic acid diethylamide) acts through the S_2 receptor and chlorpromazine blocks its effects, so powerful did the 'neuroleptic' idea and the dopamine hypothesis become, that for years pharmaceutical companies tried to produce compounds that would bind only to dopamine receptors. The purest compounds of this sort, sulpiride, remoxipride and amisulpride, appear to be good if somewhat less potent antipsychotics, which perhaps surprisingly have less than average extrapyramidal side effects, given their action on the dopamine system.

Then, in the late 1980s, clozapine was rediscovered, and with it came the recognition that a drug could be 'antipsychotic' without triggering extrapyramidal syndromes and without binding potently to the D_2 receptor. Where the trend up to the development of remoxipride was to produce compounds with increasing specificity for one receptor, clozapine seemed a step back into the past: it was a 'dirty' drug that bound to many different dopamine, noradrenergic, cholinergic, serotonergic and other receptors. Its binding to S_2 receptors was particularly striking. This has led a number of companies to bring out compounds that bind to both D_2 and S_2 receptors, hoping to find another clozapine.

What does S_2 binding do? S_2 agonists such as LSD are psychedelic or may produce dysphoria. S_2 antagonists can block the hallucinogenic effects of LSD. They can also be anxiolytic and sleep enhancing, but they have not proven useful in the treatment of psychosis, when used without concomitant D_2 blockade. S_2 antagonism may also provide an inbuilt antidote to some of the extrapyramidal side effects of D_2 antagonism.

There is an alternative possibility. A long-standing view of psychosis has seen the problem in terms of a defective filter, which allows too much stimulation in to bombard the psyche. This opens up the possibility that what 'dirty' drugs do is to dampen down more components of the filter system (located in the basal ganglia) than do cleaner compounds. If this is the case, while some neurotransmitters such as dopamine and serotonin may be particularly important, the future will lie with compounds with just the right 'dirty' profile.

A 'WHO CARES' FEELING

In the 1950s, before the idea that the antipsychotics were antischizophrenic took hold, there were a number of attempts to pinpoint what it is these drugs do – what state of mind they bring about. In general, the verdict was that they produce a feeling of detachment, of being less bothered by what had formerly been bothering.

When the drugs are working properly, takers also report beneficial effects on their ability to focus or concentrate on things. Subjects may find themselves more alert mentally, more able to focus on tasks that need doing, less in a daydream, less distracted by internal dialogues, strange thoughts or intrusive imagery. The voices or thoughts may be described as being still present but as having receded from centre stage. At least part of the person's mind has been left free to get on with other thoughts.

However, for the past two decades, under the influence of the notion that antipsychotics are antischizophrenic, interest in these drugs has focused almost exclusively on the fact that their use seems to get people out of hospital. There has been little interest in what changes they actually bring about that allow people to function out of hospital and, as a consequence, despite

40 years of use, it is difficult to be more precise about the beneficial effects of antipsychotics. The unfortunate consequence of this is that we are not able to give a good description of what we expect the drug to do and then ask the patient to let us know whether the treatment is working as it is supposed to or not. Working in this sense may be something different to getting well. Reducing tension may make some people better, but not others. At present, when someone fails to respond, our almost reflex response is to increase the dose of the drug. But this will not be of any benefit if the drug is already working in the sense of relieving tension. In such cases something else is called for – either a completely different type of drug, perhaps an antidepressant, or a behavioural or cognitive intervention.

Everybody who takes an antipsychotic is affected by them, whether they have schizophrenia or not, whether they have a mental illness of any sort or not. In affecting everyone in much the same way, antipsychotics resemble tea, coffee, nicotine or alcohol. Just like tea and coffee, they act within a few minutes and the effect usually lasts for 4–6 h. For this reason, like tea or coffee, they are often given several times a day.

Broadly speaking, more of an antipsychotic gives more of a 'who cares' feeling up to a certain level, just as more coffee gives a more stimulating effect – up to a certain level. But beyond the point at which marked extrapyramidal effects kick in, more of an antipsychotic may start to make you feel worse, just as too much coffee can.

Broadly speaking, like tea, coffee or aspirin, antipsychotics do not cure an illness. However, just as aspirin may help a range of conditions from headaches to fevers and arthritis, so also the antipsychotics, if used properly, may be helpful for a number of different conditions, including vomiting, itching and coughing as well as states of agitation. There is one exception to this, in that antipsychotics effectively cure many delirious states.

ANTIPSYCHOTICS AND THE POSITIVE SYMPTOMS OF SCHIZOPHRENIA

Antipsychotics are almost invariably given to individuals who see or hear things that are not there (hallucinations) or who have what others consider are unrealistic beliefs (delusions). These symptoms are commonly called the positive symptoms of schizophrenia, in contrast to states of social withdrawal and apathy, which are termed negative symptoms. To observers, it often appears that the voices or delusions seem to lose their grip and the person seems less likely to act on them after some days or weeks on the drugs. It is this 'clearing up' that has led to the impression that antipsychotics are anti-schizophrenic. More often than not, however, sensitive questioning reveals that the hallucinations or delusions have not disappeared entirely. It is more usual that takers of antipsychotics will still have their voices or some of their ideas, but that they are less worried by them.

Where the management of voices and delusions is concerned, a number of points should be borne in mind. One is that many so-called normal people hear voices or have what to those treating them may seem very strange beliefs. It is not a foregone conclusion that voices need to be removed or odd beliefs need to be corrected. A great deal hinges on how distressing these phenomena are to the person who has them, or how much they are intruding on the lives of others. Many a lonely person is comforted by the exchanges they have with their voices.

Another point is that there are now a variety of cognitive and behavioural methods for handling voices (Chadwick & Lowe 1990, Romme & Escher 1994). The present status of such techniques is that they may prove beneficial against a background of judicious drug treatment: they are not an alternative to drug treatment. There is one group of patients, however, whose voices often do not seem to clear, despite what may be heroic medication regimens. These are patients with voices linked to previous abuse or trauma. In such cases, a non-drug input seems essential.

ANTIPSYCHOTICS AND THE NEGATIVE SYMPTOMS OF SCHIZOPHRENIA

The newer antipsychotics are sold on the back of being better for the negative features of schizophrenia than the original agents were. These negative features are apathy, social withdrawal, as well as poverty of thought, action and speech.

There is at present, however, almost nothing in the clinical trial evidence or the receptor profiles of these drugs to support claims such as these. These new agents have receptor profiles very like that of chlorpromazine. From the start, chlorpromazine was reported as waking people up from psychoses. It got them talking in a way they had not been talking before and made them more active than they were before. The early trial evidence, in fact, suggested that chlorpromazine was better for these features of the illness than it was for the positive symptoms of psychosis.

But the common experience of both mental health workers and patients changing on to newer agents almost certainly is that these agents improve quality of life, remotivate, and are generally much more likely to be taken than the older agents. Why the mismatch between the research and the clinical evidence? The answer to this almost certainly lies in the fact that, clinically, patients are being switched from poisonous doses of older compounds to appropriate doses of newer compounds. The improvement is real, but has little to do with the new agents being better.

CLOZAPINE AND SCHIZOPHRENIA

Clozapine, marketed as Clozaril, was launched on to the US and UK markets in the late 1980s, with claims that it constituted a radical breakthrough in the treatment of schizophrenia. Its cost, at £2–4000 per annum compared with £100–400 for older antipsychotics, certainly was a radical break.

Clozapine, however, is not a new drug. It was first synthesised in 1958 (Healy 2001) and entered clinical trials in Europe during the 1960s, when it was found to be at least as good as but no better than other antipsychotics. There were two features of its use that were very different. First, it did not produce standard extrapyramidal problems and, second, it did not seem to cause tardive dyskinesia. It was this ability to produce improvements in tardive dyskinesia that more than anything else led to its re-emergence after the problems it caused had led to its removal from the market.

In the course of clozapine's early use, a number of problems were noted. Clozapine could cause a fatal malignant hyperthermia, or neuroleptic malignant syndrome. This led some early triallists to recommend it be abandoned. For this reason, it was never licensed in Japan. But the problem that caused the greatest concern was when a number of takers developed agranulocytosis – a loss of white blood cells. This, in some cases, proved fatal and led to the withdrawal of clozapine from use.

The reintroduction of clozapine around 1990 was hedged around with a number of precautions. The term of its licence encourages its use only for psychoses that are resistant to everything else. During the course of therapy, blood tests to determine white cell count must be done weekly for the first 18 weeks and fortnightly thereafter for up to a year, after which they can be spaced at monthly intervals. If the blood tests are not done, the company does not provide the drug. The cost of these blood tests was one of the reasons put forward for its high costs, but other new agents have been brought out at similar prices even though no blood tests are involved.

It appears that around 30% of individuals who are unresponsive to other antipsychotics show some improvement when taking clozapine. One reason for this improvement may stem from the fact that clozapine acts more potently on the serotonergic (5HT) and other systems, in addition to its action on dopamine receptors. As explained above, what this might amount to in practice is more effective 'filtering' or, alternatively, the addition of something of an antidepressant effect.

Another possibility stems from the fact that clozapine binds less effectively to dopamine receptors than do other antipsychotics. Accordingly it is less capable of producing D_2 'poisoning' than other antipsychotics. If the poor response of some individuals given conventional antipsychotics results from the development of side effects such as akathisia (see Ch. 2), then some individuals, who are particularly sensitive to these effects, might be expected to improve once the 'poisoning' ceases.

Whatever the reason, there is a clear benefit for some people, although at a considerable cost. The cost element for clozapine and other newer antipsychotics has led many health purchasers to put restrictions on the number of people they are prepared to have on these newer agents at any one point in time. Does greater compliance with newer agents or freedom from certain side effects warrant such a hike in costs?

While the newer antipsychotics are less likely to cause the extrapyramidal side effects of traditional antipsychotics, they are nevertheless subject to a number of other side effects, such as weight gain, excess saliva production leading to drooling, and marked sedation. In the case of clozapine, there is an increased likelihood of epileptic convulsions. The new agents also appear to share a greater likelihood of cardiac complications. The recorded death rate in patients taking clozapine is, in fact, higher than that for any other psychotropic drug.

The reputation of clozapine may be based in part on a historical accident. Had haloperidol been removed because of some problem, leaving clozapine and similar agents to dominate the market, the reintroduction of the haloperidol kind of drugs some years later would have been accompanied by stories of miraculous cures on extraordinarily low doses in patients resistant to clozapine-type antipsychotics.

This scenario suggests that the available antipsychotics fall along a spectrum, with haloperidol and risperidone at one end and clozapine and quetiapine at the other. Some patients respond to one type, where others respond to agents from the opposite end of the spectrum. Whatever the truth of the matter, there is no room for complacency in that the life expectancy of patients with schizophrenia is falling relative to the rest of the population, despite all the advances we claim to be making.

ANTIPSYCHOTIC DOSES

The success of the new antipsychotics highlights another feature of the history of the antipsychotics. From 1970 through to the mid-1990s, these agents were delivered in ever higher doses, culminating in megadose regimens. There were three reasons for this: (1) the dopamine hypothesis of schizophrenia, (2) the ongoing need for sedation and (3) a means of behaviour control.

First, the dopamine hypothesis played a part as follows. If dopamine is abnormal in schizophrenia and if the antipsychotics act on this system, then one possibility is that the failure of patients to get well is because the drug is in some way failing to get into the brain. Lack of response therefore leads to increased doses.

Second, up till 1952, the only ways in which to help patients who were highly disturbed and in need of 'controlling' for their own sake were isolation, physical restraint or sedation. The drugs most commonly used for sedation were the barbiturates. One disadvantage of barbiturates was that they put patients to sleep and it is not possible to 'work' with sleeping patients. Another is that barbiturate overdoses can be fatal. Against this background, the antipsychotics were a major step forward. They calm agitation without producing sleep. They are much safer in large doses or overdoses than the barbiturates. As a result, they replaced the barbiturates.

This has created a problem. Very agitated or distressed patients may still need, in their own interests, to be 'controlled'. As barbiturates are rarely used now, the antipsychotics have tended to be used for this purpose. But as the antipsychotics are not particularly good sedatives, this has often led to extremely large doses being used in order to achieve sedation. Many of the problems caused by antipsychotics stem from high doses used for this purpose.

This issue has come to a head quite recently with recognition that efforts to sedate difficult patients with antipsychotics given by intramuscular routes, while the patient is being restrained, may be fatal. This had led to concerns about rapid tranquillisation, with most intensive care units developing protocols for the management of emergency sedation (Pilowsky et al 1992). There is a trend toward using benzodiazepines, and in particular lorazepam, as the first line of treatment in such instances.

Third, while not truly sedative, in high doses antipsychotics do control behaviour. They do this by literally immobilising a person (see side effects). In situations of difficulty, they can be used – and often are used – for the purpose of immobilising someone who may pose a risk to themselves or others. In an emergency, this use is defensible. However, emergencies seem to occur with greater frequency under certain consultants and certain nursing staff. There is a political dimension to this question. Without the use of antipsychotics in high doses, arguably given the staff : patient ratios that may obtain on occasions in some psychiatric units today, such units would become unmanageable.

In such situations the use of immobilising doses of antipsychotics for acutely disturbed patients seems to have a 'chemical cosh' quality to it. Many takers will have had the experience of these drugs being used to 'control' them in this manner, rather than to help them. It is against this background that problems with compliance may need to be judged.

As a result of these factors, the doses of antipsychotics during the 1970s, 1980s and 1990s rose to poisonous levels. Haloperidol narcosis was common; this involves the intravenous administration of haloperidol 10 mg hourly. Flupentixol 2000 mg per day in 18-year-old girls was not uncommon. It was routine practice in some hospitals to commence all new patients, even elderly women, on haloperidol 10 mg four times daily. The evidence base points to much lower doses being optimal (Baldessarini et al 1988, Jusic & Lader 1994, Thompson 1994).

First-generation antipsychotic dose regimens

Chlorpromazine was originally used in doses of 200–400 mg per day. At 500 mg, clear extrapyramidal problems are common. Until recently, however, chlorpromazine was administered in doses of up to 5000 mg per day, with 100–200 mg haloperidol per day being used regularly. Clinical trial evidence now clearly indicates that more than 500 mg of chlorpromazine or 10 mg of haloperidol per day is unlikely to be helpful (Baldessarini et al 1988, Farde et al 1988, Rifkind et al 1991, Van Putten et al 1990). Given patience and an attitude that does not rely totally on drug treatment to bring about benefits, lower doses will produce the best outcomes at a reduced cost in side effects. Higher doses, in fact, risk making the clinical picture worse by demotivating and causing dysphoria.

Current evidence points to the usefulness of a range of doses from a high of:

> *chlorpromazine 100 mg four times a day*
> *haloperidol/trifluoperazine/flupentixol 5 mg four times a day*
> *sulpiride 200 mg four times a day*

to a low of:

> *chlorpromazine 50 mg twice daily*
> *haloperidol/trifluoperazine/flupentixol 1 mg per day*
> *sulpiride 100 mg twice daily*

Some people can tolerate much higher doses, without significant problems. Others have difficulties even at the low doses proposed here. Doses higher than these, however, should ordinarily be used only if: (1) the taker finds them clearly helpful or (2) the taker needs to be controlled (strait-jacketed) for their own good.

If 300–400 mg chlorpromazine a day or 5–10 mg haloperidol per day fails to help, the options are to add some other non-drug treatment or a different type of drug, such as a benzodiazepine or an antidepressant. An alternative may be to change to another antipsychotic agent. This rarely happens, even though for example the evidence that benzodiazepines, for example, may be helpful is actually quite good (Wolkowitz & Pickar 1991).

A consequence of the use of high-dose antipsychotic regimens in recent years has been that mental health workers have become somewhat deskilled when it comes to the management of disruptive or awkward behaviour by non-pharmacological means. It has been all too convenient to resort to a 'chemical cosh', particularly in situations of understaffing, rather than to attempt to sort out an underlying grievance or to devise a behavioural contract to contain unhelpful behaviour.

Second-generation antipsychotics

More recent antipsychotics have come on stream after the mania for megadoses of antipsychotics had passed. As a result, there is a much greater likelihood that the doses prescribed will be in line with the clinical trial evidence of what works best. This means, in general, that 1–6 mg of risperidone will be used, 10–20 mg of olanzapine, and 400–600 mg of clozapine and quetiapine.

As things stand at present, this means that nursing staff, for instance, may be happy at the prescription of risperidone 2–4 mg per day, although the same staff would have great difficulty with the use of haloperidol 2–4 mg per day,

Box 1.1 Equivalent doses of antipsychotic drugs

chlorpromazine 100 mg = haloperidol 1–2 mg
= flupentixol 1–2 mg
= trifluoperazine 1–5 mg
= sulpiride 200 mg
= quetiapine 200 mg
= olanzapine < 5 mg
= clozapine 200 mg

For depot antipsychotics, the doses are:

chlorpromazine 100 mg daily = haloperidol 25 mg i.m. every 3–4 weeks
= flupentixol 20 mg i.m. every 2 weeks
= fluphenazine 25 mg i.m. every 3–4 weeks
= zuclopenthixol 200 mg i.m. every 2 weeks

even though all the trial evidence and receptor binding data suggest that these are equivalent.

While there has been a general and welcome lowering of doses in recent years, the allopathic compulsion (mission to cure) that led to megadoses of first-generation antipsychotics has not gone away. Today, it expresses itself in drug cocktails. In the face of a patient failing to respond, care staff want to do something. Instead of raising the dose of the original compound, they now add others, in particular mood-stabilisers of one sort or the other.

Dosage equivalence

The dose of an antipsychotic that is needed generally hinges on its potency at binding to D_2 receptors. The more potent at binding, the lower the dose needed clinically. Thus 1–2 mg haloperidol is equivalent to 100 mg chlorpromazine.

Fifty years into the antipsychotic era, there is still no clear consensus on how much of one antipsychotic is equivalent to how much of another (Foster 1989). Box 1.1 therefore gives approximate equivalents of only the most commonly prescribed antipsychotics.

FLEXIBLE THERAPY

Antipsychotic therapy should aim at producing an effect that the taker identifies as being useful. Therapy should also involve helping the patient to identify signs of stress or possible triggers to the worsening of a schizophrenic, manic or paranoid illness. At such times, the optimal use of antipsychotics would be to take them 'cleverly' – to assist coping. 'Clever' self-prescribing would also involve reducing the dose, or possibly discontinuing the drug, at times when there is less stress or an illness has become more manageable.

The aim of prescribing should be to produce an antipsychotic effect at the lowest possible dose: one that does not bring about side effects and therefore does not require the additional prescription of antidotes (see Ch. 4).

Adding the different side effects of each drug to the biological differences between subjects who take the drugs means that some people will find a particular drug, such as chlorpromazine, helpful, but others will not. Some will find that it produces a sense of security or indifference to outside pressure. Others will find the same drug, in the same dose, uncomfortable. Those who dislike chlorpromazine, however, will often find another antipsychotic perfectly acceptable.

Whether an individual will settle with a particular antipsychotic or not is something they (the patient) can often tell after the first day – sometimes after the first dose. The current evidence is that those who, from the start, like what they get do well, whereas those who don't like the effects of the drug they are put on, do not do as well (May et al 1976). This suggests that test dosing and a willingness to switch around antipsychotics until the right one is found for each individual should be standard practice. It is not.

CATCH 22

Whatever their various side effects, antipsychotics should not make someone feel much worse. If they do, then too high a dose or the wrong drug is being prescribed. It seems that many patients, when they feel worse, do not think that it could be the effects of the drug: 'My doctor wouldn't have prescribed something that could make me feel worse'.

In the case of the antipsychotics, confusion is particularly likely as increased restlessness could be caused either by a worsening of the illness or by the drugs. Demotivation can be caused by the illness, by the drugs or by life. Agitation can arise as a result of experiences caused by the illness or in reaction to feeling strait-jacketed by the drug (see Ch. 2).

Within therapy settings there is a default toward blaming the disease rather than the drug. If behaviour worsens or agitation increases, doctors and nurses almost always push for an increase in the drugs on the basis that the patient has become more 'psychotic'. In contrast, the approach outlined here would encourage individuals to trust their own instincts and speak out. Ideally, if the complaint could possibly be due to the drugs, speaking out should lead to the dose being reduced or the drug changed or halted (see Section 9).

FOR HOW LONG SHOULD TREATMENT CONTINUE?

It has been common in the past for people to be prescribed antipsychotics for years. Anything from 1 to 5 years is common. Up to 20 years or more is not uncommon. If the approach outlined here were adopted, most individuals would not be on these drugs continuously for anything like these lengths of time. The best reason for continuing a treatment indefinitely would be if a particular individual finds the drugs helpful – *not just simply because mental health staff think they should continue.*

The question of dependence on and withdrawal from antipsychotics has recently come back to the fore. This was clearly recognised in the 1960s, but for 30 years after that the possibility of such problems was discounted. The current situation is that a proportion of individuals, perhaps up to a quarter or a third, will feel dramatically worse if they try to discontinue antipsychotics – even from doses as low as 1 mg of trifluoperazine or flupentixol per day taken for several months (Tranter & Healy 1998).

For the past 20 years, rapid relapse on discontinuing treatment has been seen as evidence that antipsychotics are actually antischizophrenic. The argument has been that the use of antipsychotics makes dopamine receptors more sensitive, leading to an increase in dopamine transmission when the drugs are halted. As excess dopamine transmission 'causes' schizophrenia, problems on discontinuing antipsychotics have been seen as a breakthrough of malignant schizophrenia.

However, there are other reasons why discontinuing antipsychotics may make someone feel worse. One is that antipsychotics can cause a nervousness, restlessness or agitation (see Ch. 2), which may become manifest only when the drugs are discontinued or attempts are made to reduce them. This is commonly misinterpreted by individuals as a worsening of their mental state, leading them to restart their drugs, or misinterpreted by others as the worsening of the psychosis, leading them to demand that the patient restart treatment. On questioning mental health staff, both patients and their relatives are likely to be told that antipsychotics are non-addictive. This is perfectly true, but it does not mean that they do not produce dependence and a range of problems on discontinuation.

One possible source of difficulties stems from the simultaneous discontinuation of the anticholinergics that individuals may be on to counter antipsychotic-induced side effects (see Ch. 3). Cholinergic rebound may cause a general feeling of malaise, along with poor sleep and increased dreaming. This may be a particular problem for the many individuals put on antipsychotics who have intrusive thoughts to begin with – individuals with obsessional disorders, or post-traumatic stress disorders, or borderline disorders, for example. Often in an attempt to control recurrent intrusive images or thoughts, these individuals will have pushed their antipsychotic and anticholinergic doses as high as possible. Discontinuation of drug treatment can in these cases lead to cholinergic rebound and an increase in the intensity and frequency of intrusions of the very images and thoughts for which help was sought in the first place.

However, there is a much greater problem from discontinuing the antipsychotic itself. Up to a quarter of those taking an antipsychotic drug may expect to have either motor problems or a variety of problems – from nausea, to stress sensitivity, to pain, to problems with temperature regulation. The problem seems to be greater for women than for men. This is dealt with further in Chapter 24.

The risks of withdrawal and relapse are highest in those who stop treatment abruptly, and probably in those who are stopping from higher dose levels. Discontinuing treatment should therefore probably involve a gradual tapering of dose rather than abrupt cessation. Decisions about discontinuation should probably also take into account the nature of the problems that might arise should the individual relapse, and the hostility of the environment in which the individual will have to cope without their drug shield (Gilbert et al 1995).

DEPOT ANTIPSYCHOTICS

A depot is an intramuscular injection, which lasts in the system for 2–4 weeks. The antipsychotic depot preparations are shown in Table 1.2.

For some people, depot antipsychotics are convenient. They offer round-the-clock protection without the bother of having to remember to take pills.

However, there is another aspect to depots. A great number of people who are prescribed antipsychotics do not take them. The single greatest determinant of compliance is probably the quality of the relationship between the taker and their carers. Clearly, however, a further reason must lie in the sometimes unpleasant side effects of ongoing treatment. This is particularly likely to be the case in clinics where prescribing has been insensitive – the dosages too high, the drugs continued for too long.

Far from blaming the drugs, however, there has been a tendency among mental health personnel to see the problem in terms of the patient's unreliability or lack of insight. The patient tends to be blamed rather than the drugs.

This non-compliance led to the introduction of depots. It is quite common to find individuals diagnosed as having schizophrenia or manic depression kept on depots for many years. All too often 'community care' seems to reduce to the control of individuals in the community by means of depot antipsychotics.

Finally, one of the unusual features of depot prescription is that their prescription does not lead to a discontinuation of the prescription of oral

Table 1.2 Depot antipsychotics

Generic drug name	UK trade name	US trade name
flupentixol	Depixol	–
fluphenazine	Modecate	Modecate
fluspirilene	Redeptin	–
haloperidol	Haldol	Haldol
pipothiazine	Piportil Depot	–
zuclopenthixol	Clopixol	–

antipsychotics. Many patients are prescribed both concurrently. The rationale for this is unclear. It may owe more to the neuroses of prescribers than to anything else.

Most recently, a short-acting depot has been introduced: zuclopenthixol acetate (Clopixol Acuphase). This intramuscular preparation of zuclopenthixol lasts in the system for 48–72h and is used in the management of acute disturbances.

ANTIEMETICS

Many individuals, who have never considered they had a psychological problem, let alone a psychosis, will have had antipsychotics. These will usually have been prescribed to help control travel sickness or to stop vomiting. The drugs most commonly prescribed for these reasons are shown in Table 1.3.

Table 1.3 Antipsychotics prescribed as antiemetics

Generic drug name	UK trade name
metoclopramide	Maxolon/Gastrobid Continus
promethazine	Phenergan/Avomine
alimemazine (trimeprazine)	Vallergan
prochlorperazine	Stemetil/Buccastem

These drugs all bind to dopamine receptors in the brain. They can all be used for antipsychotic purposes, although in the doses usually given little may be apparent other than an antiemetic effect. However, even at the usual doses, extrapyramidal side effects (see Ch. 2) may occur. Conversely, chlorpromazine, sulpiride and haloperidol may all be used effectively to counter vomiting.

ANTIPSYCHOTICS AND PSYCHOTHERAPY

Sadly, drug therapies and psychotherapy tend to be cast as opponents. Those who give drugs are seen as believing that the illness is a biological one and that talking makes little sense, and those who do psychotherapy view the drugs at best as a necessary evil.

In fact, early research from the 1960s indicates that group therapy in which patients help one another to express what the problems of drug therapy are and to see the consequences of failure to take medications may have hugely beneficial effects. Up until the late 1960s, the dominant view was that the drugs, rather than curing people, opened them up to a point where other therapies might then provide further benefits.

The increasing divide between pharmacotherapeutic and psychotherapeutic approaches, however, leads to problems for anyone who wants to take any non-drug approach toward psychoses. The doses at which antipsychotics are now prescribed will often lead to a demotivation or restlessness that will make any psychotherapeutic approach from simple behavioural manoeuvres through to more complex cognitive interventions all but impossible.

 User Issues

SIGNIFICANT INTERACTIONS

Alcohol

There are reports that drinking alcohol may make the emergence of antipsychotic-induced akathisia and dystonia more likely (see Ch. 2). This is probably incorrect. Alcohol may even reduce the nervousness and restlessness that some antipsychotics can cause. More sedative antipsychotics are liable to interact with alcohol to produce much more sedation than would ordinarily be the case. This seems much less true of the non-sedating antipsychotics.

Lithium

Lithium may halve plasma chlorpromazine levels. Whether it does this to other antipsychotics is uncertain. The combination of antipsychotics and lithium is used widely and, in general, appears to be safe, although there does seem to be a slightly increased risk of neuroleptic malignant syndrome or lithium encephalopathy (see Ch. 7).

Barbiturates and benzodiazepines

Any sedatives of these classes interact potently with sedative antipsychotics such as chlorpromazine and quetiapine to produce what may be a disproportionate sedation. Interactions are much less marked with other antipsychotics.

Analgesics

Sedative antipsychotics may also potentiate the sedative effects of centrally acting analgesics such as pethidine, codeine or morphine. Perhaps more importantly, many analgesics, especially opioids, can produce many of the same extrapyramidal effects as the antipsychotics (see Ch. 2).

Antidepressants

Concurrent administration of antipsychotics and tricyclic antidepressants may result in rises in the plasma concentrations of both groups of drugs. It also seems more likely to lead to weight gain. The combination of selective serotonin reuptake inhibitors (SSRIs) and antipsychotics appears to increase the likelihood of extrapyramidal side effects.

Oral contraceptives

As with analgesics, oral contraceptives can produce a number of extrapyramidal side effects, and the combination of contraceptives and antipsychotics may make these problems more likely.

User Issues

SPECIAL CONDITIONS

Pregnancy

The effects of antipsychotics on an unborn fetus are not established. In general, for the older compounds such as chlorpromazine or haloperidol, there appears to be no clear risk. For newer compounds there is simply no available information other than animal studies, which indicate potential but minimal risks of developmental abnormalities.

Breastfeeding

All antipsychotics except clozapine and quetiapine increase the amount of breast milk, making it uncomfortably superabundant in some instances. They also enter breast milk, although in lower doses than found in the mother's plasma, potentially causing side effects to the baby. It is probably, therefore, advisable to avoid breastfeeding while taking these drugs.

Driving

See the chapters on antidepressant side effects (Ch. 5) and benzodiazepines (Ch. 11).

Others

Caution should be taken in cases of known prostatic disease, glaucoma, Parkinson disease and thyroid problems.

A GENERAL NOTE

Given the amounts of these drugs that have been prescribed for almost 40 years now, under a wide range of conditions and dosage regimens, it needs to be said that these are extremely safe drugs. Any controversy surrounding them relates as much, if not more, to the way they are administered than to their intrinsic safety.

These drugs are immensely useful – *when used properly*. Proper use depends greatly on a close cooperation between taker and prescriber. The takers need to learn what particular antipsychotics can do for them – how best to use them – but also their limitations – what they do not do. A failure to recognise the limitations of antipsychotics has led in the past, and still leads, many prescribers to prescribe doses that may make conditions worse.

Side effects of the antipsychotics

INTRODUCTION

The classical antipsychotics all bind to dopamine receptors, but almost all of them bind to at least one other receptor as well, although not all to the same other receptor. People also differ. The combination of these two principles means that the side effects of an antipsychotic may differ from one individual to another.

The side effects listed here will seem fearsome. However, for most part, they are all readily reversible by reducing the dose, changing the drug, halting it or using the right antidote.

Treatment, however, may involve a trade-off. In practice it seems that many individuals are prepared to tolerate the interference with daily living that some of the side effects listed in the next few pages may cause, in exchange for peace of mind. The reason for listing these side effects is not to deter pre-scribers from prescribing or takers from taking, but rather to involve the taker in making the trade-off rather than having it imposed insensitively on them, and to give prescribers some feel for the nature of that trade-off.

Dissatisfaction about the balance between the benefits and side effects should not lead to unilateral action, except in an emergency, but rather should lead to a process of negotiating a position acceptable to the taker, their family and all practitioners who may be involved. Negotiation may involve showing this list of side effects to a relative, who perhaps believes that these drugs are curative and that, therefore, the taker should be on them regardless.

A second point is that, for the most part, the side effects listed here will clearly seem like side effects and, as such, will be irritating – but no more. There are, however, a number of effects potentially brought on by the drugs that may seem more like a worsening of the illness than side effects. It is important that takers of these medications are able to discriminate between such drug-induced effects and the illness. All too often individuals mistakenly believe that some of their problems are a consequence of an initial complaint or illness rather than a consequence of having taken drugs for that illness.

DOPAMINE SYSTEM SIDE EFFECTS

Antipsychotics all reduce the amount of dopamine activity in the brain. As Parkinson's disease involves reduced dopamine levels, they tend to produce a state that resembles Parkinson's disease. They do not, however, cause Parkinson's disease. Once they are stopped, the state clears up. For a general 'feel' of the states that may be caused, there are two books worth reading: *Ivan*, by Ivan Vaughan (1986), and *Awakenings*, by Oliver Sacks (1982). The best descriptions of the full range of problems are in a book by David Cunningham-Owens (1999) – *A Guide to the Extrapyramidal Side-Effects of Antipsychotic Drugs*.

There is general agreement now that people should, for the most part, be treated either with an antipsychotic that does not cause dopamine-related side effects or with a dose of antipsychotic that does not produce these side effects. However, this has not always been the orthodox view. For a long time, from 1960 through to 1995 or so, clinicians aimed to produce dopaminergic side effects in the belief that it was only when such effects were apparent that the treatment was likely to produce its benefits.

The side effects of akinesia, dyskinesia and dystonia are more likely to be immediately apparent, and for this reason they are listed first. However, the most important dopamine-related side effects are tardive dyskinesia, akathisia and demotivation.

User Issues

STIFFNESS/LACK OF MOVEMENT: AKINESIA

This is the central feature of Parkinson's disease. When caused by antipsychotics it is felt in a mild form as a slowing down of spontaneous movement. This may not be unpleasant. In a more severe form, the feeling may be one of being restricted, even strait-jacketed – which can be very distressing.

This slowing down may produce clumsiness. It can also lead to someone ending up just sitting motionless in the one place, in a way that makes them look like a zombie. A zombie because they may be wide awake but not moving much, not even smiling. This happens because antipsychotics may slow down all movements, and all extra or unnecessary movements are reduced in frequency – even down to facial expressions. There may also, for instance, be noticeable delays between questions being asked and answers being offered.

The effect is such that even one dose can make a healthy mental health professional look like a schizophrenic (Healy & Farquhar 1998). A good deal of the stigma now linked to mental illness is therefore tied up in the rather obvious effects of this type that the antipsychotics can produce.

If the dopamine system is blocked to the point that an individual has a lot of parkinsonian side effects, then two things may also happen. One is that the drugs may cause drooling. This seems to happen because the muscles of the face and mouth are stiffer and slower to react when saliva builds up and therefore it dribbles out in a way that it would not ordinarily. This can easily be put right by reducing the dose, but it is unpleasant to experience and to observe.

Another is that, when the person starts to walk, they may find themselves leaning forward or to one side. They may also find it difficult to start moving or, having once started, they may find it difficult to stop. These effects can all be put right quickly by lowering the dose of the drug, changing to a different drug or using an antidote (see Ch. 3).

User Issues

ABNORMAL MOVEMENTS: DYSKINESIAS

Abnormal movements are one of the most noticeable features of Parkinson disease. The pill-rolling tremor of the hand that this illness produces is perhaps the commonest of these. When brought on by antipsychotics, this tremor will be experienced as anything from a very fine tremor that is hardly noticeable to a clear shake that makes coordination difficult, causing someone, for example, to be unable to drink tea without spilling it. This can seriously interfere with social life. Tremors can also be caused by antidepressants, lithium, valproate, caffeine and bronchodilators, among other drugs. The combination of these drugs with an antipsychotic may need to be reviewed.

continued

The commonest set of abnormal movements affects the hands or arms, but the legs may also be involved. This shows itself as an inability to keep the legs still when sitting down. The muscles of the mouth and face may be also involved, as well giving a repetitive pouting of the lips and protrusion of the tongue. The jaw may be affected, leading to tooth grinding and dental problems. The entire body may also writhe or shake. This can be most obvious when sitting down.

One of the least recognised set of dyskinesias involves the respiratory muscles. When the movements of these muscles become autonomous or discoordinated the result is breathlessness, wheezing or shortness of breath. This may be long lasting or short lived, happening for instance at night. Commonly, these effects may be misinterpreted as an anxiety attack, and an SSRI or tranquilliser may be prescribed, either of which is likely to make the problem worse.

 User Issues

ABNORMAL MUSCLE TONE: DYSTONIA

The term dystonia means that some muscle has gone into spasm. Typically spasm happens abruptly. Virtually any muscle may be affected, but the muscles of the eyes, the mouth and jaws tend to be most commonly affected.

When the eyes are affected, the eyeballs roll up in the head so that only the whites of the eye can be seen, in what is called an oculogyric crisis. Needless to say, the person affected can see almost nothing. The first time this happens, the person affected and anyone else watching may be very alarmed. The spasm will usually wear off inside an hour. It can also be quickly reversed by an anticholinergic antidote (see Ch. 3).

When the mouth or larynx is affected, there can be difficulty in speaking distinctly or in eating or drinking. These conditions are readily reversed on discontinuing treatment or with an antidote, but there have been reports of serious complications. Dystonias of the larynx may also lead to a change in voice, so that the person sounds hoarse or like a Dalek. Other mouth area problems include clenching of the jaw, especially at night; this can become a serious dental problem. Another problem is trismus or lockjaw.

Spasms are the obvious form of dystonia, but pains are by far the commonest. These pains can affect the jaw, throat, muscles of the face, and either the limbs or trunk. They may lead to a mistaken diagnosis of facial pain or atypical pain syndromes of one sort or the other. Treatment should involve changing drug, rather than painkillers.

 User Issues

TARDIVE DYSKINESIA: LATE-ONSET DYSKINESIA

Tardive dyskinesia refers to a set of abnormal movements of the face and mouth, and is one of the most serious problems that antipsychotics can cause. This is a dyskinesia that may come on only several months after the drug has been started, which has led to it being called tardive (late onset). It leads to lip-smacking movements and protrusion of the tongue and chewing movements. It may extend to writhing movements of the trunk of the body.

Between 5% and 20% of people who take antipsychotics may be affected. The problem is commoner in women than men, in older rather than younger people, with higher doses of drugs rather than lower doses, and occurs with some antipsychotics rather than others. The newer agents, especially clozapine and quetiapine, are much less likely to cause a problem. The problem, however, can happen after relatively low doses given for months rather than years, and milder versions may be seen in people who have never had an antipsychotic, suggesting that in some individuals there may be a vulnerability to this kind of problem.

Unlike other abnormal movements, tardive dyskinesia may last for several months or years after the drug has been discontinued. As these movements involve the face, they may be very obvious and socially embarrassing. There are, at present, good antidotes for most of the other side effects of antipsychotics, but not for tardive dyskinesia. One option now is to switch anyone who has this problem to quetiapine or clozapine, as both have been demonstrated to suppress dyskinesias.

The occurrence of tardive dyskinesia has been the subject of legal action in the United States. The threat of further legal action led to a hiatus in the production of new antipsychotic drugs through the 1970s and 1980s (Healy 2001). The re-emergence of clozapine owes a lot to the fact that it does not cause this problem and may even lead to it clearing up. The present position is that the occurrence of tardive dyskinesia can constitute grounds for suing, if the individual has not been forewarned of the risk. The availability of clozapine and quetiapine has added a new dimension to this issue.

 User Issues

RESTLESSNESS, NERVOUSNESS, AGITATION, TURMOIL: AKATHISIA

One of the worst side effects of the antipsychotics is akathisia. This is essentially a complex, unpleasant, emotional state that often leads to visible restlessness. Throughout the 1970s and 1980s, this visible restlessness was all that most people meant when they thought of akathisia. The word akathisia refers literally to an inability to sit still, and this is what was noticed along with foot-tapping or restless legs in those who were able to sit down.

However, there may be no obvious restlessness. The problem may be apparent only subjectively, in which case an individual may feel anything from being mildly twitchy to being extremely so, so that they are unable to stay still or feel like leaping out of their skin. It may be difficult to decide from the outside whether this is normal fidgetiness or akathisia.

The term restlessness, however, does not even begin to convey all that may be involved. The very first descriptions of this problem were in normal people taking reserpine for blood pressure problems. This led to quotes such as the following: 'increased tenseness, restlessness, insomnia and a feeling of being

continued

very uncomfortable', 'the first few doses frequently made them anxious and apprehensive ... they reported increased feelings of strangeness, verbalised by statements such as "I don't feel like myself" ... or "I'm afraid of some of the unusual impulses that I have"'. Or take the case of CJ, who on the first day of treatment reacted with marked anxiety and weeping, and on the second day 'felt so terrible with such marked panic at night that the medication was cancelled' (Healy & Savage 1998).

The phenomenon therefore includes the emergence of strange and unusual impulses, often of an aggressive nature. Dysphoria is a much better technical description of what is at the heart of akathisia than restlessness is. Turmoil is probably the best everyday word to describe the state.

The implication of this is that reports of increased irritability or impulsivity from anyone taking an antipsychotic should be taken seriously. However, they rarely are, because antipsychotics are expected to reduce irritability and impulsivity – not increase it.

One study of healthy volunteers taking haloperidol, carried out by King et al (1995), found that up to 50% of subjects taking doses as low as 4 mg may feel uncomfortable, ill at ease with themselves, and unable to settle. Some find it almost impossible to remain in the room or experimental situation, but at the same time find it very difficult to explain what is wrong. These effects are probably not a million miles from the 'wired' feelings that most people will have had if they have taken too much coffee. Many psychiatrists who have tried antipsychotics have experienced this effect, and a number have written up their experiences as being close to the worst experience of their lives. We have found similar results to the King study, with the extra twist that discomfort and irritability were still clearly present in some of our volunteers up to a week later (Jones Edwards 1998). We were not unique in this; others have found similar effects (Kendler 1976).

These reactions are of obvious relevance to what may apparently be 'difficult' behaviour on the part of some people when they come into hospital. Patients who develop this problem may be seen as getting worse, and as a result they may be put on more treatment. Alternatively they may feel they have to leave hospital quickly and, if they are not obviously deluded, ward staff may consider that they have little option but to let the person leave. People leaving hospital in circumstances like this, or developing problems like this at home, are probably at high risk of suicide.

Whether in healthy volunteers or patients, the condition sometimes responds to an anticholinergic antidote, or to propranolol. One of the most effective agents appears to be red wine. This is a problem, therefore, that may literally drive a patient to drink. In other cases, halting the medication completely may be the only way to alleviate the problem. In a proportion of subjects who have been on antipsychotics for a long time, it may take several months after discontinuation of the drug for the akathisia to wear off. High-potency antipsychotics such as haloperidol or risperidone seem to be particularly likely to cause this problem. Low-potency treatments such as chlorpromazine, quetiapine or clozapine are much less likely to do so.

Akathisia may present during the first few days on treatment or it may emerge only some weeks or months later, as the drug builds up in the system. This form of tardive akathisia is a particular hazard with depot antipsychotics. Akathisia may also emerge only during attempts to discontinue antipsychotics. This may incorrectly lead both takers and prescribers to think that the taker's mental problems are getting worse.

Recently akathisia has begun to be recognised as potentially one of the most serious side effects of antipsychotics. The particular hazard lies in the fact that, from the inside, it may feel as though one's nerves have got worse. Whether the problem is an unbearable worsening that makes people contemplate anything – even suicide – in order to bring it to an end, or a milder one, if the akathisia is interpreted as a worsening of the illness despite being on treatment, this may lead to hopelessness and to the conclusion that suicide is the only way out. Some of the newer antipsychotics are now being sold explicitly on the basis that they are less likely to cause dysphoria of this type and are therefore less likely to lead to suicide.

There is a high incidence of suicide in patients with schizophrenia or psychosis. Tragically this seems commonest among younger sufferers who have recently been diagnosed and put on drug treatment. This has usually been interpreted as a fatalistic reaction on the part of intelligent sufferers, who, appalled at the prospect of what lies in front of them, opt to bring their suffering to an end as quickly as possible. This may account for some cases of suicide, but there are a number of clearly documented cases in which a successful or attempted suicide followed the development of akathisia (Drake & Ehrlich 1985). The idea of suicide in these cases was clearly out of character for the person afflicted. What appears to happen, as mentioned above, is that individuals feel worse and misattribute what is happening to a worsening of their mental state. (See Chapter 5 on antidepressants and suicide.)

A less serious version of this problem also happens relatively commonly but may not be picked up. In a number of cases, when a person in an outpatient clinic expresses thanks for the wonderful tranquillisers they are on, it turns out that these wonderful tranquillisers are the anticholinergic tablets, which were once regularly prescribed concurrently with antipsychotics to reduce side effects (see Ch. 3). The 'nerves' these antidotes tranquillise, therefore, are being caused by the so-called tranquillisers (antipsychotics) the person is taking.

 User Issues

LACK OF INTEREST: DEMOTIVATION

As the antipsychotics produce a state of indifference, a potential problem of long-term use or too high a dose is that the user may become apathetic, listless and indifferent to everything.

The relation of this side effect to Parkinson's disease can be illustrated in the following way. Before drug treatment of Parkinson's disease with L-dopa, it was often observed that people might simply sit on a chair for days on end, seemingly unable to move. However, a fire alarm might produce rapid fluent movement, indicating that often what is lacking is not the ability to move but sufficient motivation to do so.

It is known that people who take antipsychotics continuously are significantly less likely to relapse and to have to be readmitted to hospital. However, studies have suggested that they may be also less likely to get married or involved in significant relationships, to find themselves jobs, or to get on with their lives compared with individuals who have the same illness but who do not take continuous antipsychotics (e.g. Johnstone et al 1988).

continued

Another finding is that all emotions may be blunted, rather than just certain emotions that have been troubling. Many takers complain that all feelings, from joy to anger, are dulled. Not all people have this side effect. Broadly speaking, it depends on the dose being taken, although some people will be clearly affected at very modest doses.

As this is a psychological rather than a physical side effect of antipsychotics, it is in many ways far more important than the other side effects mentioned. It can be pernicious in that the person may become indifferent to being indifferent. It is also important because there are few antidotes for it – other than halting the drugs or psychostimulants.

It may, in addition, be very difficult to distinguish drug-induced demotivation from a schizophrenic or depressive demotivation, or life itself. Trying to tease out what is happening may require great skill and cooperation between the taker of the drug and the prescriber. All too often, the appearance of apathy and listlessness results in individuals, who are taking antipsychotics, also being prescribed an antidepressant – inappropriately. Antidepressants do not help this condition.

One of the things most commonly mentioned by people on stopping long-term antipsychotics is a return of interest in things, along with finding that they have more 'get up and go' and that everything is not impossibly difficult to undertake any more. This can lead to problems if an unwary individual throws themselves into things too much and becomes stressed or overloaded as a consequence. It can also be somewhat frightening as feelings such as anger, temper outbursts or a more vivid appreciation of the sexuality of others may re-emerge in all their potential awkwardness.

 User Issues

HORMONAL CHANGES

All antipsychotics, except clozapine and quetiapine, by binding to D_2 receptors, increase the level of the hormone prolactin. As the name suggests, this hormone is central to lactation. As a consequence, taking an antipsychotic can in some cases lead to women who are already lactating having a much more profuse supply of milk. It can result in lactation in women who are not lactating. It can also lead to an increase in breast size in all women, in some cases producing changes from a 34A to a 38C, for example.

Increased prolactin levels can also lead to some men having a mild degree of breast swelling. This is completely reversible and usually disappears quickly once the drug is halted. In rare instances in men, there may even be the production of small amounts of milk.

Partly because of their effect on prolactin secretion, the antipsychotics are also liable to cause disturbances in menstrual regularity and may even lead to menses ceasing altogether. This can lead to a belief that one is infertile and to unprotected sexual intercourse. However, pregnancy is still possible in these circumstances. Given that this situation may be brought about by the use of an antipsychotic in low doses for anxiety (which is quite common owing to concerns about benzodiazepine prescribing), this perhaps brings home what is often forgotten: that every prescription involves a trade-off between a benefit and a risk.

There are a number of other effects of antipsychotics on sexual functioning that are not caused by their effects on prolactin; these are outlined below and in Section 7. On the positive side, antipsychotics may lead to a decrease in the intensity of period pains.

OTHER DOPAMINE-RELATED SIDE EFFECTS

There are many aspects of parkinsonian states that are still poorly understood and often unrecognised. One of these is that Parkinson disease is sometimes accompanied by painful sensory symptoms. Other features include change in the oiliness of the skin or hair. Similar changes may also occur with antipsychotics. The risk is that they will be dismissed as impossible. The general effect of all these changes is to produce a great deal of what is now seen as a 'schizophrenic look'.

OTHER SIDE EFFECTS

Dopamine-related side effects may be found with all antipsychotics, but they are more common with some antipsychotics than with others. They are least common with chlorpromazine, clozapine and quetiapine. However, a number of other side effects are more likely to occur with chlorpromazine or quetiapine, and yet other side effects are common to all antipsychotics but unrelated to dopamine.

 User Issues

WEIGHT GAIN

This is a very common side effect of all antipsychotics. The precise reason for this is uncertain. It may in part stem from a reduction in activity consequent on akinesia or demotivation with no compensatory reduction in appetite. It may stem from the increase in thirst that most antipsychotics cause, which is slaked by high-calorie drinks. However, there also appears to be some stimulation of appetite and/or a reduction in metabolic rate. An S_2 antagonistic action appears to make weight gain more likely (see Section 4), as do actions on the histamine system. Broadly speaking, olanzapine and clozapine cause the most marked weight gain and cause it most commonly. Chlorpromazine and others can cause equally large amounts of weight gain, but seem to do this much less often.

This 'cosmetic' consequence of treatment is sometimes considered trivial by prescribers, who believe that the dopamine-related side effects mentioned above are likely to be of much greater concern to patients. However, surveys of patients indicate that weight gain is their most important concern, and when prescribers are asked what would worry them most if they had to take treatment, weight gain also comes out as the most important side effect.

continued

In most cases the weight gain is mild, but in a substantial proportion of cases there may be a gain of 2–3 stones, and in some cases the gain may be 5 stones or more. This may lead to attempts to lose weight by dieting or to instruction from a general practitioner to lose weight. Dieting alone is rarely successful in cases of antipsychotic-induced weight gain, and this failure may lead to considerable frustration and guilt if it is not realised that the drugs are responsible for the problem.

Marked weight gain is a sufficiently serious side effect to warrant a consideration of the prescription of appetite suppressants, such as a stimulant or fenfluramine, to assist weight reduction programmes or the fat absorption blocking agent orlistat (Xenical). However, in my experience, many physicians and even antipsychotic takers themselves are reluctant to take a 'chemical' way out. Many seem to think that weight gain is in some way the fault of the taker.

 User Issues

SYMPATHETIC SYSTEM EFFECTS

Chlorpromazine, clozapine, olanzapine and quetiapine also bind to receptors in the sympathetic system, producing sedation and a lowering of blood pressure (hypotension).

The drop in blood pressure on antipsychotics is ordinarily not marked. In most cases, the only awareness that an individual will have of this is a slight exaggeration of the tendency that we all have to feel faint when we leap off a chair or jump out of bed. However, in some cases the drop in blood pressure may be quite substantial and may lead to actual fainting or falling, leading to bruising or cuts and, in the elderly, to fractures. The frequency with which this happens is unknown, but if it is suspected it would be good grounds for halting the drug.

The combined effects of potential sedation and serious hypotension make high-dose chlorpromazine, or quetiapine, olanzapine or clozapine given acutely, hazardous in situations where the level of observation is low. Patients, even on psychiatric wards with adequate staff levels, may be at risk of damaging falls or accidents. Elderly individuals in residential homes may run an equivalent risk from much lower doses.

An action on the sympathetic system may also lead to palpitations – an awareness of the heart beating quickly or irregularly. This is usually not serious, although it may feel very alarming. This range of effects on the cardiovascular system means that there are hazards to any precipitate administration of large amounts of these drugs, as reports of sudden death after large amounts of antipsychotics in patients being restrained perhaps indicate.

Another effect in men, that may in part be mediated through the sympathetic system, may be an inability to sustain an erection. This, as with the other symptoms above, is reversed once the drug is halted. For a more detailed consideration, see Section 7.

Finally, sympathetic system effects may produce difficulties in the urinary system. This may range from an uncomfortable fullness of the bladder, to difficulties in passing water (being slower to start and taking longer to stop), to complete urinary retention. In the past this was described as an anticholinergic effect of these drugs, but it is now clear that it is sympathetic in origin. While this problem may be worse in older men with prostate problems, it can happen to anyone – even young women.

 User Issues

ANTICHOLINERGIC EFFECTS

Chlorpromazine also has prominent anticholinergic effects, as do a number of the other antipsychotics. The commonest anticholinergic effect is a dry mouth. In some cases this may be quite severe. There may also be a nasal drying, which some people find uncomfortable.

Anticholinergic effects may also lead to stomach upsets and constipation. Another effect may be blurring of vision. Any apparent worsening of eyesight, therefore, when on these drugs, should not lead the person to seek an eye test until the drugs have been discontinued.

Ordinarily, antipsychotics are given to people in order to reduce agitation, to suppress delusional beliefs and to abolish hallucinations. However, in some cases, particularly in the elderly, the anticholinergic effects of chlorpromazine, for instance, may cause agitation, confusion and hallucinations.

Mild anticholinergic side effects usually wear off after a few days on the drug. If they are sufficiently marked to make someone clearly uncomfortable and do not clear up after a few days, the drug should be changed or discontinued.

 User Issues

THIRST: COMPULSIVE DRINKING

Up to 20% of individuals on long-term antipsychotics drink excessive volumes of fluid. This may be either water, high-calorie soft drinks, or tea and coffee. It is not clear whether this is caused by the dry mouth some antipsychotics can induce, or whether they can also cause repetitive drinking apart from this, or whether drinking is a means of washing the drugs out of the system.

Excess drinking may cause problems if allied to cigarette smoking. Many hospitalised or community-based individuals on chronic antipsychotics smoke more than the average. The reasons may be that communal smoking provides something to do in an otherwise boring day. Another possibility is that smoking may ameliorate some of the side effects of antipsychotics. Combined with excess drinking, this can cause a problem in that nicotine reduces the volume of urine produced, potentially leading to water intoxication with convulsions and disorientation. There has been an increasing number of reports of this syndrome, particularly in learning difficulty settings.

User Issues

SEDATION AND AROUSAL

Although not nearly as sedating as the barbiturates, the sedative effects of antipsychotics with effects on the sympathetic system may be extremely useful in some cases, particularly to help sleep at night. In other cases the taker may prefer to have a non-sedating antipsychotic. The sedation may be quite marked and interfere with normal activities such as driving a car.

Given the widespread belief that antipsychotics generally are sedative, the effects of these drugs on levels of arousal are contradictory and sometimes surprising. When given in low doses, it may be necessary to restrict the prescription of antipsychotics to the morning as, if given in the evening, they may interfere with sleep.

Even when given in somewhat larger doses at night, they may permit sleep but yet give a very unsatisfying sleep. A common report of people who discontinue these drugs is that they sleep more soundly off the drugs.

These effects vary from individual to individual and from drug to drug. The very same dose of an antipsychotic given to one individual in the evening may lead to sleeplessness, whereas another person may be sedated by it. Both chlorpromazine and thioridazine are more sedative that other antipsychotics, as mentioned above, by virtue of their action on the sympathetic system. It is very common because of this to find chlorpromazine used for years as a night-time aid to sleep.

 User Issues

SEXUAL SIDE EFFECTS

There has been a certain coyness on the part of both prescribers and takers to look closely at the sexual side effects of antipsychotics. From the limited surveys that have been done, it seems that there may be sexual side effects in up to 50% of individuals taking antipsychotics. Coyness therefore seems misguided, particularly as such side effects are likely to influence whether someone is prepared to continue with treatment.

The most commonly reported side effects in men are an inability to sustain erections or a delay in or inability to ejaculate. These effects may occur in up to 50% of men taking antipsychotics but most probably relate to dosage, so that at lower doses they are less likely to be present. The opposite effect of involuntary and sustained erections (priapism) has also been reported, as have involuntary ejaculations.

Also very common is a decrease in libido (sex drive). This is probably part and parcel of a general demotivation syndrome (see above). A change in the quality of orgasms has been reported, although exactly what kind of change has not been specified clearly.

In women, decreased libido, change in the quality of orgasm and anorgasmia have also been reported, but in general there is even less awareness of what the impact of antipsychotics is on female sexual functioning (Sullivan & Lukoff 1990). (See Section 7.)

User Issues

SKIN RASHES

All drugs may cause skin rashes of one sort or another. These are commonly allergic reactions. In the case of a marked reaction, the drug should be stopped. The rash will usually clear up in 24–48 h. A different antipsychotic should then be taken, if one is still needed.

Chlorpromazine may also cause two other skin problems. The most dramatic of these is photosensitivity. This involves an exaggerated tendency to burn when exposed to sunlight. It can lead to subjects getting severely sunburnt when exposed to even relatively mild sunlight for any length of time. Blocking creams can help with this, but if it is marked the drug should probably be stopped. For this reason chlorpromazine probably should not be given during the summer. Even in spring and autumn, care should be taken. There is an obligation here on staff closely involved with patients in or out of hospital to draw attention to this problem and advise on sunblocks, etc.

Another skin problem caused by chlorpromazine is an uncomfortable itchiness and dryness of the skin. This is probably related to the tendency of chlorpromazine to produce jaundice, a side effect found only with chlorpromazine. This has nothing to do with hepatitis or infection of any sort. Its precise cause is uncertain. It usually starts some weeks after the drug has been started and the only treatment is to discontinue the drug. It does not appear to be serious.

User Issues

AGGRESSION AND IMPATIENCE

Antipsychotics are so often given to control aggression that, for many prescribers, it is rather difficult to believe that they could also cause aggression. One way that this can happen is through the production of akathisia. However, a common report from takers is that they feel more impatient, irritable, and liable to fly off the handle. Whether all of this can be put down to akathisia is not clear. Whatever the cause, while there are no studies showing that antipsychotics can cause aggression or impatience, drug companies clearly believe this can happen. It has been listed as a side effect on the data sheet of a number of these drugs.

User Issues

NEUROLEPTIC MALIGNANT SYNDROME

Neuroleptic malignant syndrome (NMS) is a state in which the individual becomes stiff and feverish. The condition may be fatal if not caught quickly. NMS is probably closely related to catatonia, which also comes in fatal or malignant forms (Healy 2001).

continued

Severe forms of NMS are not common. Milder forms may occur and resolve spontaneously. The severe forms are most likely to happen in individuals taking higher doses of antipsychotics together with a variety of other drugs at the same time, and they seem most likely if the individual develops an additional low-grade infection or other physical problem. This type of reaction is commoner in elderly individuals, perhaps because they are prone to dementing or parkinsonian conditions. However, even for patients on a number of different drugs who also develop a fever, the incidence of severe forms of this complication is low.

Treatment until recently involved discontinuing all drugs and inpatient hospital observation to monitor for dehydration. There has been a recent revolution in treatment, with current recommendations that lorazepam in doses of up to 15–20 mg a day be used as the first line of treatment. If this fails, electroconvulsive therapy appears to produce a rapid response in most cases.

User Issues

SECOND-GENERATION ANTIPSYCHOTIC SIDE EFFECTS

The use of clozapine in recent years has been associated with cardiovascular instability in individuals during the early stages of treatment. It is common to find signs of a reduction in blood pressure and of an increase in heart rate, as well as symptoms of faintness, flushing and palpitations. This may continue so that some individuals may feel they are having panic attacks on these drugs. For these reasons treatment is started at very low doses and increased slowly. Other newer agents, such as quetiapine, are similarly titrated up slowly for this reason.

Another unusual problem on clozapine is bed-wetting. This may occur in one in five patients starting clozapine. The mechanism at present is somewhat uncertain, but it seems that there is a serotonin input into the bladder and that SSRIs may actually increase bladder distensibility or capacity, at least temporarily, whereas clozapine does the opposite.

This rather unusual side effect has been included for two reasons. One is to warn people that it may happen. A second reason is to draw attention to the fact that many unusual side effects may happen on a drug, some of which will not appear in any textbook and some of which may be unknown to the professionals involved in an individual's care. It is important to create an atmosphere that facilitates the reporting of problems, particularly those that seem unlikely to stem from treatment. It is also important to maintain an open mind as to whether problems that are reported may indeed stem from treatment. At the very least, they are being reported because the person is having problems with some aspect of their treatment.

The newer antipsychotics are too recently released to be certain what idiosyncratic side effects they may have. Olanzapine and clozapine have been associated with the appearance of diabetes, and this may manifest itself in thirst and the frequent passage of urine. Other surprises may wait in store.

User Issues

CARDIOVASCULAR CONDITIONS

The effects of antipsychotics on the cardiovascular system are at present the subject of close scrutiny. Pimozide was one of the first to cause concern. In high doses it led to a lengthening of the Q-T interval in the heart, potentially causing arrhythmias. Thioridazine has similar effects. It has led to a number of reported deaths and has recently been relabelled with warnings to indicate the risk.

The problems came to the forefront with the new antipsychotic sertindole. The Q-T interval changes produced by this drug led to its suspension from the market and to the recognition that many other antipsychotics and antidepressants have similar effects. The problem is that no one is clear on what is a safe level of Q-T interval lengthening.

In addition to these well documented problems, there is a growing number of others. The dose of clozapine has to be titrated up slowly because of precipitous blood pressure falls and the possibility of cardiac arrhythmias. If there is a previous history of cardiac abnormalities or of coronary thrombosis, this may become a consideration. A drug with less clear-cut cardiac effects, such as haloperidol, can be prescribed instead, but even then caution should be taken not to put anyone on too large a dose initially.

Beyond these effects there are others. Clozapine and some other newer agents appear to cause myocarditis, which can be fatal. Many of these agents also increase blood lipid levels. While most takers will have none of these problems, there probably should be a greater level of routine cardiac screening in anyone taking an antipsychotic than has been customary up till now.

User Issues

EPILEPSY

All antipsychotics may trigger epileptic convulsions in susceptible individuals. This, however, is rare. Haloperidol seems less likely to trigger this problem than chlorpromazine or clozapine. Clozapine is particularly likely to lead to convulsions.

Management of side effects

There are a number of groups of drugs that can be used to manage some of the side effects of the antipsychotics. These include the anticholinergic drugs, benzodiazepines, propranolol, psychostimulants and calcium channel antagonists.

ANTICHOLINERGICS

The anticholinergics (Table 3.1) are the drugs most used, often appropriately but equally often not so appropriately. This group of agents antagonise the action of the neurotransmitter acetylcholine (ACh) at one of its receptors, the muscarinic receptor.

Jean Martin Charcot was the first to use atropine in the form of belladonna to treat Parkinson's disease in the 1880s. Anticholinergic agents have been used ever since for parkinsonian problems, although they have largely been superseded now by the use of L-dopa and dopamine agonists. However, before L-dopa came on stream with a recognition that most antipsychotics cause parkinsonian symptoms, the anticholinergics were pressed into routine use to alleviate these side effects.

They have not been replaced for this purpose with modern antiparkinsonian treatments, owing to a probably ungrounded suspicion that more directly acting dopamine agonists such as L-dopa might make schizophrenia worse. The evidence for this is not strong, and there is a good deal of evidence to suggest that psychostimulants can usefully reverse many of the parkinsonian problems of the antipsychotics (see Section 3). There may be a place for testing out other new antiparkinsonian treatments also.

Table 3.1 Anticholinergic drugs

Generic drug name	UK trade name	US trade name
trihexyphenidyl (benzhexol)	Artane/Broflex	Artane
benztropine	Cogentin	Cogentin
orphenadrine	Disipal/Biorphen	Disipal
procyclidine	Kemadrin/Arpicolon	Kemadrin
biperiden	Akineton	Akineton

From the 1970s onwards, the anticholinergic drugs were almost certainly used too routinely (Barnes 1990). In many instances it became common practice to co-prescribe an anticholinergic agent with an antipsychotic from the start, even before side effects had appeared. The rationale for this was a belief that the emergence of side effects might compromise an individual's willingness to continue with medication. But in many cases an early prescription of an anticholinergic will have meant that hospital staff or a general practitioner was not called out of hours by a distressed patient, who might otherwise have been paralysed by a dystonic reaction or had some other side effect.

 User Issues

ANTICHOLINERGIC SIDE EFFECTS

In the past, when much larger doses of antipsychotics were prescribed, the occurrence of parkinsonian side effects were all but inevitable and the co-prescription of anticholinergic agents could be defended on this basis. Today, with the emphasis on much lower antipsychotic doses, and agents less likely to induce parkinsonism, the routine prescription of anticholinergic agents is less defensible, particularly as these agents bring their own problems and risks. The common side effects are shown in Box 3.1.

Until recently, this list of side effects would have included urinary difficulties, with a feeling of uncomfortable bladder fullness and possible retention. This, however, now seems more likely to stem from effects on the sympathetic system.

In addition, there is some evidence that the concurrent taking of anticholinergics may increase the risk for two of the most serious complications of antipsychotic therapy: tardive dyskinesia and neuroleptic malignant syndrome.

A further consequence of the regular, unthinking use of anticholinergics has been that all antipsychotic-induced side effects are routinely treated with these drugs, whereas only some side effects benefit. The stiffness, tremor and acute muscular spasm brought about by antipsychotics will often respond to anticholinergic antidotes – sometimes with gratifyingly dramatic speed. In some instances, akathisia may also respond. However, many cases of akathisia and most dyskinesias, in particular tardive dyskinesia, do not respond.

Box 3.1 Common side effects of anticholinergics

◆ Dry mouth

◆ Stomach upset and constipation

◆ Dizziness

◆ Blurred vision (and a possible onset of glaucoma in susceptible individuals)

◆ Theoretically, difficulties with having an erection might be expected (see Section 7), but in practice this does not seem to be a problem.

◆ An anterograde amnesia, so that subjects appear not to take in and retain things that happen while on these drugs. Similar problems are produced by alcohol and benzodiazepines, so that elderly subjects, in particular, taking both anticholinergic agents and a benzodiazepines hypnotic, for instance, may have quite marked impairments of memory. This may be marked enough to lead to worries about dementia.

◆ Dissociative reactions (see Ch. 5). These may include acute confusion and disorientation.

It seems increasingly reasonable to suggest that antipsychotics should be prescribed in such a way that side effects do not emerge, that is, low doses should be prescribed from the start and there should be a willingness to change antipsychotics to find one that does not cause side effects. If such an approach is taken, there should be a considerable reduction in the amount of anticholinergics needed.

At the risk of repeating a point too often, I will mention that one of the saddest things I find in clinical practice is to have a patient come and thank me for the marvellous tranquillisers they have been put on – only to realise that they are referring to their anticholinergic antidote.

There is a further intriguing possibility. For the past three decades the anticholinergic effects of antidepressants have been portrayed as a bad thing. In fact, any trials done of anticholinergic agents in depression point strongly to the fact that this action may be antidepressant. This is not surprising because the anticholinergics are euphoriant (Healy 2001).

CALCIUM CHANNEL BLOCKERS

There has been some recent interest in the effects that a group of compounds called the calcium channel blockers may have on antipsychotic side effects. These drugs include diltiazem, nifedipine and verapamil. Claims have been made for their usefulness in mania, in states of agitation, for alcohol and opiate withdrawal, in limiting the damage done by strokes (see Ch. 19) and in reversing certain side effects induced by antipsychotics (Barrow & Childs 1986).

These compounds have been used to treat angina, hypertension and disorders of cardiac rhythm for years. In general they cause dilatation of blood vessels, and it is this that probably underlies their antianginal effects as well as their effects on blood pressure. They are widely used and well tolerated.

Calcium channels are associated with many receptors – dopamine, noradrenaline and serotonin – either as part of the receptor or lying adjacent to it. Modulating calcium entry through these channels offers a means of fine-tuning conventional neurotransmitter function. It has become clear also that calcium channel blockers act to damp down spontaneous electrical discharges in the heart or brain. This is what underlies their antiarrhythmic action in the heart, and possibly provides the basis for an anticonvulsant effect in the brain. This damping down of spontaneous discharges may be what accounts for their effects on tardive dyskinesia and akathisia.

In the course of using calcium channel blockers, a number of researchers have noted that takers of these drugs say that these compounds are also tranquillising – in a manner that has not yet been clearly specified.

PSYCHOSTIMULANTS

As mentioned above, another group of drugs with potential usefulness in treating the side effects of the antipsychotics is the stimulants. For many years these drugs were avoided assiduously in anyone with psychosis in the belief that they might trigger psychosis. With the demise of the dopamine hypothesis of schizophrenia, the way is open to renewing the investigation of the usefulness of these drugs and other dopamine agonists such as amantadine. This group is dealt with further in Section 3.

BENZODIAZEPINES

A number of cases of akathisia appear to respond to benzodiazepines, as does neuroleptic malignant syndrome (see Ch. 2) and some dystonias. At present lorazepam is assuming a status in many units not unlike that formerly occupied by the anticholinergics: it is almost routinely prescribed in the early phases of treatment. This use is possibly excessive.

BETA-BLOCKERS AND ANTIHISTAMINES

These are occasionally given for akathisia (Ayd 1995, Bezchlinbnyk-Butler & Jeffries 1995).

References

Ayd FJ (1995) Lexicon of psychiatry, neurology and the neurosciences. Baltimore, MD: Williams & Wilkins.

Baldessarini RJ, Cohen BM, Teicher MH (1988) Significance of antipsychotic doses and plasma levels in the pharmacological management of the psychoses. Archives of General Psychiatry 45: 79–91.

Barnes TRE (1990) Comment on the WHO consensus statement. British Journal of Psychiatry 156: 413–414.

Barrow N, Childs A (1986) Antitardive-dyskinesia effect of verapamil. American Journal of Psychiatry 143: 1485.

Belmaker RH, Wald D (1977) Haloperidol in normals. British Journal of Psychiatry 131: 222–223.

Bezchlinbnyk-Butler KZ, Jeffries JJ (1995) Clinical handbook of psychotropic drugs. Toronto: Hogrefe & Huber.

Chadwick PJ, Lowe CF (1990) Measurement and modification of delusional beliefs. British Journal of Clinical Psychology 26: 257–265.

Cunningham-Owens DG (1999) A guide to the extrapyramidal side-effects of antipsychotic drugs. Cambridge: Cambridge University Press.

Drake RE and Ehrlich J (1985) Suicide attempts associated with akathisia. American Journal of Psychiatry 142: 499–501.

Farde L, Wiesel FA, Halldin C, Sedvall G (1988) Central D_2 dopamine receptor occupancy in schizophrenic patients treated with antipsychotic drugs. Archives of General Psychiatry 45: 71–76.

Foster P (1989) Antipsychotic equivalence. Pharmaceutical Journal 431–432.

Gilbert PL, Harris J, McAdams LA, Jeste DV (1995) Antipsychotic withdrawal in schizophrenic patients: a review of the literature. Archives of General Psychiatry 52: 173–188.

Healy D (1990) Schizophrenia: basic, reactive, release and defect processes. Human Psychopharmacology 4(5): 101–121.

Healy D (1991) D_1 and D_2 and D_3. British Journal of Psychiatry 159: 319–324.

Healy D (2000) Sitting on it. OpenMind March: 18.

Healy D (2001) The creation of psychopharmacology. Cambridge, MA: Harvard University Press.

Healy D, Farquhar G (1998) The immediate effects of droperidol. Human Psychopharmacology 13: 113–120.

Healy D, Savage M (1998) Reserpine exhumed. British Journal of Psychiatry 172: 376–378.

Johnstone EC, Crow TJ, Frith CD, Owens DG (1988) The Northwick Park 'functional' psychosis study: diagnosis and treatment. Lancet ii: 119–125.

Jones Edwards G (1998) An eye-opener. OpenMind September: 12, 13, 19.

Jones Edwards G (2000) On the receiving end. New Therapist 7: 40–43.

Jusic N, Lader M (1994) Post-mortem antipsychotic drug concentrations and unexplained deaths. British Journal of Psychiatry 165: 787–791.

Kendler KS (1976) A medical student's experience with akathisia. American Journal of Psychiatry 133: 454.

King DJ, Burke M, Lucas RA (1995) Antipsychotic drug-induced dysphoria. British Journal of Psychiatry 167: 480–482.

May PR, Van Putten T, Yale C et al (1976) Predicting individual responses to drug treatment in schizophrenia. Journal of Nervous and Mental Diseases 162: 177–183.

Pilowsky LS, Ring H, Shine PJ, Battersby M, Lader M (1992) Rapid tranquillisation. British Journal of Psychiatry 160: 831–835.

Rifkind A, Doddi S, Karagigi B, Borenstein M, Wachspress M (1991) Dosage of haloperidol for schizophrenia. Archives of General Psychiatry 48: 166–170.

Romme MAJ, Escher S (1994) Accepting voices. London: MIND Publications.

Sacks O (1982) Awakenings. London: Picador.

Sullivan G, Lukoff D (1990) Sexual side effects of antipsychotic medication: evaluation and interventions. Hospital and Community Psychiatry 41: 1238–1241.

Swazey JP (1974) Chlorpromazine and psychiatry. Cambridge, MA: MIT Press.

Thompson C (1994) The use of high-dose antipsychotic medication. British Journal of Psychiatry 164: 448–458.

Tranter R, Healy D (1998) Neuroleptic discontinuation syndromes. Journal of Psychopharmacology 12: 306–311.

Van Putten T, Marder SR, Mintz J (1990) A controlled dose comparison of haloperidol in newly admitted schizophrenic patients. Archives of General Psychiatry 47: 754–758.

Vaughan I (1986) Ivan. London: Paparmac.

Wolkowitz OM, Pickar DM (1991) Benzodiazepines in the treatment of schizophrenia: a review of reappraisal. American Journal of Psychiatry 148: 714–726.

Management of affective disorders

SECTION CONTENTS

The antidepressants

INTRODUCTION

It is perhaps more difficult to specify exactly what antidepressants do than it is to say just what any other drug that acts on the brain does. In the following pages, I employ an ulcer model of depression in an attempt to clarify some of the issues, but this model seriously simplifies both ulcers and depression, and this should be borne in mind.

Part of the problem in trying to say what antidepressants do lies in trying to agree what depression is. The terms mood and emotions are notoriously difficult to define. One way to define them is in relation to each other – to compare, for instance, the relation of mood to emotions with the relation between climate and weather, or the relation between the pedal and the keys of the piano. The climate sets the frame within which weather varies, but it does not itself change much. The pedals colour the tone of a melody. In the same way, mood sets the frame within which emotions operate. Mood disorders are like a change in climate rather than emotional outbursts stemming from particular problems. The antidepressants seem to act to reset climatic controls rather than acting on a particular piece of bad weather.

At times there can be considerable difficulty in distinguishing antidepressants from anxiolytics or antipsychotics. Part of the problem lies in our changing views of depression brought about by the development of antidepressants in the first instance. However, the marketing imperatives that dictate drug company strategies also come to the fore here. This latter issue is taken up further in Section 10.

While it is difficult to specify exactly what it is that antidepressants do, it is possible to describe their side effects fairly well and the risks associated with both taking them or not taking them. These are laid out in detail. There are a great number of different antidepressants, most of which have slightly different side effects. For most people, it probably makes little difference which antidepressant they have, but for a significant proportion of people it may make a considerable difference in terms of discomfort or adverse outcomes.

HISTORY

Tricyclic and MAOI antidepressants

The tricyclic antidepressant, imipramine, and the monoamine oxidase inhibitor (MAOI), iproniazid, were discovered in 1957 by Roland Kuhn and Nathan Kline respectively (Healy 1997). What was discovered, however, was not just a drug but a disorder that the drug treated (Kuhn 1990, Sandler 1990). There was no preconceived idea that these drugs should be antidepressant. Indeed, Kuhn thought he was testing out a new antipsychotic when he first gave imipramine to patients. Furthermore, there were a great number of stimulants available at the time, such as the amphetamines, but these did not appear particularly helpful for depression. What Kuhn and Kline did then, as much as find the compounds themselves, was to make visible a condition that responded to these compounds. It is this condition, variously called biological or major depression, which is in many respects the source of difficulties in specifying what the antidepressants do. We still do not know the nature of depression or its boundaries.

In 1965, the Medical Research Council (MRC) reported the outcome of a large multicentre study to compare the MAOI, phenelzine, with imipramine, electroconvulsive therapy (ECT) and placebo. Imipramine and ECT came out as superior to placebo and phenelzine, with phenelzine being no better than placebo. This, together with the recognition of the cheese effect of MAOIs (see side effects), which was emerging at the same time, put paid to the MAOIs, leaving the tricyclics as the dominant antidepressants for more than two decades.

There was, however, a flaw to the MRC study in that too low a dose of phenelzine was used: 45 mg in contrast to the 90 or 120 mg that is more customary now. Studies that have used a more adequate dose have subsequently found the MAOIs to be as effective for major depressive disorder as the tricyclics. It remains the case, however, that there are some people who respond to MAOIs but who do not respond to tricyclic antidepressants. Sometimes patients with a clear-cut case of major depressive disorder, who might be expected to respond to a tricyclic do not do so, despite changing the drug several times and having lengthy trials at adequate doses. When given an MAOI, however, there may be a prompt response. The reverse also appears to hold true.

The selective serotonin reuptake inhibitors (SSRIs)

In the early 1960s it was discovered that tricyclic antidepressants blocked the reuptake of the neurotransmitters, noradrenaline and serotonin. Subsequently, it was demonstrated that the first two tricyclics, amitriptyline and imipramine, broke down in the body to nortriptyline and desipramine, which both turned out to be antidepressants. This suggested that these were, in fact, the real antidepressants, rather than imipramine and amitriptyline.

Nortriptyline and desipramine both block noradrenaline but not serotonin uptake. The logical conclusion was that depression involved a disturbance of noradrenaline rather than serotonin function. This observation led to the catecholamine hypothesis of depression. It also led to a belief that the production of further antidepressants should focus on producing compounds that acted specifically on the noradrenergic system.

However, in a marvellous example of ignoring the theories of how things work and focusing instead on whether they work, Arvid Carlsson from the Karolinska Institute in Sweden noted that, while it appeared that nortriptyline and desipramine must be the core antidepressants, clinicians appeared to prefer amitriptyline and imipramine (Carlsson & Healy 1996). Looking at these compounds, Carlsson pinpointed the inhibition of serotonin reuptake as the one thing amitriptyline and imipramine did which nortriptyline and desipramine did not. He proposed, accordingly, that drugs that selectively blocked serotonin reuptake should be produced. This led to the production of zimelidine in the early 1980s. This worked but had to be withdrawn because of side effects. It has been succeeded by fluvoxamine, fluoxetine, sertraline, citalopram and paroxetine.

There is, however, no good indication that blocking serotonin reuptake is necessary for an antidepressant action. There is, for example, no correlation between how effective these drugs are at blocking serotonin reuptake and how quickly or how effectively they cure depression. The reason why so many of these compounds are being produced has probably more to do with marketing and legal issues than with 'science'. The term SSRI (selective serotonin reuptake inhibitor) was coined by investigators working with paroxetine. This seemed like a good marketing angle and was exploited first by SmithKline Beecham, but use of the term spread thereafter to cover all the drugs in the group, even though, strictly speaking, none of them is selective to the serotonin (5HT) system.

It is worth briefly considering the SSRI story a bit more in order to bring out the difficulties in specifying what antidepressants do. Before zimelidine, clomipramine was the tricyclic antidepressant that inhibited 5HT reuptake most effectively. This had been produced by Geigy in the 1960s, but it seemed no more effective than other antidepressants and appeared, if anything, to have more side effects – so much so that it was not licensed for release in the USA until 1990. This left the company with a marketing problem. Their answer was to produce an intravenous preparation of clomipramine and to encourage prescribers to give it in large doses intravenously. The outcome of this was a discovery that clomipramine seemed to be in some way anxiolytic: it was found to be useful in phobic and obsessional states (Beaumont & Healy 1993).

Are SSRIs then in some way anxiolytic rather than or in addition to being antidepressant? If blocking serotonin reuptake is anxiolytic, this might explain why clinicians prefer tricyclic antidepressants that also block 5HT uptake to those that do not, as most depressed patients are anxious as well as depressed (Healy 1991).

There is a further possibility. Given that we now know that most cases of depression resolve with time anyway, perhaps treatment with an anxiolytic might promote recovery in most cases. Anxiolytics might, in other words, be antidepressants. There is a considerable amount of evidence that treatment with agents that reduce anxiety or agitation may be all that is necessary to improve many patients with depression. It is on this basis that benzodiazepines and antipsychotics may be of benefit in depression. Many clinicians, however, would think that there is something more to antidepressants such as imipramine or phenelzine than just an anxiolytic effect, but exactly what antidepressants do over and above alleviate anxiety or enhance energy levels has been difficult to specify.

ANTIDEPRESSANT DRUGS

Table 4.1 lists the major classes of antidepressants.

A number of other treatments for bipolar disorders or the prophylaxis of recurrent affective disorders are also used in depression (see Chs 6 & 7). In addition, benzodiazepines such as diazepam and alprazolam, as well as antipsychotics such as flupentixol, are used. These often work, but whether they are antidepressants in the same sense as ECT, imipramine or phenelzine is a matter of dispute. The serotonin S_{1a} agonist, buspirone, has in addition been marketed as antidepressant, and other compounds from this group look as though they may also emerge as antidepressants (see Ch. 12).

Table 4.1 The antidepressants

Generic drug name	UK trade name	US trade name
Tricyclic antidepressants		
amitriptyline	Tryptizol/Lentizol	Elavil/Endep
imipramine	Tofranil	Tofranil
nortriptyline	Allegron	Aventyl
protriptyline	Concordin	Vivactil
desipramine	Pertofran/Norpramin	Pertofrane/Norpramin
clomipramine	Anafranil	Anafranil
dothiepin (dosulepin)	Prothiaden	–
lofepramine	Gamanil/Lomont	–
doxepin	Sinequan	Adapin/Sinequan
trimipramine	Surmontil	Surmontil
Monoamine oxidase inhibitors (MAOIs)		
phenelzine	Nardil	Nardil
tranylcypromine	Parnate	Parnate
moclobemide	Mannerix/Aurorix	–
Serotonin reuptake inhibitors		
citalopram	Cipramil	Celexa
fluvoxamine	Faverin	Luvox
fluoxetine	Prozac	Prozac
paroxetine	Seroxat	Paxil
sertraline	Lustral	Zoloft
venlafaxine	Efexor	Efexor
Other antidepressants		
bupropion	(Zyban – smoking cessation)	Welbutrin
maprotiline	Ludiomil	Ludiomil
mianserin	–	–
mirtazapine	Zispin	Remeron
nefazodone	Dutonin	Serzone
L-tryptophan	Optimax	Trofan
reboxetine	Edronax	–
trazodone	Molipaxin	Desyrel

Finally, ECT is also used. The mechanism of action of ECT and its use clinically are not discussed in this chapter. ECT has a clear role when antidepressants fail to work, for mania, catatonia and some cases of schizophrenia.

DEPRESSION

In the case of the antipsychotics and the benzodiazepines, discovery was uncomplicated because these drugs bring about clear changes that are noticeable to the taker and to others within an hour. In the case of the antidepressants, the discovery happened only when these drugs were given to a particular group of patients, and even then it took several weeks of treatment

Box 4.1 Core symptoms of depression

◆ Loss of energy

◆ Loss of interest

◆ Feeling physically run down, below par or ill

◆ Poor concentration

◆ Altered appetite

◆ Altered sleep

◆ A slowing of physical and mental functions

before the effect became apparent. The antidepressants were not discovered because they rather obviously made sad people happy. A particular kind of depression and the drugs had to be discovered at the same time.

The illness has been called vital, biological or endogenous depression, or melancholia. This is a state characterised by the symptoms shown in Box 4.1.

These core symptoms are predominantly physical in character. For most people who get the disorder, it is like having mild influenza. For some it is more severe.

In addition to the core symptoms, a number of other physical problems may come with a depression. These include:

◆ heartburn

◆ indigestion

◆ constipation

◆ ulcers of the gut

◆ dry skin, hair and mouth

◆ pins and needles

◆ aches and pains around the body

◆ headaches

◆ altered periods

In addition to these physical symptoms, there is also sadness, hopelessness, guilt and suicidal ideas. However, going through this checklist of symptoms should bring home the point that the condition that the first antidepressants treated was not ordinary or even severe sadness, guilt or hopelessness. What they treated was something different from what most people think of as depression. Indeed, the term depression was introduced for this condition only in the early years of the 20th century. The question of what antidepressants treat has become more complicated since the introduction of the SSRIs; see below.

In cases of classical depression for which antidepressants are helpful there will be some of the above physical symptoms. However, in most cases there will also be some of the following psychological symptoms:

- hopelessness
- helplessness
- guilt
- ruminations
- suicidal ideas or a wish to be dead
- anxiety

The older antidepressants are commonly of little use for individuals who have these psychological symptoms but not any of the preceding physical symptoms. They were not discovered as 'anti-psychological problem pills'. This issue had become clouded somewhat by the increasing use of SSRIs in anxiety states, in lieu of diazepam (Valium) (see Section 4). The 'cases of Valium' who are now 'cases of Prozac' get labelled as depressed now, but many people being labelled now as depressed would until recently have been diagnosed as anxious. The fact that anxious people are also unhappy makes it easier to make this jump.

Reactive and endogenous depression

These terms were once very common. It was thought that 'reactive' depression, which comes on after a life event, is a mild psychological problem that should not be treated with antidepressants. As a contrast to reactive depression, it was also common to hear talk of endogenous depression, which was supposedly a more severe biological illness, one that was not triggered by life events and that was accordingly appropriately treated with pills.

These ideas are largely a consequence of the development of ECT and the tricyclic antidepressants: it appeared that the more severe depressions, and in particular those with clear physical features, responded to these treatments whereas the response of states of anxious misery or morbid distress was much less convincing. The former became known as endogenous depressions. They were presumed to arise by virtue of some biochemical change in the brain. The latter were the reactive or neurotic depressions. These were presumed to arise in response to life crises and, accordingly, many have assumed that treatment with antidepressants must be inappropriate in these milder depressions.

Current research suggests that these views are wrong. Depressions with physical features, the so-called endogenous depressions, are now known to be triggered by life events just as often as neurotic depressions. Antidepressants are helpful for many seemingly mild depressions, provided the condition is not just one of misery. In current psychiatric practice the terms endogenous and reactive depression have fallen out of use and have been replaced by major depressive disorder and by dysthymia, which refers to a chronic low-grade misery.

Recent developments

Since 1980 there has been an increasing recognition of the post-traumatic stress disorders, of which grief reactions to the loss of a loved one are the most common. Others include the shocks that may be consequent on traffic accidents, rape, public disasters, etc. These states are considered further in the chapter on anxiety. Their relevance here is that, although they are primarily anxiety disorders, they may involve serious mood changes, leading to an abrupt descent into the blackest of depressions. Typically these mood changes are briefer than major depressive disorder and do not have the same physical character.

Psychiatrically the post-traumatic stress disorders are most likely to cause a problem when the trauma has occurred in childhood and has given rise to what is termed a borderline personality organisation. This state often leads to repeated suicidal acts or self-injurious behaviour and states of profound desperation (Healy 1993). Is this a mood disorder? For the most part, antidepressants are not helpful in these disorders and may indeed make the condition worse. This issue is complex in that someone who is grieving or traumatised may later go on to become depressed in a way that will respond to antidepressants.

Another set of developments has been the demonstration that a number of brief focused psychotherapies – in particular interpersonal therapy and cognitive therapy – can bring about a clear response in depressions that would also be expected to respond to antidepressants (Williams 1990). The fact that the same depressions respond to a number of very different types of psychotherapeutic intervention suggests that there is not just one right way to treat a depression. It might be better, therefore, to regard the different treatments as offering antidepressant principles. There are considerable differences between the tricyclic, MAOI and SSRI antidepressants, which suggest that they may also act according to quite different principles.

Finally, it can be argued that the patients with depression who ended up in hospital during the 1950s, 1960s and 1970s were in many respects atypical. This is significant, because it was from amongst this subject group that the volunteers for clinical studies on the antidepressants were drawn. Today it is recognised that most patients with depression that could respond to antidepressants are being seen by general practitioners rather than psychiatrists, in a ratio of over 20 to 1. Studying this larger group has led to the conclusion that depression often resolves spontaneously without physical treatments, with the average time to response being somewhere around 14 weeks (Healy 1990).

THE ULCER MODEL OF DEPRESSION AND ANTIDEPRESSANTS

Ulcers and their treatment provide a helpful model for the effects that antidepressants have on depression. For example, if one considers the question that often seems to puzzle people, 'How can an illness come on after stress or life events', it is clear in the case of ulcers that a very real physical illness can come on after stress. Ulcers, however, are not just a psychological problem and they do not necessarily clear up once the stress goes away or one learns to manage it. They are appropriately treated with drugs. In part, this may be because other factors intervene such as *Helicobacter pylori*, to lead to chronicity.

Initially many antiulcer drugs have little or no effect on an ulcer. The pain remains and there seems to be little improvement. If persisted with, however, after one or two weeks the pain of the ulcer begins to resolve as the wound closes over. As the pain clears up, the anxiety that goes with having an ulcer also clears up – a virtuous circle can be set in place.

The effects that many, but not all, antidepressants have on hopelessness, guilt and suicidal thoughts are rather like the effect that antiulcer pills have on anxiety. Once the core physical problems have cleared, the associated psychological reactions also clear up. In much the same way that no one would give antiulcer drugs to patients who are anxious but who do not have an ulcer, so also there should be some caution about giving antidepressants for sadness and unhappiness if patients do not have the kind of brain 'ulcer' I am calling depression.

Considering depression in terms of a brain ulcer also allows us to offer answers to questions such as how long should treatment continue, should drugs be combined with psychotherapy, and do antidepressants cure?

For how long should treatment continue?

Current research suggests that it is prudent for the patient to stay on an antidepressant for at least 3 months, and probably for 6 months, after they have started feeling well (British Association for Psychopharmacology 1993). This is much the same advice that is given to patients who have ulcers. This is because the period when ulcers are most likely to reopen or recur seems to be during the 3–6-month period after initial recovery.

This does not mean that halting antidepressants immediately after recovery would necessarily lead to relapse. In many cases stopping can be done successfully. However, the risks of relapse are far less if the patient is prepared to go on with the antidepressant for 3–6 months afterwards. The risks of relapse seem to increase according to the number of previous episodes an individual has had and to the severity of those episodes. If there have been a number of clear-cut previous episodes, severe enough to warrant hospitalisation, current opinion would lean toward possibly permanent ongoing treatment. In the case of ulcers, frequent relapse seems to be associated with the presence of an organism called *H. pylori*, and quite different treatment to the usual antiulcer treatment is called for. Something comparable probably applies in depression, but at present we have little idea of what that is or how to help.

Drugs or psychotherapy?

The ulcer model brings out one further aspect of the use of antidepressants. Provided they are not too severe, it is often possible to treat ulcers without recourse to physical treatments at all. By eating a lot of small, bland meals throughout the day rather than large, hot and spicy meals, along with avoiding smoking and alcohol as well as relaxing, ulcers can often be cured without any drugs at all. This seems to be because ulcers, just like wounds on the hand, heal naturally unless there is something interfering with the healing. Exactly the same thing seems to be true for 'biological' depressions, and, indeed, relapse rates in one-off cases of depression seem to be lowest in patients who recover with support only and without any formal psychotherapy or pharmacotherapy. Even though depression may be a physical disorder, it now seems that many cases can be treated without pills, either by activity or with a number of newly developed therapies, of which cognitive and interpersonal therapy are the best known.

Regarding the treatment of depression without pills, two points can be made. One is that it is not always the case that ulcers can be treated without pills. If the ulcer is located on the posterior wall of the gut or if the individual has higher than average gastric acid levels or an infection with *H. pylori*, the ulcer is liable to be slower to heal or more likely to reopen. Chronic ongoing stress also interferes with spontaneous recovery. In many cases, treatment with antiulcer drugs is necessary. Indeed it may even still be necessary to proceed to surgical intervention.

Much the same seems to be true of depression. Recent evidence suggests that the majority of depressive disorders that could respond to antidepressants clear up themselves eventually. Most of them seem to last for anything between 1 week and 3 months. Some, however, can last for longer than this, sometimes over a year, and a small proportion of these may become relatively permanent states of depression or involve a constant cycling between depression and elation.

The second point is that, in the case of ulcers, relaxing and taking bland meals as well as taking an antiulcer pill is the quickest and most certain way to treat the ulcer. In the same way, combining antidepressants and the latest techniques for handling depression psychologically is probably quicker and more likely to lead to cure than only taking antidepressants or having cognitive therapy without pills, for example. There are strong suggestions that the combination of treatments is likely to be the most effective means of preventing any relapse (Healy 1997).

Do antidepressants cure?

Many people think that antidepressants and ECT do not cure any thing, that they only suppress problems or blunt reactions to some trauma until the individual has a chance to recover. However, the effect of antidepressants on depression, in this regard, is rather like the effect of antiulcer pills on ulcers. Many people who are treated for an ulcer will only ever have that one ulcer. The pills cure it. In the same way, with depression, many people only ever have one serious episode.

The other way of putting this question is: 'Does depression ever truly clear up?' The answer is – yes, it does. However, just like ulcers and influenza, depression is a disorder that, even if this episode is cured, may recur. There are some suggestions that recurrence is more likely if the initial episode was treated inadequately. Current estimates are that perhaps up to half of us have at least one episode of biological depression during our life, although this may be so physical or so mild that it may not be clearly recognised as a 'depression' by many of us.

While antidepressants do cure most episodes of depression, some people go on to have chronic depression, and others to have regular episodes of depression – in some cases alternating with elation. It is probable that a variety of physical factors, such as mildly abnormal endocrine status, and psychological factors, such as pre-existing impairment of self-esteem, make this more likely.

Does psychotherapy cure any better than antidepressants? The answer to this appears to be no. Even if a depression has been cured with the latest techniques, it may relapse in just the same way following psychotherapies. In this regard depression, just like ulcers, seems to be a physical illness that clears up but may also come back. For the most part, it is not an illness like coronary artery disease or rheumatoid arthritis which, once you have it, can never really be cured. However, patients with manic–depressive illness, for example, have a life-long condition, as do patients with dysthymia who are recognised as having a chronic predisposition to misery, often present from an early age.

Finally, antidepressants also resemble antiulcer pills in two other ways. One is that just as there are a number of quite different ways to treat an ulcer – you can reduce acid levels, or coat the ulcer, or kill *H. pylori* – so also are there a number of different ways to get depressions better. The tricyclic antidepressants do so by acting like old-fashioned tonics in many respects: they improve sleep and appetite. The SSRIs do so by being serenics, or anxiolytic – they produce a mellow state, which works for some people. The MAOIs and other drugs selective to the noradrenergic system help by being more energising than the other drugs.

In addition, while both antidepressants and antiulcer treatments often cure the illness they treat, on both treatments relapse is possible even while the individual is on active treatment. This links into the vexed question of dependence.

WHAT DO ANTIDEPRESSANTS DO?

The principal theories about what the antidepressants do to biological systems in the brain have focused on their effects on the neurotransmitters, noradrenaline and serotonin (5HT). The first of these theories, the catecholamine hypothesis of depression, was put forward in 1965. It was based on the idea that drugs that lower noradrenaline or 5HT in the brain seemed to trigger depression, and the then known antidepressants appeared to increase the levels of these neurotransmitters. This hypothesis and its derivatives have dominated thinking on the mode of action of antidepressants, particularly the theories that are put forward in popular books on depression or antidepressants or in articles from magazines such as *Cosmopolitan* or *Esquire*. The truth, however, is that despite more than three decades of work there still is no convincing theory about what antidepressants do. To suggest that there is one would be misleading.

This lack of a convincing rationale for what antidepressants do leads some people to have doubts about taking them. It should be borne in mind, however, that the questions of whether antidepressants work and how they work are quite separate. In the case of most drugs, we have no good idea how they work but convincing indications that they do work. This situation comes about because most drugs are developed by chance rather than by rational design – although many psychiatrists and drug companies would have us believe otherwise. So, although there is little agreement about what the antidepressants do, there is compelling evidence that they work and a good case can be made that, in many cases, they cure.

Clinically, for the first 2 weeks of treatment, the standard view is that antidepressants do very little except cause side effects. The change that then occurs seems to creep up on people rather than to sweep in on them. It seems to be rather like the kind of change that goes with influenza clearing up, rather than the instant and dramatic changes brought about, for instance, by antianginal tablets in cases of angina, or by bronchodilators in the case of asthma. What usually happens is that there is a slow increase in energy, a slow return of interest, a mild increase in appetite and an improvement in sleep. These occur gradually rather than clearly and they may be patchy, for example with one good night's sleep followed by a poor one the night after. Rather like a slow change of season – to return to the climate analogy used earlier.

For the most part, improvements in the sadness, hopelessness, guilt and suicidal thoughts that may go with depression seem to occur as a reaction to changes in things such as sleep, energy and interest. They often, therefore, take somewhat longer to become established. Sometimes sleep improves, and energy and interest increase, but the individual may remain demoralised. The temptation in such cases is to increase the dose of the antidepressant; this rarely produces the hoped for benefits.

Having made these points, we have recently given antidepressants to healthy volunteers – with surprising results. First, when the drug suited an individual, it was possible to make perfectly normal people 'better than well'. In the case of the SSRIs this involved making a person more serene or mellow. For some people this can be unhelpful; for others it seemed to be something they appreciated. In the case of drugs active on the noradrenergic system, when these drugs were appreciated it was because they produced what the taker saw as a useful increase in energy and drive. And all these effects were visible within 48 h.

A number of lessons fall out of this. One is that calling these drugs antidepressants is in some sense misleading. These drugs have effects on a wide variety of conditions and even on normal people. The second is that there is probably a roughly 50 : 50 chance that a person put on a drug by their doctor will be put on the wrong drug for them. This means that the first few weeks of treatment should be monitored carefully. Finally, these effects will be visible long before 2 weeks are up. What happens at the 2–3-week stage is that the depression breaks up. But long before that it may be possible for someone to work out whether the pill they are on is suiting them or not.

Aside from the issue of what brain systems they work on, there are a number of ways in which the antidepressants differ from other psychotropic drugs.

First, unlike any other drugs that act on the brain, whether tea or coffee, nicotine or alcohol, antipsychotics, minor tranquillisers or marijuana, the traditional view is that the antidepressants do not have an immediately obvious action, within 30 min or so. The only thing antidepressants obviously do within 30 min is to produce side effects. The lifting of a depressed mood, in contrast, typically takes up to 2 weeks and sometimes longer to begin to appear.

Because tea or tranquillisers act within 30 min and their effects wear off in a few hours, it is usual to take them several times every day. It seems sufficient, however, to take antidepressants once a day. For this reason they are often now given in one dose, last thing at night or first thing in the morning.

Another unusual feature of the antidepressants is that the dominant view is that they only do anything to people who are depressed. This is not true for tea, coffee, antipsychotics and everything else, which have much the same actions in people with or without mental disorders. Beneath these apparent differences, however, lies a complex set of effects.

While it may often take several weeks to 'break up' a depression, the effects of an antidepressant will often be apparent within 1–2 days, if looked for. These may range from the tonic effects of some tricyclic antidepressants, which lead to an almost immediate improvement in sleep and appetite, to the anxiolytic or serenic effects with SSRIs, to drive-enhancing effects that can be seen with agents selective to the noradrenergic system. This is very obvious when these drugs are given to healthy volunteers, when the right effect for the right person may in fact even produce a better-than-well effect in a totally normal person. On an SSRI, for instance, normal individuals may become mellow, and this may suit them.

These effects, however, are rather subtle compared with the effects of tea, alcohol, benzodiazepines or antipsychotics and, because of this, few people ask what is this drug doing to get a depressed person well, or what do we want a drug to do to get this person well. The assumption is that all antidepressants do much the same thing regardless of which brain system they work on. Nothing could be further from the truth.

A further unusual feature of the antidepressants is that, broadly speaking, it is not the case that some of an antidepressant does a little bit of good and more of it does more good – as is the case with tea or coffee. It seems to be that, if one takes a dose below a certain threshold, nothing much may happen apart from side effects, and that doses greatly in excess of the threshold do not seem to operate any more effectively or any more quickly than does the threshold dose. Indeed, higher doses are simply more likely to cause further side effects.

Finally, antidepressants differ from the other drugs in psychiatric use in that in overdose many older antidepressants can be fatal in relatively small amounts, although this is much less the case with some of the more recently produced compounds.

ANTIDEPRESSANTS: FIRST CHOICE OR LAST RESORT?

Given that many depressions heal naturally, and given that psychotherapy can help, should people take antidepressants at all? Those who would argue that you should not take them commonly put forward three different objections. One is that antidepressants alter brain chemistry and this cannot be a good idea. Another is that antidepressants block messages in the brain and this cannot be a good idea. The third is that the use of antidepressants will interfere with the development of natural coping mechanisms.

Antidepressants and brain chemistry

Antidepressants do act on receptors in the brain. Not only this, but they alter far more brain receptors than do drugs such as diazepam, for example. Quite mysteriously, they even bring about changes in brain receptors on which the drugs themselves do not act. Could this predispose individuals who take these pills to further episodes of depression, by making them chemically unstable?

The answer to this is, for most people, no. Unlike other drugs that act on the brain, antidepressants act 'weakly' on the brain receptors they bind to. They neither vigorously act on nor comprehensively block anything. The changes they bring about tend to be within the range of changes that are happening during the day anyway: brain receptors and enzymes fluctuate in levels according to a circadian rhythm. This is quite different to the effects of coffee, tranquillisers or alcohol, for example, which push the brain systems they act on well beyond the normal range of circadian variation.

A further important point is that the illness itself also brings about changes in brain functioning. For example, it is known that depression causes an increase in levels of the stress hormone, cortisol. What has recently become clear is that prolonged increases of cortisol concentration reset the central mechanisms controlling cortisol levels to a higher setting. This in turn is liable to lead to raised cortisol level even when the person is not depressed. Increased cortisol synthesis may even, in time, lead to brain cell loss and premature ageing. Chronically raised cortisol levels will lead to far more comprehensive and long-lasting changes in brain receptors than antidepressants ever bring about.

Whether through cortisol or some other mechanism, ongoing depression predisposes to future relapses of a depressive episode and to increasing severity of that episode. It is also likely to increase the risk for tumours and infections. Indeed, a dramatic recent discovery has been that the presence of depressive symptoms after a heart attack is a significant factor in determining recovery or otherwise from the attack: the presence of depressive symptoms greatly increases the likelihood of death in the following 12-month period (Frasure-Smith et al 1993). Therefore, leaving the illness untreated is not as natural or as healthy as it might sound.

Again, the ulcer model may shed some light on this. Leaving an ulcer untreated for too long can lead to extensive scarring in the area around the ulcer. Even if the ulcer then heals, this scar tissue, by distorting the natural shape of the stomach and duodenum, can make future ulcers more likely and slow their recovery.

Do antidepressants block important messages?

Another reason given for not taking antidepressants is based loosely on the biochemical theories of how they work. The argument goes that they block impulses flowing from one brain cell to another. This never sounds like a good idea to anyone. However, chemical messages and psychological messages are not the same thing. As we age there are many fewer neurotransmitters whizzing around our brains, but psychologically we remain the same.

Antidepressants and coping

A third argument goes: if antidepressants suppress or otherwise bring a halt to a depressive episode, surely the individual will not learn the coping skills that are necessary to handle depression and will therefore remain vulnerable to yet further depressive episodes. These latter depressive episodes will then increasingly have to be chemically controlled.

Regarding the question of whether antidepressants interfere with the development of natural coping mechanisms, the following points can be made. Depression is a demoralising disorder. It tends to be particularly demoralising the longer and more severe it is. Demoralisation is not something that antidepressants clear up. It typically resolves when the underlying depression resolves. At least, it does so when the underlying depression has not been particularly severe or long lasting.

We spring back naturally. Springing back does not come about because we have developed new coping skills. We simply do not need to be anxious and demoralised once normality has returned. We are less likely to spring back in this way if the underlying depression has lasted for a long time or has been severe. In this case, antidepressants may clear up the sleep and appetite disturbances and improve energy levels but leave the person miserable, unhappy and with an impairment of self-esteem that may be more or less permanent. This impaired self-esteem will also make further serious and lengthy depressions more likely, as, should the person ever become mildly clinically depressed again, their impaired self-esteem will summate rapidly with the depression, leading to a very rapid evolution to severe depression.

Therefore, everything possible should be done to avoid demoralisation. The best method of doing this is to ensure that the depression a person has is as brief and as mild as possible and, in particular, that they are not exposed to a severe or long-lasting disorder. The best advice, therefore, is that, at the first hint that the disorder is not going to be brief and self-resolving, some intervention is called for in order to preserve current coping skills and to prevent them from being lost in the face of increasing demoralisation. This may be either a cognitive or interpersonal therapy, or other behavioural approach or antidepressants. Most importantly, it should be something rather than nothing.

Having made this point, however, the point also needs to be made that people who take antidepressants and whose depressions resolve should not conclude that the restoration of the self-confidence they have had is down to their antidepressant alone. Thinking this could lead on to a belief that one had to keep on taking the antidepressants in order to remain stable, or to a belief that one is more vulnerable than the average person to further depression. Halting antidepressants, if this were the case, could be seen as the potential removal of a crutch and it could become quite threatening. Such an idea of what antidepressants do would rob a person of confidence in their own resources to handle further episodes of depression – and even to handle episodes of interpersonal difficulties in general.

All too often, prescribers of antidepressants seem to have assumed that, just because antidepressants were not supposed to cause a physical dependence or withdrawal symptoms, there was no problem with prescribing them for lengthy spells. What we have all too often failed to realise is that depression causes a loss of self-esteem and that antidepressants do not necessarily put this right. If it comes right, it comes right in the way that anxiety clears up after an ulcer resolves. If it does not come right, some consideration should be given to a psychological intervention rather than simply to more or longer courses of an antidepressant. On top of this, it has now become clearer that some people may become physically dependent on antidepressants, in particular the SSRIs.

Return to normality

One of the hardest things for people to do after they have been depressed, whether or not they have been treated with antidepressants, but particularly if they have been, is to let themselves get normally depressed after they halt the drugs. We seem to assume that, because we have been cured, we should not get depressed again. The first hint of a poor spell after stopping antidepressants may cause a serious panic.

But, in fact, returning to normal means returning to the normal ups and downs of life. What has to be relearnt is an ability to live with these ups and downs – as they cannot be stopped. Even on antidepressants, the normal ups and downs should continue. The greatest block to recovery may often be the person's own idea of what it means to be well: treatment should make me into someone who never has any ups or downs again.

What if there is no response?

Before concluding that there will be no response to an antidepressant, a subject should have been taking a full dose of the antidepressant they have been put on for up to 6 weeks – provided there are no indications that the drug is not suiting them. If there is then definitely no response, the options are:

- To change to another type of antidepressant, if there is any indication that the current antidepressant is not suiting.
- To go to a higher dose, as some people do not seem to absorb the drugs as well or there may be other biological reasons why a higher dose is necessary (see doses).
- To add in a psychological therapy. Paradoxically, many resistant 'biological' depressions seem to need the addition of psychological interventions.
- To have a combination of antidepressants, for example a tricyclic along with an MAOI or lithium, or an SSRI with mianserin or lithium. This is termed an augmentation strategy.
- To discontinue antidepressants completely on the premise that, although the person is very miserable and demoralised, they do not have the kind of problem that responds to antidepressants. In this case, psychotherapy will be necessary.
- To have ECT. This remains the most effective treatment for depression. Today it is usually used as a treatment of last resort. But, in fact, ECT has fewer side effects than many of the other treatments. It is used, for example, in the frail elderly or after heart attacks, where antidepressants may be contraindicated. As a treatment of last resort, however, ECT is sometimes given inappropriately to individuals who have failed to respond to medication but who should never have been given antidepressants in the first instance. This can only lead to ECT getting a bad name.

STARTING AND STOPPING

Tricyclic antidepressants

The usual dose of a tricyclic antidepressant is 150 mg per day. In some cases, it is possible to start at 75 mg daily and increase to 150 mg within a few days. For others it is necessary to start at 25 mg per day and work up slowly. The more anxious the person, the slower the dose escalation. There is a trend toward giving the entire 150 mg in one dose, usually last thing at night.

If there is no response to 150 mg a day, in some cases the dose may be put up higher, to anything up to 300 mg daily, depending on side effects. For most non-responders such an increase will make no difference, but in some cases there is a failure to absorb the drug and larger doses are needed to produce the normal blood levels. Other factors that hinder recovery may be overcome by a higher dose. These include high levels of the stress hormone cortisol, concurrent infections, concurrent treatment with contraceptives and obesity.

At present, all the clinical trial evidence suggests that there is little point being on less than 75 mg a day of a tricyclic for full-blown depression. A little bit of an antidepressant just is not a little bit antidepressing. However, in clinical practice, tricyclics such as dothiepin (dosulepin) are often given in a 25-mg night-time dose and they work – at least in the sense of improving sleep in what may be cases of mild depression or anxiety.

For four decades the received wisdom was that antidepressants are non-addictive, and for many people there may be essentially little or no withdrawal reaction. Rebound effects, such as cholinergic rebound, which may produce increased dreaming at night for one or two nights but little more, were recognised. Aside from these rebound effects, stemming from the action on the cholinergic system, it is now clearer that a smaller number of individuals again may become more classically physically dependent on these drugs, and on halting may have difficulties lasting for a few days or even up to several weeks. These dependence reactions have been associated mostly with the SSRIs, but many tricyclics also act on the serotonin system (see Section 8).

MAOIs

In the case of the MAOI, phenelzine, the effective dose is between 60 and 120 mg per day. For tranylcypromine, it is 20–40 mg a day. For moclobemide, the dose is 600–900 mg daily, in divided doses. These drugs are usually prescribed first thing in the morning rather than last thing at night, as they may be mildly stimulant and interfere with sleep.

Withdrawal from a MAOI poses the same issues as withdrawal from a tricyclic, although phenelzine has something of a reputation of being more difficult to get off, for reasons that have never been clearly pinpointed.

SSRIs

The SSRIs have had a convenience factor that may have accounted in part for their success: the possibility of treatment with a single pill per day (except for fluvoxamine). This has clear advantages, but also disadvantages. It is clear that many people cannot immediately tolerate the amount in even one pill; this is particularly true for people who are anxious. Company representatives warn physicians about the hazards of serotonin pick-up syndromes, even though officially the companies deny that this happens. This has led to a widespread practice of co-administering benzodiazepines for the first few weeks of treatment.

If starting an SSRI is more convenient on average than starting other anti-depressants, stopping them poses greater problems. It is now clear that SSRIs may lead to significant physical dependence in 10–20% of takers. The commonest symptoms of this are dizziness, headache, sweating, fatigue and nausea, but a wide variety of problems can occur from electric sensations shooting up and down limbs, to depersonalisation and muscle pain (Taylor 1999). Indeed, the picture may so resemble depression that, in early SSRI trials, the problems that occurred on stopping the drugs were interpreted as illness relapse rather than withdrawal (Glenmullen 2000, Rosenbaum et al 2000). Alternatively, someone who does not suspect withdrawal from their pills may wonder whether they have caught influenza.

No one knows at present the precise figure for the number of people affected by significant withdrawal problems. Women seem more likely to be affected than men – just as women seem more prone to tardive dyskinesia than men. The greatest difficulty with the withdrawal scenario is that it is as likely to affect a person put on SSRIs for a relatively short period of time with a minor complaint that could have been handled without drugs as it is to affect someone on them for a longer time with a more severe problem. This kind of physical dependence needs to be distinguished from addiction: antidepressants do not cause addiction. This important point is developed further in Section 8.

Withdrawal is probably related to the phenomenon of 'poop-out', first described with the SSRIs, where these drugs appear to stop working. This is most probably mediated by the same mechanisms that lead to problems on discontinuation.

Managing withdrawal

The recommendations for managing withdrawal are standard for all psychotropic drug groups. In all cases, antidepressants of whatever class should be tapered rather than discontinued abruptly. In cases of established or suspected withdrawal, the taper should be even slower. There are then options of switching the individual to a tricyclic with a lesser degree of serotonin reuptake inhibition, such as imipramine, and then tapering that even further. Another option is to use fluoxetine, which comes in a liquid form, allowing the dose to be lowered much further. The long half-life of fluoxetine, ordinarily an inconvenience, can be useful here.

Some of the unexplored aspects of these problems concern the best ways to manage the psychological aspects of the withdrawal process. Some of us in situations like this, not unreasonably, get what amounts to a withdrawal phobia, so that the slightest variation from normal plunges us into turmoil. There are good grounds for believing that a cognitive approach to managing this phobia, just like any other phobia, might pay off.

5

Side effects of antidepressants

INTRODUCTION

For the first 2 weeks of taking an antidepressant, there may be little other than side effects. If the pill is ultimately going to be suitable for the person taking it, these will generally be mild. In some cases, however, they may be irritating or even intolerable. The first point is that an antidepressant should cause only tolerable side effects. If treatment makes someone clearly worse, it should be stopped until advice has been sought and until that advice clearly addresses the problem in hand.

There may be difficulty in distinguishing the effects of treatment from some of the symptoms of the illness. Both drugs and illness may cause a dry mouth, headache, indigestion, increased anxiety, sleeplessness or sedation, for example, and even suicidality.

There is a further unusual aspect to the side effects of antidepressants. When individuals are severely depressed, they are often much less sensitive to the effects of anything. They cannot smell, taste or hear as acutely as before, for example. It is also common to find that sleeping pills do not help the insomnia that goes with depression – even three or four times the recommended dose may not bring about sleep. The same people, a few weeks later when they have recovered, may be knocked out by a low dose of the same sleeping pill. All of these points, however, are less likely to apply to patients with a milder form of depression, who are now most likely to be prescribed antidepressants. And, while some people are less sensitive to side effects when they are depressed, others seem to be more sensitive. It is very difficult, therefore, to predict the side effects that an antidepressant will have.

The side effects listed on the next pages are the typical ones. Some of these occur in everyone to some extent, depending on the particular compound they are on, but they are usually mild and wear off after a few days. Even if they are severe, it should be noted that these side effects are almost all reversible and will halt almost immediately on stopping the drugs.

As with the antipsychotics, there are two sorts of side effects to note: those that seem more like side effects, such as a dry mouth or sedation, and those that may feel like a worsening of the illness – like feeling more nervous or feeling strange and unreal, or even hearing voices. These latter side effects are the ones that need careful judgement and may pose the greatest risks.

 User Issues

THE OBVIOUS SIDE EFFECTS OF ANTIDEPRESSANTS

Sedation

Many of the tricyclic antidepressants, especially amitriptyline and trimipramine, as well as mianserin and mirtazapine are sedative when first taken. This sedation is quite like the effect of some of the older antihistamines

continued

(travel sickness pills). Just as with the antihistamines, about one-third of people who take these drugs are clearly sedated, while two-thirds are either slightly sedated or not sedated at all. Sedative effects may be quite unpleasant to begin with, but they usually wear off in the course of a few days. In a minority of people, the sedation may persist, in which case the drug should be stopped, particularly if driving or work is compromised.

In the case of the SSRIs, there may be a paradoxical coexistence of feeling drowsy or fatigued, along with an inability to sleep. Even more clearly with the SSRIs, some people may be drowsy on them while others are unable to sleep, so that for some the dose should be given in the morning and for others in the evening.

Arousal

In some people, rather than cause sedation, tricyclics may bring about an alerting effect, which can make sleep impossible. In this case it makes more sense to take the pill first thing in the morning rather than last thing at night. This is a problem more likely to happen with tricyclic antidepressants with preferential actions on noradrenergic systems, such as desipramine or nortriptyline, or with reboxetine.

MAOIs are more likely than tricyclics to cause arousal. For this reason they are usually given in the morning rather than at night. However, MAOIs may be heavily sedating in some cases and have to be given last thing at night.

In most individuals the SSRIs usually have minimal effects on arousal or sedation. A proportion of people, however, are somewhat stimulated by them, whereas others are clearly sedated. Even more unusually, the SSRIs appear sometimes to cause a subjective drowsiness while at the same time bringing about what is normally seen as a more 'alert' performance on tests of cognitive function.

Dry mouth

An almost universal side effect of antidepressants is that they cause a dry mouth. This will usually be mild and after the initial effects wear off may be unnoticeable, unless the taker has to talk at length, when there is a tendency for the mouth to become dry anyway. Occasionally, it may be severe to the point of feeling that the tongue is stuck to the roof of the mouth or that the inside of the mouth feels like sandpaper. The nose may also be affected so that it feels dry and congested.

For the most part, a dry mouth is a relatively minor inconvenience. It can, however, be a more serious problem for some individuals as saliva protects against tooth decay and its lack may lead to an aggravation of dental caries. This is likely to be a hazard only with some of the tricyclic antidepressants.

It has been traditional to put dry mouth down to the anticholinergic properties of antidepressants. However, the SSRIs, which have been supposed to have little or no anticholinergic effects, also produce a dry mouth.

Fainting

Tricyclic antidepressants, MAOIs, mianserin and mirtazapine all lower blood pressure. This is apt to show up most clearly on getting out of bed or standing up from a chair. For most of us, abrupt changes in posture like this can produce a feeling of faintness or a hint of seeing stars. On treatment, this may become marginally more exaggerated or it may become very marked so that a minor change of posture may cause quite a significant drop in blood pressure, and may cause a subject to topple over, potentially leading to serious falls and injuries. This is a particular hazard in older individuals for whom changes in posture are even more likely to cause a drop in blood pressure.

Palpitations

Palpitations are one of the more unsettling effects of an antidepressant. Finding one's heart beating irregularly or thumping in one's chest is alarming. Despite being alarming, palpitations are usually harmless. The commonest cause comes from the heart trying to compensate for a drop in blood pressure by putting out more blood. There may be a real hazard, however, for individuals who have pre-existing heart trouble; these individuals should be assessed with greater care. In some cases, the drug may also be causing a problem that might require treatment with another compound.

Urinary difficulties

All antidepressants can cause trouble with urination. In the mildest cases, the subject will be aware that there is a slight delay before passing water. There may also be a feeling of distension around the bladder area, which causes a feeling of fullness just above the pubic bone. This may be uncomfortable and even painful. Textbooks usually list these symptoms as affecting only men, but they also affect women – even young women. Occasionally the problem may be more marked to the point of having clear difficulty in passing water or even urinary retention. This latter is most common in older men with enlarged prostate glands.

While this side-effect is usually put down to the anticholinergic properties of tricyclic antidepressants, there also appears to be a serotonin (5HT) input to the bladder, so that SSRIs may lead to something of an increase in bladder capacity and antipsychotics that block serotonin S_2 receptors, such as clozapine, may lead to a decrease. With the release of reboxetine, which has no anticholinergic effects, it has become clearer that the greatest problems stem from the action of any of these drugs on the noradrenergic system.

Sweating

It is not uncommon for antidepressants, especially tricyclics, to produce sweating. This is particularly common in hot weather. It may be most noticeable at night, when it can lead to waking up to find the sheets drenched. Increased perspiration may also be a feature of the serotonin syndrome (see below).

Shake or tremor

In some cases, individuals on an antidepressant may find they have a shake of their hand or arm. This is commonest on high doses. If it happens, it may mean that the dose is too high. In some individuals, because of differences in rates of absorption, the usual clinical dose may be too high and may need lowering. A shake is one hint that this may be the case.

Essentially, antidepressants – and in particular the SSRIs – can cause all the problems that the antipsychotics cause, from dyskinesias, to dystonias, to akathisia and parkinsonian features (see Ch. 2). All these problems are likely to be more obvious when SSRIs are combined with antipsychotics, lithium, valproate, analgesics or oral contraceptives.

continued

Twitch or jerk

All antidepressants can cause twitches or jerky movements (myoclonus) of the head, arms or legs. These seem to be commoner in the legs at night but may affect any part of the body at any time. This is a side effect of antidepressants rarely noted in any books, but it happens to a significant extent in up to 10% of takers. It may be commoner with drugs active on the serotonin system. It usually stops on switching to another treatment.

Tooth grinding (bruxism) and jaw locking (trismus)

Another rarely described side effect is tooth grinding. This is something many of us do during sleep anyway. Some antidepressants, in particular the SSRIs, may lead to tooth grinding during the day. This may get so intense as to cause marked gum pain. Those who can remove dentures do so, but at the cost of embarrassment. Occasionally the problem may be sufficiently severe to lead to a grinding down of the teeth. There may be two distinct components to the problem: (1) abnormal movement of the jaw (a dyskinesia) and (2) an increase in tone of the jaw muscles (dystonia).

In mild forms, this increased tone may be painful and, confusingly, may be experienced simply as a pain in the jaw area. In more severe forms, it can lead to lockjaw (trismus). The problems may also affect the throat, and may be experienced as an acute sore throat (pharyngitis), leading the taker to believe they have a throat infection. In other cases there may be difficulty swallowing, as though the throat is constricted. Another variation on the phenomena is forced yawning.

Up to 50% of the takers of an SSRI may experience some of these problems during the first week of treatment. Tooth grinding is the more likely to persist. This has the potential to lead on to tardive dyskinesia and perhaps should lead to treatment being halted.

Headache

Headaches are a common feature of depression and therefore it may be difficult to be sure whether an antidepressant has caused them. The kind of headache caused by the pills is usually slightly different to the one found in depression itself. Typically, it is a muzziness or feeling of painful fullness rather than the aching tension type of headache that most of us have had at some point or other. It may not be possible to distinguish these headaches, however, and if a new headache comes on after starting an antidepressant, or the old one seems to get worse, it may be wise to seek advice.

In rare instances antidepressants may trigger migrainous headaches – headaches that have a throbbing, pulsating character which usually affects one side or other of the head and which may be accompanied by disturbances of vision and/or nausea and vomiting. The reason for this appears to be because most of these drugs act on the serotonin system, which regulates blood flow through the head and brain. Whether the ordinary kind of headache or a migraine, headaches will almost certainly be harmless. The issue is whether they are too uncomfortable to put up with, rather than whether they are serious.

In a small proportion of cases, the headache may be more serious. This applies particularly to individuals who are on MAOIs and who have eaten food containing tyramine (see Cheese effect below). It may also apply to individuals who are taking lithium (see Ch. 7). Headaches are also likely to be more serious when they occur in someone taking combinations of treatments, such as antidepressants and antipsychotics, antidepressants with lithium, or lithium with antipsychotics.

Blurred vision

A further side effect of most antidepressants is blurred vision. This is particularly likely to happen on tricyclics, which have the most marked anticholinergic effects, but eyesight disturbances also happen with SSRIs. While this is listed as one of the obvious side effects of antidepressants, it is surprising how often it leads people to make appointments to get their eyes checked. It is important not to have an eye appointment for failing eyesight and a possible change of glasses until after the drug has been discontinued, at which point, if there is still a problem, advice should be sought.

Occasionally, individuals prone to glaucoma will have their condition exacerbated and it will be necessary to prescribe an antidepressant with minimal or no anticholinergic effects. For those who do not know they are prone to glaucoma, the condition, if it is aggravated, presents with acutely painful eyes. It must be stressed, however, that this is a rare occurrence.

Weight gain

Depression often leads to a loss of appetite and a loss of weight. Treatment with antidepressants can therefore be expected, by restoring appetite, to lead to some weight gain in all of us. For some individuals, however, there is a far more serious weight gain than this. They may put on up to a stone or two extra for reasons that are not fully understood. Weight gain may be aggravated in individuals who are also taking lithium (see Ch. 7) and antipsychotics (see Ch. 2).

Until recently there was no option as regards the issue of weight gain because all the antidepressants in use were liable to cause the problem. The SSRIs, however, do provide an option. In the short term, in general, these drugs have an appetite-suppressing property. In some cases they may cause nausea and even vomiting. The nausea generally subsides within a few days but a mild suppression of appetite, as opposed to the mild increase that may be brought about by tricyclics, may remain. Over time, however, weight gain on SSRIs may occur as a delayed-onset effect and, indeed, may be dramatic.

While weight gain may seem like an obvious side effect of drug treatment, many individuals seem to be unaware that their drugs may be causing them weight gain and, accordingly, they may try to diet strenuously, abetted by their general practitioner. Their inability to lose weight in the expected way may be quite demoralising.

Nausea

All antidepressants may cause nausea. They may also cause indigestion, constipation and a bloated feeling. The SSRIs, however, are far more likely to cause nausea and indigestion than other agents. Up to 25% of people who take these drugs may feel as though they are sea-sick. This usually wears off after a few days. In some cases, however, it may be quite severe, may lead to vomiting and may not wear off. In such cases the drugs have to be stopped.

The addition of lithium to another antidepressant is particularly liable to lead to nausea. It seems that nausea in many of these instances is brought about by a sensitisation of serotonin receptors in the gut.

continued

Rashes and infections

All drugs may cause idiosyncratic hypersensitivity reactions. The commonest sign of such a reaction is a skin rash. Such reactions are usually not harmful and go quickly once the drug has been stopped. A more serious problem is recurrent fevers, with a sore throat and painful mouth. This may also be a hypersensitivity reaction. It may be necessary to take a blood test to check the white blood cell count to establish what is happening. Treatment may have led to a lowering of the white cell count, which predisposes to infection. The antidepressant most noted for this is mianserin, but there is evidence that other antidepressants may have this effect, especially in the elderly.

 User Issues

THE AMBIGUOUS SIDE EFFECTS OF ANTIDEPRESSANTS

Depersonalisation

Depersonalisation refers to an experience of feeling strange and unusual, almost as though you are not really yourself anymore, or that you are operating in a kind of a dream or haze. It refers to the unreal feeling that many of us may have at interviews or other stressful situations where part of us seems to be functioning automatically and not under full control. Depersonalisation and derealisation are the commonest dissociative reactions.

Derealisation

Derealisation refers to a similar set of feelings and perceptions seen in depersonalisation, but in this case they apply to the world rather than to the self. This is a state in which the world seems strange or unreal; everything may seem far away or staged in some way – as though life is being watched rather than lived.

These feelings happen in anxiety states but they also happen commonly in depression as well. If, however, they start for the first time after taking an antidepressant or get clearly worse, treatment should be discontinued. The sensations will go within hours, or at the most days, after stopping treatment. They are not serious, although, like palpitations, they may be very unsettling experiences.

The danger of these dissociative experiences lies in the fact that they may be interpreted by either the person taking the antidepressant or others as evidence that the illness is getting worse or that brain damage of some sort has been caused that may be permanent. If misinterpreted, such reactions can lead on to suicide (see below). This risk, and the fact that a drug causing such reactions is most unlikely to cure depression, provide grounds for switching treatment to something else.

Other dissociative reactions have also been reported. These include:

- A feeling that time is standing still
- Déjà vu experiences
- Prominent nightmares
- Out-of-body experiences
- Amnesia. In some cases an individual on antidepressants may find their memory clearly impaired. Subsequently, on discontinuing the drug, they

may find it difficult to remember what it was like to be on it and a number of the things that happened to them while they were on treatment.

◆ Auditory or visual hallucinations. These are more likely in the elderly but can happen to anyone. They are not serious. They clear up once the drug is discontinued. The problem arises should the experience prompt someone to think that their illness must be getting worse because 'everyone knows voices are a sign of lunacy'.

Confusion or disorientation

Also rare and serious is the occurrence in some individuals, especially older people, of confusion. This is probably quite closely related to depersonalisation. In the case of depersonalisation, individuals ordinarily know that things are not quite right, yet are able to operate normally and appear to outsiders to be quite normal. One step further along this path lies confusion, when it becomes obvious that something is not quite right. An affected subject may get to the stage of being disoriented and, as a consequence, quite agitated in a way that puts them at risk to themselves or to others.

Added to this is the fact that in rare instances, again especially in the elderly, tricyclic antidepressants and MAOIs can cause hallucinations. Combined with a confusional reaction, the occurrence of hallucinations may produce a picture of what looks like an almost full-blown insanity. The fact that it all clears up quickly once the drugs are stopped indicates that what is involved is a side effect of treatment rather than any change in the individual's mental balance.

Sexual side effects

The issue of sexual side effects of psychotropic medication is dealt with more fully in Section 7. As with the antipsychotics, there is a general coyness about enquiring about the effects of antidepressants on sexual functioning, and hence information is limited.

In men, antidepressants may cause difficulties in sustaining an erection or in ejaculating. Estimates have been creeping up recently, with suggestions that up to 50% of those on tricyclics or MAOIs and more than 50% of those on SSRIs have notable effects. The distress that this causes is also unclear, but presumably it will lead some people to discontinue treatment. In some cases, however, delayed ejaculation can be helpful for men and there is a growing use of SSRIs for this purpose.

There is a further unusual effect on ejaculation, which is retrograde ejaculation. In this case, owing to altered sphincter tone, the seminal fluid passes backwards into the bladder on ejaculation rather than forward in the usual manner. This effect may only be noticed later when the affected person notices that their urine is more cloudy than usual.

The antidepressant for which all these effects are most clearly documented is clomipramine, which can cause difficulties in up to 80% of men taking it. For the most part, however, when this is being taken to ameliorate obsessional symptoms (see Ch. 10), most takers appear happy with the trade-off between an easing of their symptoms and changes in their sexual functioning, which can be managed by, for example, weekend breaks from treatment. On withdrawal, clomipramine may produce the opposite: repeated unwelcome ejaculations/orgasms, in both men and women. Clomipramine appears to produce these effects mainly through an action on serotonin reuptake.

continued

Not surprisingly, therefore, the SSRIs produce similar effects. Effects can range from an inhibition of erection and/or ejaculation to just the opposite.

Another side effect is priapism: sustained erection of the penis. If mild, this may be a welcome development, but in some cases the erection produced may be so full as to be painful or may be so sustained (12–24 h) that it causes permanent damage to the tissues of the penis. In such cases, surgical relief may be required. The antidepressant most likely to cause this is trazodone. The effect is thought to be mediated through both noradrenergic and serotonergic receptors.

Effects on erectile functioning are the most obvious of the effects on the sexual system. What is much less clear is the effect of antidepressants on interest in sex (libido). A reduction in libido is a common feature of depression, and reduced libido often seems to be one of the last things to return to normal, when a depression clears up. Over and above this, however, there is some evidence that antidepressants may in a minority of cases actually reduce libido further, although compounds that act on serotonergic receptors such as trazodone and nefazodone may do the opposite and enhance libido.

The effects of antidepressants on sexual functioning in women are somewhat more clear than the effects of antipsychotics. The SSRIs and clomipramine are liable to cause a failure of orgasm in women in exactly the same way as they inhibit ejaculation in men. There is no reason to believe that it occurs any less frequently in women than in men.

As with men, trazodone and nefazodone are likely to lead to an increased libido in women. The effects of other antidepressants on libido are less clear in that libido is commonly lost in the course of a depressive disorder and restored when the disorder clears up; whether a particular compound delays the recovery of libido or not has been very difficult to gauge against the background of depression.

Other possible changes involve disturbances to:

◆ the frequency and/or intensity of periods
◆ changes in breast size and/or tenderness

The reason for including the sexual side effects of antidepressants in this section is because any impairments of sexual functioning are all too liable to be interpreted by depressed individuals as personal failings, providing further evidence of their inadequacy. All sexual side effects appear to be reversible on discontinuation of the drugs. Even increasing libido in a subject who is not expecting it may cause problems.

Emotional blunting

There are good grounds for arguing that the SSRIs are primarily serenics – agents that produce an anxiolytic effect (see Ch. 12). They make individuals less reactive to triggers from the environment. When this works, it produces a mellow or docile state, a sanguine frame of mind. In many cases, however, either too much of this effect is produced or the effect is not appreciated by the taker, with complaints that the treatment is making them emotionally dead or emotionally blunted.

This can be noticed in people who have failed to respond to treatment who report that they still cannot eat or sleep but that they have at least stopped crying. In people who have recovered, it is common to hear complaints that everything would be great if they could only cry at sad movies or songs (Hoehn-Saric et al 1990).

Restlessness, agitation and turmoil: akathisia

This side effect, common with antipsychotics, was thought to be uncommon with antidepressants but is being increasingly recognised and thought to be significant (see Suicide below). It may occur within hours of starting an antidepressant or take up to 2 weeks to appear.

It is traditional to translate akathisia into the lay term 'restlessness', but this does not begin to convey all that may be involved. The very first descriptions of this problem were in normal people taking reserpine for blood pressure problems. This led to quotes such as the following: 'increased tenseness, restlessness, insomnia and a feeling of being very uncomfortable', 'the first few doses frequently made them anxious and apprehensive … they reported increased feelings of strangeness, verbalised by statements such as "I don't feel like myself" … or "I'm afraid of some of the unusual impulses that I have"'. Or take the case of CJ, who on the first day of treatment reacted with marked anxiety and weeping and on the second day 'felt so terrible with such marked panic at night that the medication was cancelled' (Healy & Savage 1998). These quotes make it clear that a word such as turmoil is probably a much closer description of what is involved than just restlessness.

This kind of turmoil seems most liable to happen in subjects who are anxious or agitated to begin with. It is particularly marked when antidepressants are given to patients who have panic disorder. Such patients may be made much worse if put immediately on a high dose, such as 75 mg at night of a tricyclic antidepressant, increasing after a day or two to 150 mg. In the case of highly anxious patients it seems better to start a lower dose and to work slowly up to a higher dose.

In addition to inner turmoil, this state may manifest itself on the outside as apparent tension rather than restlessness. The critical point is the inner subjective aspect of what is happening (there is another word for abnormal restless movements happening outside the subject's control – dyskinesia). The difference between akathisia and dyskinesia is that one comes with a clear sense of turmoil or tension (akathisia), whereas the other is less likely to.

A more classical antipsychotic-like akathisia, with obvious foot movements, also appears to happen on antidepressants, especially with the SSRIs. The drug for which this has been most clearly described is fluoxetine, but it probably applies to most tricyclics and to other SSRIs also (Cunningham-Owens 1999, Sachdev 1996).

Antidepressants and suicide

Depression brings with it a risk of suicide. There is no generally accepted theory of why depressed individuals commit suicide. It has been widely noted that one of the times people are most likely to attempt to kill themselves has been around 10–14 days after starting antidepressant treatment. The rationale sometimes given for this is that depression causes both a slowing up (psychomotor retardation) of the affected individual and suicidal ideation. Antidepressants are then supposed to clear up the retardation before they have effects on suicidal thoughts. This, it is argued, leads to individuals having the necessary drive and energy to effect their own demise, in a way that was not possible when they were extremely slowed up in themselves.

continued

While this may be true in some instances, recent developments suggest that this is not the only reason why individuals may commit suicide while on antidepressants. It now seems likely that the occurrence of restlessness or tension or dissociative reactions while on antidepressants may lead to suicide attempts. Patients who are not depressed or suicidal, or healthy volunteers put on antidepressants, can become suicidal.

There is some dispute as to why this should be the case. In the case of depressed patients, it might be argued that subjects on antidepressants who find themselves feeling depersonalised or in turmoil sometimes reason that what is happening is that their nerves are getting worse. As this happens despite their being on treatment, they conclude that they are incurable and that there is no option other than suicide. This is particularly likely to be the case in instances where the turmoil is quite intense – as it may be. This rationale may even apply if the subject believes the drugs to be responsible for their feeling worse and discontinues treatment, only to find no immediate relief. In this case, an individual may conclude (incorrectly) that the drug has done permanent damage to their nervous system. An increasing number of cases of this sort are being recognised. Impairments of sexual functioning of one sort or another are a further side effect that could conceivably produce a similar outcome (Creaney et al 1991, Healy 1994, Jick et al 1995). However, this scenario does not account for healthy individuals becoming suicidal on SSRIs (Healy 2000). It may not be simply a mistake or a misinterpretation.

The SSRIs and other newer agents are clearly safer in overdose than the older tricyclic compounds, and this initially led to hopes that their use might be associated with a lower incidence of successful suicide. However, a number of studies have cast doubt on this. In particular a large study by Jick and colleagues (1995), tracking the outcomes of 172 000 subjects treated by their general practitioner, found a higher rate of successful suicides (by any method) in subjects taking newer as opposed to older antidepressants. This could not be explained by supposing that the more severely depressed patients had been given the newer drugs (Jick et al 1995). More recently a study by Donovan et al (2000) showed that patients on SSRIs are considerably more likely to be assessed in casualty departments following self-harm or overdose attempts than are patients taking tricyclics.

The serotonin syndrome

Antidepressants, and in particular the SSRIs, may produce a picture that has similarities to the neuroleptic malignant syndrome (NMS) described in Chapter 2 (Lejoyeux et al 1994, Sternbach 1991). A group of side effects, which all appear to stem from an excess of serotonin, occurs in this condition. The occurrence of any one of these side effects on their own is not a cause for alarm; it is their conjunction that constitutes the serotonin syndrome which, although not as serious as NMS, does need urgent attention.

The commonest feature of the syndrome is myoclonus (jerks and twitches), which occurs in up to 40%. Tremors of the tongue or fingers occur in 25%, as does shivering and sweating. Up to 20% of subjects may be confused, agitated or restless. In 15% there may be evidence of hyperreflexia and in 10% diarrhoea. Little is known of the subjective nature of the state, at present.

At least three of these symptoms should be present before making a diagnosis. Unlike NMS, this condition often simply responds to halting treatment. It is not clear how often the condition actually occurs – and simply clears up without anything specific being done. However, the condition may also be more serious, requiring hospitalisation, and a small number of fatalities have been suspected.

As the name implies, it is thought that the disorder stems from an excess of serotonin. It probably first began to occur when individuals were put on a combination of MAOIs and tricyclic antidepressants, especially those such as clomipramine which inhibit serotonin reuptake. It appears to have become more common with the recent availability of more potent SSRIs. Combining these with other drugs that act on the serotonin system and/or MAOIs appears liable to trigger the state.

The combination of MAOIs and tricyclics or SSRIs is generally reserved for patients with depressive conditions that are resistant to monotherapy. Where undertaken, there are some indications that moclobemide may be a safer bet than the older MAOIs, and citalopram or paroxetine safer than other SSRIs or tricyclics on the basis that they affect fewer neurotransmitter systems.

Antidepressants and manic reactions

Intuitively it would seem that drugs that elevate mood could go too far and precipitate someone into a manic state. However, ECT and lithium are both antidepressants and at the same time are antimanic. Why should this not also be true for antidepressants? This issue is treated in more detail in the sections on mania and lithium (Chs 6 & 7).

Quite apart from mania proper, another possibility is that antidepressants will disinhibit or induce an emotional dysregulation or lability that may be mistaken for mania. It is also important to distinguish between a manic episode proper and the hyperactivity that may stem from mild confusion or a stimulant effect from one of the older MAOIs in particular. Such reactions require treatment to be halted and should clear up quickly following discontinuation.

Antidepressants and psychotic reactions

A relatively rare side effect of antidepressants, and perhaps of those with an action on the serotonin system in particular, is that certain susceptible individuals may decompensate and develop a psychotic reaction. Such reactions have been noted in the clinical trials of all SSRIs.

 User Issues

EFFECTS SPECIAL TO THE MAOIs

The cheese effect

A particular hazard of the older MAOIs is the cheese effect. This was first noticed as dangerous increases in blood pressure following an intake of cheese in people taking MAOIs. The signs of the problem are headaches, neck stiffness, perspiration, flushing or vomiting. As increased blood pressure can potentially cause a stroke, there was concern. Indeed fatalities on MAOIs have been put down to just such a mechanism, although there is some dispute about this. Cheese contains a substance called tyramine. This is normally broken down in the gut by MAO, so that it does not get into the

continued

body. The MAOIs prevent this breakdown and hence tyramine enters the body and leads to increases in blood pressure.

This means that anyone on an MAOI needs to avoid tyramine-containing foods. This includes all cheeses, except cottage and cream cheese and Danish brie and Danish camembert, as well as pizzas, which usually have mozarella cheese as an ingredient, or pasta dishes with parmesan cheese on them.

Other foods containing tyramine include:

◆ avocado
◆ bananas
◆ caviare
◆ canned figs
◆ pickled herring
◆ liver
◆ smoked or fermented sausages, including peperoni and salami
◆ yeast extracts, including bovril, marmite and oxo
◆ broad bean pods, which are sometimes eaten when beans are young

Almost all wines and beers contain some tyramine. This is particularly the case for Chianti wines. In general it is advised that only fresh food should be eaten. If there is any hint that food such as meat, eggs or poultry may be going off, it should be avoided; game, for example, cannot be eaten.

For the most part, except for some cheeses, pickled herrings and caviare sausages, the amounts of tyramine in the other foods listed above are unlikely to cause significant problems. But, adopting the principle that it is better to be safe than sorry, all the above are usually held to be unsafe. However, the combined effect of avoiding all the foods listed above is a considerable interference with normal living, and for this reason the MAOIs are not usually used as the antidepressant of first choice. They tend now to be used most commonly in individuals who do not tolerate the side effects of tricyclics or who do not respond to tricyclics.

While all the above foods may cause trouble, they do not usually do so. There is no need for anyone to rush to hospital if they are on an MAOI and have suddenly realised that they have just been having cheese and wine. Unless there is a clear feeling of illness, such as the onset of a headache or temperature, or a stiffness of the neck, the odds are that there will be no harmful effect.

Moclobemide, which is termed a reversible inhibitor of MAO, appears to be relatively free of the cheese effect. Large amounts of tyramine will displace the drug from the enzyme, which means that above a certain level the tyramine is metabolised. As a result, even cheese and wine in normal quantities can be taken safely – it would take extraordinary quantities to cause a problem.

 User Issues

SPECIAL CONDITIONS

Pregnancy

At present there seems no good evidence that the older tricyclic or MAOI antidepressants cause a significantly increased risk of abnormalities in the fetus. There appears, therefore, to be no pressing need to discontinue treatment in someone who becomes pregnant. If pregnancy is being contemplated, however, or if there is no clear need to continue with treatment, it may be wiser to stop treatment. Rebound reactions have been noted in infants born to mothers taking antidepressants at the time of labour. These include restlessness, irritability and insomnia, lasting for a few days.

The situation is somewhat different for lithium (see Ch. 6). It is also different for the SSRIs. There is much less experience with these compounds and hence the risks are less certain. There has been a hitherto inconclusive debate about possible teratogenic effects of SSRIs on the fetus.

Both tricyclics and MAOIs enter breast milk in small amounts but appear to be of no risk to babies being breastfed. Fluoxetine and citalopram are contraindicated in breastfeeding, and both paroxetine and sertraline come with warnings.

Cardiac conditions

A further complication of antidepressant treatment, which can now be avoided because of the range of drugs available, concerns the possible effects of these drugs on the heart. For all of us, tricyclic and MAOI antidepressants can be shown to have demonstrable effects on the electrical conduction of the heart. Such effects are not necessarily harmful and, indeed, in a number of therapeutic situations where the heart is not working properly such effects can be helpful.

However, in individuals who have compromised cardiac function, who have recently had a heart attack, who have angina or disturbances of cardiac rhythmicity, the effects of these antidepressants are unpredictable. These individuals should have their heart investigated and the potential effects of an antidepressant on it determined before a course of treatment is started. These problems can usually be overcome by the choice of an alternative antidepressant.

Epilepsy

A further complication of tricyclics that has been overcome by the newer agents concerns their interaction with epileptic disorders. Owing to their effects on electrical conductivity, the tricyclic and MAOI antidepressants alter electrical thresholds. In the case of epilepsy this can actually be beneficial and make the occurrence of an epileptic fit less likely.

However, there can be a problem when the drugs are halted. The changing electrical thresholds that occur at this point in time may trigger a seizure. As halting can be accidental, as, for example, forgetting to take the drugs one night, this issue may be a problem for subjects with epilepsy. The SSRIs seem to be relatively free of this complicating factor.

Overdoses

In general, despite the fearsome list of side effects just covered, anti-depressants rarely cause problems when handled properly. The exception is in the case of overdosage. By far the most important danger with antidepressants stems not from taking a tricyclic antidepressant in the presence of an unsuspected cardiac condition or accidentally combining an MAOI with cheese or wine but rather from overdosage. Antidepressants differ from most other drugs in psychiatric use in that they are liable to be fatal in overdose. This was particularly the case with older tricyclic and MAOI

continued

antidepressants. Overdoses with a relatively modest amount of these pills can kill. Death is by interference with cardiac conduction, causing the heart to beat irregularly or to stop, or is brought about by causing convulsions. There is much less risk with the newer antidepressants.

Driving

With the development of the less sedative SSRIs concern began to be noted about the possible behavioural toxicity of older antidepressants, and in particular their possible role in causing road traffic accidents (O'Hanlon 1995). The first point to note here is that untreated severe depressions probably pose a greater hazard in the main than do the effects of treatment. Second is that the risks associated with taking the older compounds have not yet been established. Third, there can be considerable interindividual variability in the effects of drugs on a performance such as driving. Finally, any such risks seem likely to be of much less practical importance than the risks posed by drinking and driving.

Having made these points, individuals on a cocktail of drugs, or those who are clearly sedated by their drugs, or those who have just started a drug regimen, should probably be advised not to drive or at least should assess responsibly whether their performance is affected. This applies particularly to the driver of heavy goods vehicles or those driving coaches or other passenger-carrying vehicles. While the legal responsibility to issue such warnings may strictly lie with the medical prescriber, in practice those who may be best placed to judge the extent of any risks, apart from the patient, may be friends, relatives or keyworkers.

INTERACTIONS

Important interactions between antidepressants and other drugs are outlined in Box 5.1.

Box 5.1 Antidepressants and drug interactions

- ◆ Barbiturates, benzodiazepines, alcohol and antipsychotics may all increase the sedative effects of antidepressants.
- ◆ Barbiturates, steroid hormones and oral contraceptives may all lower the plasma levels of tricyclic antidepressants.
- ◆ Combinations of antidepressants and antipsychotics may increase the risk of antipsychotic-type side effects.
- ◆ MAOIs may react badly with a number of other drugs. These include cough medicines, pain relievers and cold cures, particularly those containing ephedrine. The MAOIs may also interact seriously with pethidine as well as with a number of anaesthetics given for surgery or even for dental work. It is generally safer to halt the drugs in these instances, or at least to inform the anaesthetist.
- ◆ MAOIs appear to enhance the effects of insulin and oral hypoglycaemic drugs. This may require either a change of antidepressant or a reduction in the dose of insulin or the hypoglycaemic agent.

Management of mania

INTRODUCTION

Mania is, for practical purposes, the mirror image of depression. The majority of people affected present with an elated, euphoric mood. They may be grandiose in their attitudes and beliefs, and disinhibited in their behaviour. However, some may be irritable rather than elated and euphoric, and paranoid rather than grandiose. Common to both groups is an increased level of activity, so that hyperactivity is perhaps the most consistent diagnostic feature of mania. In addition, there is typically an increase in appetites and a decrease in time spent asleep.

In 1850, Falret and Baillarger independently described a bipolar disorder in which affected individuals cycled between periods of elation or mania and depression. This was variously called *folie circulaire* or *folie de deux périodes*. It forms the basis for what is now recognised as manic–depressive disorder (Pichot 1996). In 1896, Emil Kraepelin divided the major psychiatric illnesses into manic–depressive illness and schizophrenia. The former was primarily a disorder of mood, the latter a disturbance of cognitive functions. The former usually followed an episodic course with individuals recovering to normal between episodes. The latter was more likely to become a chronic illness, with a majority of affected individuals not ever fully recovering. These distinctions have broadly speaking held to this day (Healy 1997).

Within the manic–depressive group, Kraepelin included all mood disorders, whether or not the person oscillated between manic and depressive poles. For this reason, some psychiatrists will diagnose individuals who only have recurrent depressive moods as having manic–depressive illness. Others would distinguish between bipolar and unipolar mood disorders. In a bipolar disorder an affected individual will present with evidence of having at some point had episodes of both mania and depression. In contrast, unipolar disorders are those illnesses in which there appear to be only depressive episodes. Unipolar mania is rare.

At present there is little to distinguish bipolar from unipolar disorders, other than episodes of mania. When they are depressed, both groups look indistinguishable, both respond to the same treatments, and there are at present no biological markers that reliably pick out the one group from the other. In part the problem may be that, in practice, one never knows whether one is dealing with a true unipolar disorder or a bipolar disorder that has hitherto presented only with depressive episodes.

Somewhere between one-third and one-half of moderate to severe depressions appear to be associated with an episode of mania at some point during a subject's lifetime (Healy 1997). The difficulties in being precise lie in the fact that many episodes of 'biological' depression may be so mild as to go unnoticed by a general practitioner. Depending on the patient for an accurate history may be a mistake. This is one condition where the patient's partner, parents or children may have a more accurate view of how serious or sustained periods of overactivity and possible disinhibition were. There are also episodes of hypomania, which can be diagnosed retrospectively based on a clear history of a sustained period of several weeks during which the subject was elated, overactive and perhaps somewhat disinhibited but during which the individual's behaviour led neither to a diagnosis nor to hospitalisation. In the United States a distinction is drawn between bipolar 1 disorders, where an individual has been hospitalised for a manic episode at some point, and bipolar 2 disorders, where there is a history suggestive of a period of elation but this is not confirmed by a hospital admission. Some clinicians even talk about bipolar spectrum disorders and suggest that up to 5% of the population may be affected.

There are two issues that arise in any consideration of the management of manic episodes: one is the active treatment of the manic episode itself, dealt with in this chapter, and the other is the prevention of further episodes of either mania or depression, considered in Chapter 7.

LITHIUM

At present, the most specific treatment for mania is generally held to be lithium. It appears to bring about a more specific resolution of manic episodes than does treatment with antipsychotic drugs. Lithium is used both as a specific treatment for episodes of mania and in the prophylaxis (prevention) of further episodes of either mania or depression. The questions of dosage and side effects of lithium are covered in the section on prophylaxis (see Ch. 7).

Treatment with lithium involves a physical screen of the patient beforehand, which takes some days. Because the effects of lithium are slower in onset than those of antipsychotics, and because the use of lithium involves a commitment to ongoing therapy which the patient may not be able to make in the acute stage of a manic illness, the antipsychotics are typically used as a first line of treatment in mania.

In contrast to the effects of antipsychotics in mania, there has always been a substantial body of opinion that has claimed lithium brings about a more specific response in mania. According to this view, patients will sometimes need to be controlled with antipsychotics for the first days in hospital but, if they are prescribed lithium also, the mania will resolve much more specifically and cleanly than it would on antipsychotics alone – usually somewhere around day 10 after therapeutic blood levels have been reached (Healy & Williams 1989, Small et al 1988).

Lithium also appears to have antidepressant properties. This is somewhat more controversial, but a number of studies have shown that major depressive disorders respond to lithium, if treated with adequate doses. Another line of evidence points towards an antidepressant effect of lithium: lithium augmentation treatment for refractory depressions. In cases of depression that prove resistant to conventional antidepressants, it is common practice now to add lithium to the treatment the person is already taking. It appears that, in up to 50% of cases, the addition of lithium will bring about a response over the course of 2–3 weeks' treatment.

Antipsychotics

In practice antipsychotics, and in particular haloperidol or chlorpromazine, are often the first line of treatment for mania (see Ch. 1). In part this stems from the often pressing need to contain the behaviour of individuals with mania, and antipsychotics in moderate to large doses do this relatively quickly. Some of the largest clinical doses of antipsychotics are used for just this purpose.

But, aside from immediate control, antipsychotics are often the only treatment given for an episode of mania. There is some dispute as to whether antipsychotics are specific treatments for mania, or whether they simply contain the disorder until it resolves spontaneously. A number of authorities have argued that, because antipsychotics are helpful in manic states, mania must involve a disturbance of dopamine neurotransmission. If this were the case, then antipsychotics would be a specific treatment for mania, but this argument is a circular one (Healy & Williams 1989).

An alternative is that antipsychotics are of some therapeutic usefulness in mania without being specifically therapeutic. Just as attempts to engage depressed individuals in programmes of motivated activity will often bring about or assist a cure, so conversely the demotivating and immobilising effects of antipsychotics could be expected to assist the resolution of a manic episode by 'taking the wind out of the sails' of affected individuals. Indeed, it can be argued that antipsychotics may play a similar role to that which light plays in the treatment of depression. Arguably, when light therapy works for depression, it does so by activating the sufferer. The opposite treatment for mania might involve putting a patient in a darkened room in order to deactivate them. In practice, large doses of antipsychotics may have a somewhat similar effect to being put in a darkened room.

A fall-back position would be that antipsychotics simply contain manic behaviour non-specifically, by virtue of their chemical strait-jacketing effect, until such time as the episode burns itself out. This issue is not without importance for a number of reasons. One is that antipsychotics may have serious long-term consequences (see Ch. 2). Another is that the long-term treatment of a recurrent bipolar disorder requires engaging patients in the management of their own condition. This is something they are likely to be less willing to do if they have been the victims of some of the regimes that may be inflicted on them in hospital. In recent years a number of individuals have formed 'survivor' groups for those who have been through psychiatric treatment. Many of these individuals are people who have had manic episodes.

The second-generation antipsychotics have introduced a new dimension into the treatment of mania. Clozapine, quetiapine and olanzapine are tricyclic agents from a class of drugs, many of which are antidepressant. It may well be that many of the 'schizophrenic' patients who do best on clozapine are schizoaffective or even have mood disorders misdiagnosed as schizophrenia. The success of clozapine with this kind of patient has led the companies producing olanzapine and quetiapine to undertake trials in mood disorders, and in particular for treatment-resistant mood disorders. These may be effective for mania precisely because their marked sedative effects compared with haloperidol mean that much lower doses are used.

CARBAMAZEPINE

Carbamazepine (Tegretol, Teril) came into widespread use for epileptic disorders, and in particular for temporal lobe epilepsy, in the 1960s. Compared with the barbiturates, which were then the first line of treatment, it was less sedating and non-addictive. In the late 1960s Japanese psychiatrists noticed that patients being treated with carbamazepine showed a lightening in their personalities which suggested an effect on mood in some way. It was also noticed that patients with mood disorders and convulsions treated with carbamazepine did well. This led to a series of trials confirming its usefulness in the management of bipolar mood disorders.

In addition to a use in epilepsy and mood disorders, carbamazepine is also used for a number of other purposes. It is used as a first line of treatment for trigeminal neuralgia. It has also been recommended for what is termed episodic dyscontrol syndrome. This term refers to outbursts of behaviour that appear to occur for no obvious reason. It has been argued that such outbursts in some cases may actually be epileptic episodes without the normal convulsions, rather than just temper tantrums. On this basis carbamazepine has been used with some evidence of efficacy. In practice, however, electroencephalography is rarely done to check for epilepsy, and carbamazepine is used on a trial basis: if it seems to help it is continued, and if not it is stopped.

The place of carbamazepine in the first-line treatment of mania, as opposed to the prophylaxis of bipolar disorders, is less established. Combined with antipsychotics, it is used for mania that does not respond to lithium. It is also used for mania and bipolar disorders characterised by dysphoria (irritability and paranoia) rather than elation, and for rapidly cycling affective disorders.

 User Issues

SIDE EFFECTS OF CARBAMAZEPINE

The main side effects are dizziness, discoordination, double vision and lethargy. Dry mouth, nausea, and diarrhoea or constipation may occur. It may cause sedation and may also produce skin rashes in up to 15% of takers.

In general, a plasma level of between 4 and 12 μg/L is aimed at. Typically the actual dose that is needed to produce such a level may vary considerably. It is customary to start individuals off on a dose of 200 mg per day and increase very slowly – usually 200 mg per week. A dose of 800–1200 mg per day seems the commonest.

Carbamazepine may cause a fall in white cell counts and predispose to the development of fever and sore throats as a consequence. If there are signs of fever, sore throat or infection of any sort, a white cell check should be done; if this is low it may be necessary to discontinue treatment. In general blood counts and liver function tests should be done monthly while carbamazepine is being taken.

Carbamazepine induces liver enzymes. As a consequence a number of other treatments/medications may be metabolised more rapidly. Notable among these is the contraceptive pill. This may mean that a number of treatments, and in particular the pill, do not work as well as before. Haloperidol and lithium may also be affected. Carbamazepine also blocks calcium channel entry and, accordingly, it should be used cautiously with calcium entry blockers.

SODIUM VALPROATE

Sodium valproate is another agent that was used in the first instance for the management of epilepsy. It is formulated in different ways in Europe,

Britain and the United States: sodium valproate (Epilim), semisodium valproate (Depakote), valproic acid (Convulex) and valpromide. In the United States, where it is used more frequently than elsewhere in the management of affective disorders, sodium valproate has come into use as an alternative to lithium and, indeed, has replaced carbamazepine as the first alternative to lithium.

Sodium valproate is used both for the management of acute episodes of mania and for prophylaxis of the recurrent episodes of a bipolar disorder. In acute mania, doses in the order of 1200–2400 mg are used. There are some suggestions that, as with carbamazepine, episodes of mania characterised by dysphoria and irritability rather than euphoria may respond better to sodium valproate (Balfour & Bryson 1994).

 User Issues

SIDE EFFECTS OF VALPROATE

The side effects of valproate are weight gain (up to 50%), weakness (up to 30%), tiredness or drowsiness (30%), a fine tremor (5–10%), and hair loss or hair change (10%). Older preparations of valproate were associated with nausea in up to 40% and with vomiting or abdominal pain in up to 25%. More recently developed preparations are enteric-coated and this has resulted in a lower incidence of nausea. Menstrual irregularities can occur with valproate and there are suggestions of teratogenic effects on the developing fetus.

Valproate inhibits liver enzymes and this can lead to increases in co-administered drugs. For the most part, the co-administered drugs that have been looked at have been other anticonvulsants, but there also appear to be interactions with anticoagulants and salicylates.

LAMOTRIGINE

Based on the effectiveness of valproate and carbamazepine, a number of other anticonvulsants have been tried in both mania and for the prophylaxis of bipolar disorders. Among these have been lamotrigine (Lamictal). Lamotrigine in contrast to the others, however, is possibly more effective for depressive states than for mania. This may be because it produces a sense of well-being rather than the sedation the others produce. This is dealt with in greater detail in Chapter 7. Lamotrigine also requires a slow titration upwards of its dose, and this makes it unsuitable for front-line use for mania.

GABAPENTIN

As with lamotrigine, this anticonvulsant (Neurontin) has also come into use in bipolar mood disorders. It does not appear to be a stand-alone treatment for mania, although it may be useful in conjunction with antipsychotics, and appears to have a role in the prophylaxis of mood disorders. Its use is considered in greater detail in Chapter 7.

TOPIRAMATE AND VIGABATRIN

Topiramate (Topamax) and vigabatrin (Sabril) are two other anticonvulsants that in recent years have been tried in the management of mania and for the prophylaxis of recurrent mood disorders. At present, the data suggest a significant burden of side effects, including sleep disturbances, slurred speech, discoordination, and impairment of concentration and memory, along with other problems in the case of topiramate, and disinhibition or emotional dysregulation and possible psychotic decompensation in the case of vigabatrin. These drugs are unlikely to find a place in the regular treatment of bipolar disorders. The evidence of these two drugs suggests that a simple anticonvulsant action per se does not mean that a drug will be mood stabilising. The anticonvulsants that are helpful must therefore be doing something other than being anticonvulsant.

ACETAZOLAMIDE

This is another anticonvulsant that acts to inhibit an enzyme called carbonic anhydrase. It is rarely used and there have only been a few reports claiming that it may be useful. In particular, however, these reports have claimed that acetazolamide is of some use for the kind of dreamy confusional psychoses that may occur postpartum or perimenstrually.

ELECTROCONVULSIVE THERAPY (ECT)

There has also been a tradition that ECT is both antimanic and antidepressant. In the case of mania, there are very few manic episodes that fail to respond to either lithium or antipsychotics and, accordingly, for a long time there was no satisfactory research evidence that ECT is specifically beneficial in mania. The rationale for using it, until recently, stemmed from the fact it was used widely in the era before lithium and antipsychotics were introduced, and was noted to be useful. In recent years this situation has been remedied. It is now clear that ECT is as specific and as effective as lithium in the treatment of mania (Fink 2000).

There may be an independent effect of ECT on mania, but there is another aspect of the problem that should be noted. There is another bipolar disorder, which comes in overactive and underactive forms: catatonia. There is very good evidence that up to 15% of patients with rapidly cycling or mixed affective states or dysphoric mania may, in addition to mania, have catatonic signs. ECT is the most effective treatment for catatonia. In cases that do not respond readily to lithium or antipsychotics, ECT should be thought of for this reason.

BENZODIAZEPINES

In part, perhaps because the prevalence of catatonic features is so high in bipolar mood disorders, benzodiazepines such as clonazepam and lorazepam are used widely in the management of manic states in North America. As a first line of treatment for catatonia, benzodiazepines and barbiturates bring about a response in 60% of cases. The use of these drugs may therefore make sense in the early stages of treatment of mania.

DO ANTIDEPRESSANTS CAUSE MANIA?

There has been a belief for many years that tricyclic or MAOI antidepressants cause mania. It seems intuitively obvious that this should be the case. However, against this intuition is the fact that lithium, ECT and carbamazepine appear in some respects to be both antidepressant and antimanic. Based on this, one might wonder whether all agents that were antidepressants should not also be antimanic. At present the only studies of tricyclic antidepressants given in mania suggest that they too may be antimanic (Angst 1985). Why, then, is there a belief that antidepressants may cause mania?

This arises partly because all mental health professionals have seen people taking antidepressants become elated. However, a number of studies recently have indicated that there has always been a natural incidence of manic episodes following episodes of depression, even before the availability of the antidepressants or ECT. The implication of this is that individuals recovering from a depression may swing into mania. The opposite also appears to be true in that a number of subjects recovering from mania appear to get depressed. Many manic patients treated with antipsychotics appear to become depressed, but there is good clinical trial evidence that most antipsychotics can also be used to treat many cases of depression. Ordinarily such swings into mania and swings into depression tend to be relatively short lived and mild (Balfour & Bryson 1994).

The effects of ECT and antidepressants in affective disorders appear to be to abort what might be lengthy depressive episodes much more rapidly than would otherwise have been the case. This may lead to the occurrence of a manic swing earlier than would have happened. Such swings occur even on ECT or lithium, which are effective antimanic treatments.

We tend to attribute, however, anything that happens to individuals who are on medication to the effects of the medication. Because of this there is a natural tendency to attribute episodes of mania that may occur on antidepressants to the action of those antidepressants, even though it is possible that tricyclic antidepressants and even MAOIs might be antimanic agents also.

There are two other factors that tend to obscure the picture. In the case of the tricyclic antidepressants there may be dissociative reactions. These are episodes of confusion, agitation and possible hyperactivity (see Ch. 5). They are more likely in an elderly group of patients. This agitation and hyperactivity may be diagnosed as mania and the inference drawn that the drugs have caused this mania. However, such reactions ordinarily resolve rapidly once the offending drug is withdrawn, whereas a true manic episode should last somewhat longer.

In the case of the MAOIs, in some instances there may be a stimulant effect resembling that produced by amphetamines. This will also resemble mania. It differs from mania, in that the state wears off once the MAOI is discontinued.

7

Prophylaxis of recurrent mood disorders

HISTORY OF PROPHYLAXIS

There are suggestions from as early as the second century AD that spring waters that were alkaline and high in lithium salts were known to be of use in the treatment of overactive states such as mania (Johnson 1984, 1987, Schou 1992).

Lithium itself was isolated first by August Arfwedson in 1817. It was named lithium because it was found in stone – lithos being the Greek for stone. During the 1850s alkaline compounds such as lithium developed a reputation for treating rheumatic disorders and gout by interfering with the precipitation of uric acid in the blood and joints, and lithium was available in many countries through the 1970s for the treatment of rheumatism.

In the 1850s, mania and melancholia were often seen as being part of the same family of diseases as gout, and this led to the use of lithium for these conditions also. As early as 1880, the use of lithium in this manner led Carl Lange to demonstrate that it had a role in preventing episodes of periodic depression. William Hammond in New York found the same thing.

Surprisingly, however, despite these discoveries, lithium slipped out of use for mood disorders and had to be rediscovered in 1949. In part this was because of its side effects. In the middle of the nineteenth century, several investigators took lithium and noted that it caused increased urine flow, tremor of the hands and difficulties with memory or concentration, which led to wariness regarding its use. Later, in the 1930s, it was used as part of a salt restriction diet in the United States, and in many cases it caused such clear-cut toxicity that the Food and Drug Administration banned its use.

In 1949, following observations that lithium had a tranquillising effect on laboratory animals, John Cade, in Australia, gave it to manic, depressive and schizophrenic patients. He noted that it was particularly beneficial in mania. Cade's observations were followed up by Mogens Schou, who confirmed in clinical trials that lithium was beneficial in patients with mania. This led to its subsequent spread for use in the treatment of mania.

The adoption of lithium by the psychiatric community, however, was slow and has remained patchy. Several reasons have been given for this. One is that the compound can have serious side effects. Blood lithium levels have to be determined regularly in order to ensure that the side effects do not outweigh its benefits. A second reason put forward has been that lithium as an elemental compound is widely available and therefore no drug company stands to make much money out of it. It has certainly not been marketed as aggressively as other compounds. Awareness of its usefulness has depended almost entirely on the research and evangelism of Mogens Schou.

In the early 1960s, studies from the UK and Denmark appeared, which supported Lange's 1880 claim that lithium may be useful in the prevention of recurrent episodes of mania or depression. The claims for the prophylactic effects of lithium caused a storm of controversy which, in fact, may have helped the spread of lithium. One of the arguments of critics was that the results that showed people doing well on lithium and poorly off it might be explained in terms of a lithium withdrawal syndrome. This argument was dismissed by lithium's supporters at the time, but it now seems that there is indeed a dependence syndrome.

Lithium was not available in Japan during the 1960s. It was this that led to an interest to try carbamazepine in manic and other mood disorders, and to the discovery that this drug had a prophylactic effect of some sort. The effects of valproate on mood were discovered in France in the 1960s at a time before the use of lithium had become widespread in France.

In the 1980s, an appreciation of the effects of valproate and carbamazepine led to the suggestion that anticonvulsants might help mood disorders in much the same way as they helped convulsive disorders – by reducing kindling. The notion was that each episode of a mood disorder kindled a further episode, in the same way as each epileptic fit increases the vulnerability to the next fit. This hypothesis led on to the systematic testing of every new anticonvulsant that has emerged on the market to see whether it might do something useful.

There are two ways in which an anticonvulsant might help. One would be by acting to reduce kindling, in which case all anticonvulsants should help – although they do not appear to. The other would be by virtue of each anticonvulsant doing something else that is potentially useful. For instance, valproate is somewhat sedative, gabapentin is anxiolytic, carbamazepine is anti-irritability or anti-impulsive, and lamotrigine produces a sense of well-being. If they all act in different ways, conceivably they should suit different patients. At present there is no clear answer on this one.

Linked into the emergence of the psychotropic properties of these anticonvulsant drugs, there has been a trend to reinterpret many chronic personality disorders as mood disorders. Borderline, emotionally unstable and explosive personality disorders, it has been argued, involve an affective dysregulation at their core, and sustained treatment with a 'mood stabiliser' might help. There has also been a tendency to argue that any patient with a recurrent mood disorder should be taken off antidepressants and put on mood stabilisers instead.

The other side of this coin is that there has been an increasing awareness of the larger picture to be treated, as opposed to the particular episode of mania or depression currently presenting – an awareness that, while an antidepressant may help in the short term, in the longer term it may not be a good idea to focus on clearing up this episode without first taking the larger picture into account.

Table 7.1 Mood stabilisers

Generic drug name	UK trade name	US trade name
lithium carbonate	Camcolit/Priadel/Liskonum	Eskalith/Lithobid
lithium citrate	Priadel liquid/Litarex/Li-liquid	–
carbamazepine	Tegretol/Teril CR	Tegretol
sodium valproate	Epilim	Depakene
semisodium valproate	Depakote	Depakote
valproic acid	Convulex	Depakote
lamotrigine	Lamictal	Lamictal
gabapentin	Neurontin	Neurontin

It is by no means clear, however, that drugs such as gabapentin are mood stabilisers (Table 7.1) in the same sense as lithium is. Gabapentin is far more anxiolytic than many of the other compounds being considered here. It is therefore not a surprise that patients with borderline personality problems respond to it. We end up in a circular argument, however, if their response to a 'mood stabiliser' such as gabapentin is taken to show that, in actual fact, they have a mood disorder. The Japanese distinguish between mood stabilisers and psyche stabilisers. This may be the kind of distinction we will need to make more often.

LITHIUM

Unfortunately we have no idea how lithium works. It affects such a large number of physiological processes that the surprise, perhaps, is that it acts so widely throughout the body and yet is relatively specific in its therapeutic effects to one group of disorders. At present lithium is used regularly in the treatment of manic states. It is sometimes used to treat depression, often in conjunction with other antidepressants, as part of a strategy called lithium augmentation. It is perhaps used most commonly, however, to prevent recurrent episodes of mania or depression.

Since the early 1960s there has been a clear body of evidence pointing to a role for lithium in the prevention of episodes of mania and depression in bipolar affective disorders (that is affective disorders where subjects are liable to attacks of both mania and depression). Many individuals who have been treated in hospital for mania are maintained on lithium for years or even decades afterwards in order to prevent recurrences in what is known to be a recurrent disorder.

There is a considerable amount of evidence also indicating a role for lithium in recurrent depression. The current wisdom is that lithium is indicated if there are as many as two episodes per year or three episodes of depression over the course of 2 years. The efficacy of lithium, however, seems to fall off once there are more than four episodes of a depressive disorder a year, and it does not seem to help in what are called rapidly cycling mood disorders, where there are four or more episodes of a mood disorder of any sort per year.

Dosage

Unlike most other drugs used in psychiatry, there is a very clear window for lithium levels in the blood, below which level the drug appears not to work and above which its toxic effects outweigh its benefits.

In general, in the acute treatment of mania or depression, a plasma level in the range of 0.9–1.4 mmol/L is needed. There is, however, a wide range in the amount of lithium that may be needed to produce these blood levels. Anything from 150 to 4200 mg per day may be needed. Because of this, dosages are usually determined by screening blood levels. For the prophylaxis (prevention) of affective episodes, the current wisdom is that blood levels between 0.4 and 0.8 mmol/L are adequate (Abou-Saleh 1987).

Because of the dynamics of lithium in the blood, when determining blood levels it is usual to take a blood test 12 h after the last dose of lithium taken. It is usually necessary also to wait for 7 days after a change of dose to give plasma levels time to settle down at a new steady-state level before taking the next blood sample.

Because of its side effects, and in particular its effects on the kidney, there was until recently a tradition of giving lithium in divided doses during the day. Takers would be prescribed lithium tablets to take three or four times per day. Concern about kidney toxicity also led to the production of slow-release preparations of lithium. These are preparations where the capsule is taken but lithium is released steadily from it during the course of the day so that more even plasma levels are supposedly produced. It had become customary as well to give these slow-release preparations in a divided dose: half in the morning and half in the evening.

However, there has recently been a change in the received wisdom. It now appears from animal studies that a single pulse of lithium, giving a high plasma level at one point in the day and falling off to a lower steady-state level, may be less toxic to the kidneys than having a moderate level the whole time. The kidney appears to tolerate brief surges of lithium better than sustained moderate doses. The implication of this is that lithium should perhaps be given as a single dose at one point in the day, and indeed that slow-release preparations possibly offer no more advantages than the conventional preparations.

 User Issues

LITHIUM WITHDRAWAL AND DEPENDENCE

At present one of the most contentious issues in lithium treatment is whether there may, for some people, be a withdrawal syndrome on discontinuing treatment. In clinical practice, people who have just stopped their treatment seem to relapse with striking frequency. But is this because they had begun to go high and therefore stopped – after the new illness episode had started? This has led to a series of vigorous disputes.

While it is difficult to control for all the factors that may be involved, the consensus of opinion on this issue at present would appear to be that some people, perhaps up to a third or a half, may have a withdrawal problem. This can be minimised by tapering the dose slowly (Goodwin 1994).

One of the consequences of this is that lithium is probably best suited to those who will take it regularly. Early discontinuation may bring forward the next illness episode. By some estimates, it is necessary to take lithium for over 2 years regularly in order actually to reduce the frequency of episodes.

 User Issues

SIDE EFFECTS OF LITHIUM

There is a considerable rate of non-compliance with lithium. The usual reasons given are that takers have intolerable side effects. The ones most commonly cited are weight gain, poor memory, tremor, thirst and tiredness. Other reasons cited are that takers miss the highs that they normally get when not on lithium, or that they feel well and therefore see no need to continue with treatment. Or else people discontinue because they are bothered by the idea of drug treatment itself.

Tremor

Individuals taking lithium may develop a fine rapid tremor. This is in itself harmless, although it may interfere with daily living by causing tea to spill from cups that are full, for example. It will usually clear up when the lithium is discontinued, and can be helped by the addition of a beta-blocker such as propranolol (see Ch. 13).

Thirst

Lithium causes people to feel thirsty and drink a lot. In actual fact, what has been caused is an inability to concentrate urine which leads to the passing of greater volumes of urine than normal. It is this loss of water that subsequently leads to thirst. The reason why water is lost is that lithium antagonises the action of a hormone called vasopressin or antidiuretic hormone (ADH), which acts on the kidney to promote the reabsorption of water from urine. Inhibiting ADH leads to an inability to concentrate urine, with a consequent loss of body water and thirst.

Urinary frequency

The action of lithium to block ADH leads to the passing of large volumes of urine during both day and night. One of lithium's most troublesome complaints is having to get up during the night to pass water. Up to 50% of those on lithium have this side effect. It is normally reversible once the lithium is stopped, but a small proportion may develop an incapacity to concentrate urine further when lithium is discontinued: the frequent drinking and frequent passing of urine will continue.

Dry mouth

As lithium leads to fluid loss and thirst, so also it leads to a dry mouth. Paradoxically, however, despite the fact that one of the symptoms of lithium is a dry mouth, lithium leads to an increased production of saliva. It may also lead to an enlargement of the salivary glands.

continued

Kidney problems

In a small proportion of people lithium can produce chronic kidney problems of a more serious kind. These are commoner in individuals who have been exposed to toxic doses of lithium at some point or other. At present the precise nature of the renal condition is uncertain, although it appears to involve the destruction of some kidney cells and a permanent impairment of the ability to concentrate urine.

Kidney function should therefore be tested before commencing a patient on lithium, and yearly thereafter. In particular, renal function should be tested in people who develop urinary frequency, especially frequency by night. In such subjects the plasma level of lithium that should be aimed at is in the range of 0.4–0.6 mmol/L.

Ordinarily, a simple blood test for urea and creatinine is a sufficient screening procedure. In order to avoid kidney toxicity, it is important to attempt strenuously to avoid inadvertent overdosing; see Overdose and Interactions below.

Weight gain

Up to 50% of people who are put on lithium gain weight – up to a stone or more. The reasons for this weight gain are not entirely clear. One factor may be the thirst induced by lithium. Thirsty individuals, who drink anything other than just simple water, are likely to be consuming more calories than they would otherwise do. In cases of thirst, people taking lithium should stick to water only, if possible.

It is also possible, however, that lithium increases appetite by reducing the effectiveness of insulin in the body. This could lead to low blood sugar levels, which stimulates appetite centres in the brain. This, however, is unclear. Another possibility, at present unproven, is that lithium may lower basal metabolic rates, which means that less food is burnt off as energy during the day.

Diarrhoea

Diarrhoea is commonly found in individuals first taking lithium. Some people may continue to have somewhat looser stools than they would otherwise have, for as long as they remain on the drug. In a minority of individuals taking lithium there may be constipation.

Diarrhoea is also a symptom of lithium toxicity. If an individual who has not been having diarrhoea from their lithium develops diarrhoea, lithium toxicity should be thought of. In the case of toxicity, the diarrhoea is likely to be accompanied by nausea, vomiting and a tremor (see section on Overdose).

Abdominal discomfort

Up to one-third of people taking lithium have a certain amount of abdominal discomfort for the first few weeks or months of treatment. In occasional cases this may be severe and will lead to the need to discontinue the drug. Also found is a sensation of bloating or painfulness in the lower abdominal area, one cause of which may be having a fuller than usual bladder owing to the effects of lithium on water concentration.

Loss of appetite and bad taste

Lithium, in occasional cases, may cause a loss of taste for food with a consequent loss of appetite.

Discoordination

A rarely mentioned but important side effect of lithium is that it may cause episodic discoordination or muscle weakness. Although rarely mentioned, it seems that this side effect is not infrequent. As one individual writing on psychiatric drugs has put it, the first thing she knew about lithium discoordination was when she fell down the stairs. What appears to happen is that there is a brief momentary loss of coordination and/or muscle strength. This leads to a feeling that a fall is imminent, a feeling that is often described as feeling dizzy or faint but in actual fact is neither dizziness nor faintness (Blaska 1990).

Skin and hair changes

Lithium may cause a variety of skin rashes, eruptions or irritations. The commonest problems are a simple skin rash, pustules, acne. Occasionally there are more exfoliative irritations that, in the extreme, may amount to psoriasis. These usually clear up once the drug is stopped but recur once it is restarted. They appear to happen because of an accumulation of lithium in the skin and sensitivity to that accumulation. In the normal course of events a tetracycline antibiotic would be given for an acne, but tetracyclines are contraindicated with lithium because of potential kidney problems.

In about 5% of people there may be quite marked hair loss on lithium. This will usually clear up of its own accord even while staying on the lithium, but occasionally it will resolve only once the drug has been discontinued.

Quite rarely there are changes in the texture of the nails, with pitting in the nails. This is a sign of a possible predisposition to psoriasis and perhaps should lead to a discontinuation of treatment.

Heart

In general lithium has no adverse effects on the heart. In occasional cases where there is a pre-existing cardiac problem, there may be some difficulties. Palpitations or shortness of breath, which develop while a person is taking lithium, should, however, be investigated for this reason.

White cells

Lithium increases the number of white cells in the blood. This will not be noticed by individuals taking lithium. It may sometimes be noticed by another doctor, leading them to wonder whether the person in question has an infection, as infections also lead to an increased white cell count.

Hypothyroidism

Lithium can occasionally lead to hypothyroidism – underactivity of the thyroid gland. The signs of this are dry skin, dry hair, hoarseness, weight gain, hair loss, sluggishness, constipation and sensitivity to the cold. On blood tests there are low thyroid hormone (T4 and T3) levels and increased TSH (thyroid-stimulating hormone) levels, and the thyroid gland may enlarge to produce a goitre. The likelihood of either hypothyroidism or goitre is increased in women over the age of 45 years and in individuals who have thyroid antibodies (these are naturally present in up to 9% of the population).

When screening for kidney functioning before commencing on lithium, it is routine practice also to monitor thyroid function. Both should be repeated anything from 3-monthly to yearly.

continued

Hyperparathyroidism (overactivity of the parathyroid gland)

Generally speaking lithium leads to an increase in serum parathyroid hormone levels. This may in very rare instances lead to excessive calcium levels of the blood, the symptoms of which are quite like the side effects of lithium itself: thirst, increased urine, loss of appetite and nausea.

Tiredness

A relatively common complaint of patients on lithium is tiredness. In some instances this may be quite marked. Tiredness can be difficult to assess, as it is also possible that a recurrent depressive disorder may give rise to tiredness. Trying to tease apart what is caused by depression and what by lithium may be rather difficult.

Tension and restlessness

In a small proportion of cases, lithium may give rise to tense, restless feelings. It may be difficult to decide whether lithium is causing the problem or not. One reason for this is that a taker of lithium may also be on antidepressants or antipsychotics, which can cause tension or restlessness (see Chs 2 & 4). A further reason, of course, is that tense restlessness may be part and parcel of a depressive disorder, or may occur naturally anyway.

Concentration and memory problems

There are a number of reports that lithium can interfere with memory and concentration. Again this is difficult to judge as disturbances of memory and concentration occur in depression anyway. On the other hand, in volunteer subjects taking lithium, difficulties with memory and concentration have also been reported to occur.

Confusion and distractibility

A prominent toxic effect of lithium is confusion and distractibility. Normally, toxic effects occur when the lithium level goes over 1.5 mmol/L, but it is possible to have central nervous system toxicity in the presence of essentially normal plasma levels of lithium. In cases of toxicity, confusion and distractibility are likely to be accompanied by nausea and vomiting as well as a variety of involuntary movements such as tremor.

This toxicity is most likely to occur if the subject has recently been put on some other drugs, particularly antipsychotics. It may also occur if they have developed an increased temperature or decreased their fluid intake because of an infection, and have become dehydrated. It can even happen if dehydration occurs because of an altered salt intake.

Headache

Recurrent headaches are a rare side effect of lithium. If they occur, they should be treated seriously. They may indicate raised intracranial pressure. This clears up once the lithium is discontinued but must be detected as early as possible.

Sexual functioning

Owing to a general difficulty in enquiring about or volunteering information about sexual functioning, little is known of the effects of lithium in this respect. There is some suggestion that lithium may inhibit sexual interest, and in men may reduce the ability to maintain an erection or to have an ejaculation. This awaits further investigation.

User Issues

LITHIUM OVERDOSE

Lithium becomes toxic at levels over 1.5 mmol/L. There is a real risk of enduring damage when the levels are more than 2 mmol/L. The side effects most commonly found in toxic doses are nausea, vomiting, diarrhoea and tremor.

Toxic levels may occur without the individual overdosing as such. Dehydration from excessive perspiration, a high temperature consequent on an infection, or restricted fluid intake may lead to a raised plasma level. In addition, other drugs may combine to increase plasma levels; see Interactions below. Inadvertent overdosage may come about simply by altering salt intake. Therefore, as regards salt in food, it is advisable to have as regular an amount as possible. In occasional cases toxicity seems to occur even in the presence of an apparently normal lithium level.

The treatment for toxic levels is primarily for the individual to take large volumes of isotonic saline (water with salt added to the level normally found in blood). This is preferably given by an intravenous method. If lithium levels exceed 4 mmol/L, dialysis is usually indicated.

User Issues

CONTRAINDICATIONS TO LITHIUM THERAPY

Lithium is contraindicated or should be taken with caution in:

◆ Pregnancy. At present, the situation with regard to lithium and toxicity to the fetus is uncertain. Animal studies and studies on babies who have been delivered by mothers who have been on lithium both at the time of conception and throughout gestation suggest that there may be a very small increased risk. The most likely side effect of taking lithium during pregnancy appears to be a slightly increased risk of heart defects in the child. At present there is no reliable estimate of how likely these are. Later in the course of pregnancy, there are other arguments against taking lithium. At this point the risk to the fetus is minimal, but it becomes difficult to determine exactly what plasma lithium levels mean, given that pregnancy brings about a large increase in body water. There is also an increased clearance of lithium through the kidneys.
There is furthermore a risk of causing lithium intoxication both to the mother and to the baby after delivery, as the extra body water shrinks rapidly on delivery and may cause, as a consequence, a marked increase in plasma lithium levels. For these reasons, if possible, it may be prudent to discontinue lithium during pregnancy.
◆ Breastfeeding. Lithium does get into breast milk. At present it seems that there is no risk to children reared on breast milk containing lithium. They seem to develop normally. If breastfeeding on lithium, it may make sense to take lithium once a day only and to ensure that feeds have taken place before the lithium dose, and that they do not take place during the 4–6 h after the dose so as to ensure the lowest possible level of lithium in breast milk. Another possibility is to use a breast pump to collect milk at the safest times.
◆ Cardiac conditions
◆ Neurological disorders, such as Parkinson disease, Huntington disease or any other organic neurological condition.

continued

- ◆ Kidney disease
- ◆ Thyroid disease
- ◆ Ulcerative colitis or irritable bowel syndrome
- ◆ Psoriasis, acne or hair loss
- ◆ Systemic lupus erythematosus
- ◆ Cataracts

User Issues

DRUG INTERACTIONS

Diuretics

Diuretics lead to water loss, which may lead to an increase in lithium plasma levels and accidental lithium toxicity. If it is necessary to use diuretics, the lithium dose may have to be reduced. Theoretically the best diuretic to use with lithium is amiloride.

Painkillers

Lithium should also be combined cautiously with most common painkillers, including aspirin, diclofenac, fenbufen, fenoprofen, flurbiprofen, ibuprofen, indomethacin, mefenamic acid, naproxen, phenylbutazone, piroxicam and tiaprofenic acid. These are all widely available over the counter for headaches, colds and flu. They are also commonly used in the treatment of arthritic conditions. Most of them lead to increased lithium levels and therefore to the potential of lithium toxicity.

For mild and occasional aches, pains and fever the best painkiller or anti-inflammatory agent to use is probably paracetamol. For more severe painful or rheumatoid conditions it appears that the best non-steroidal treatment is sulindac, which appears, if anything, to lower lithium levels. All the others are usable but their use would require extra monitoring of plasma lithium levels to ensure that toxicity is not inadvertently induced.

Others

Lithium antagonises the effects of most social drugs. The effects of alcohol, cocaine, amphetamines and other stimulants are all reduced. Tea and coffee, however, and related drugs such as theophylline, which are used for asthma, may lead to a lowering of lithium levels.

Lithium may also interact with calcium channel blockers, used to treat angina, hypertension or cardiac arrhythmias and with angiotensin-converting enzyme (ACE) inhibitors, used in the treatment of hypertension.

CARBAMAZEPINE

Carbamazepine was the first alternative to lithium as a possible prophylactic agent. Its use was discovered by Teruo Okuma in Japan (Okuma 2000). Both lithium and carbamazepine seem to have some anti-irritability action, so that carbamazepine is used in the management of aggression, in what are sometimes called episodic dyscontrol syndromes, and lithium has also been shown to be useful in aggression. Carbamazepine is commonly used and can be remarkably beneficial for chronic neuropathic pain syndromes, especially trigeminal neuralgia.

It seems unlikely that common anti-irritability actions are what underpin the benefits of both carbamazepine and lithium in recurrent mood disorders, as the two drugs seem to be useful for different patients, with claims that lithium is more useful for the classical and purer forms of bipolar mood disorder and carbamazepine for more irritable, dysphoric forms of mania. Aside from its prophylactic action, carbamazepine, like lithium, seems to be more useful for manic than depressive states.

 User Issues

SIDE EFFECTS OF CARBAMAZEPINE

Carbamazepine has a considerable list of side effects. These include dizziness, unsteadiness, drowsiness, nausea, visual disturbances, cardiac abnormalities and confusion. For those not suited to it, this can be an unpleasant drug to take. Carbamazepine can also cause a variety of metabolic and blood disorders: low white cell counts, anaemia, hypothyroidism, low sodium levels. It can interact adversely with many other drugs such as oral contraceptives, antidepressants, tranquillisers, hypnotics, lamotrigine and others, although not usually lithium or valproate.

At present, the evidence suggests that in the more classical forms of manic–depressive illness the effects of lithium are superior (Greil et al 1997). Carbamazepine has also taken something of a backseat to other more recent anticonvulsants. Its efficacy in some forms of aggression and especially for pain syndromes is, however, undoubted.

VALPROATE

Valproic acid was an oil used as a butter substitute in Germany during the Second World War. Afterwards it was used as a solvent for a variety of medicines. In this form its anticonvulsant properties were discovered in the early 1960s. Pierre Lambert discovered its mood-stabilising properties later in the 1960s (Comité Lyonnais 2000). Its anticonvulsant effects appear to stem from a blockage of voltage-dependent sodium conductance channels.

The use of valproate increased dramatically during the 1990s. This started from a vigorous promotion of semisodium valproate (Depakote – see Table 7.1) in the United States. Sodium valproate (Epilim) and valproic acid (Convulex) were also used, primarily in countries or places where semisodium valproate was not available. The reason for this dramatic increase is not completely clear. It has proven extremely difficult to run controlled trials of either valproate or other anticonvulsants in patients with bipolar syndromes or other recurrent mood disorders, as randomising patients at high risk of suicide to placebo for possibly several years to demonstrate a reduction in the rate of recurrences is extremely difficult. Instead, agents such as valproate have been through trials in mania or depression and their use as prophylactic agents has spread from there. Valproate has a clear antimanic action, possibly in large part because of its initial sedative effects.

User Issues

SIDE EFFECTS OF VALPROATE

The common side effects are nausea, stomach cramps and diarrhoea, tremor, lethargy and weight gain. Up to one in six takers find that their hair thins or changes in texture, often becoming curly. This latter may be related to zinc deficiency, and in many places it is common to co-prescribe zinc with valproate. Valproate also commonly leads to irregular menses in up to half of the women taking it, as well as gynaecomastia, polycystic ovaries (in over a third of women) and an increase in testosterone levels in nearly a fifth of women. There is, in addition, a higher rate of birth defects reported than would be expected by chance, especially neural tube problems.

As with other anticonvulsants, there may be lethargy, tremor, discoordination and slurred speech. These side effects and others are more likely in combination with antidepressants or antipsychotics. In addition, facial flushing, skin rashes and a variety of blood abnormalities including anaemia are possible. Bruising of any sort should be investigated, and possibly lead to discontinuation. Valproate has been reported to trigger systemic lupus erythematosus reactions.

Dosages used in patients with mood disorders exceed those used for anticonvulsant therapy, and range from 1200 to 2400 mg per day.

Valproate is contraindicated in anyone with liver disease, and therefore should be used with caution in individuals with alcohol or other substance dependency. It should be used with great caution in either children or the elderly, and probably should not be used in pregnancy. As with other anticonvulsants, valproate is being used increasingly widely in borderline personality disorders, post-traumatic stress disorders, panic disorder and for pain syndromes.

LAMOTRIGINE

Just as with carbamazepine and valproate, lamotrigine began as an anticonvulsant. It appears to act by blocking sodium channels on nerve cells, and does so to an ever greater extent the more the cell is in use. Reports from clinical practice that lamotrigine seemed to induce a sense of well-being led to trials in depression, with evidence that it worked. Lamotrigine seems to be antidepressant rather than antimanic. It is now used widely, especially in North America, in the management of recurrent mood disorders.

The usual dose is 100–200 mg daily, with the dose built up by 25-mg increments every 2 weeks. Doses up to 500 mg per day are used in some centres.

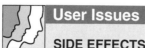

User Issues

SIDE EFFECTS OF LAMOTRIGINE

The side effects of lamotrigine in the first weeks of therapy are rashes and fevers. The greatest hazard is a skin condition called Stevens–Johnson syndrome. This occurs more often in children and adolescents than in adults, and is more likely when the dosage is increased quickly. It is in order to avoid triggering this reaction that lamotrigine is usually increased slowly over a few weeks of treatment. The skin problem is noticeable as a tingling or itch before it develops into a rash. If caught early, there is little problem. Left too late, the condition has been fatal. The occurrence of any rash in the first weeks of treatment should lead to an evaluation and possibly discontinuation of treatment.

These skin reactions are hypersensitivity reactions. However, hypersensitivity can occur without an obvious skin reaction. The signs in this case are fever, swollen lymph glands, puffiness of the face and abnormalities of liver function. Other side effects include headaches, dizziness, lack of coordination, nausea, blurred vision, and either drowsiness or insomnia.

Combinations with valproate are likely to lead to an increase in lamotrigine levels and consequent toxicity. Carbamazepine, in contrast, lowers lamotrigine levels. When added to another anticonvulsant, in addition to changes in the dosage levels, there may also be a multiplication of neuropsychiatric side effects, with blurred vision, discoordination and other similar side effects becoming more common.

When lamotrigine works well it should be relatively free of side effects and should produce a sense of well-being. If this is not happening, treatment should be reconsidered.

GABAPENTIN

Unlike lamotrigine or valproate, gabapentin has never been shown to be effective in clinical trials for either mania or depression. Despite this, its use for recurrent mood disorders has increased dramatically, outstripping that for lamotrigine and carbamazepine combined in many places. In many cases, this use seems to be because of its anxiolytic profile of action, which appears to be appreciated by many patients. This raises the possibility that gabapentin is benzodiazepine-like and is psyche stabilising rather than mood stabilising in the conventional sense. Whether it might also produce dependency is unclear at present. What is clear is that many patients with substance abuse problems and chronic personality-based problems – as well as many others – are being treated with it, and are apparently doing well. Some of these groups are possibly predisposed to having dependence problems of one sort or another, and an issue for the future will be to establish whether there are significant dependency-associated problems with gabapentin.

User Issues

SIDE EFFECTS OF GABAPENTIN

In contrast to valproate and lamotrigine, gabapentin appears to work on calcium channels. Its common side effects are drowsiness, dizziness, discoordination, visual disturbances, headaches, tremor, nausea and vomiting, slurred speech and throat pains of various sorts. Pancreatitis, liver problems and Stevens–Johnson syndrome have also been reported. Many people taking it, however, find it almost free of side effects and quite agreeable.

The usual dose of gabapentin for convulsive disorders is up to 900 mg per day, but up to 3600 mg has been used in mood disorders. Withdrawal reactions have been reported and therefore tapering should be gradual. 'Poop-out' – an apparent loss of effect – has also been reported.

PRESCRIBING ISSUES

There is a trend, especially in North America to put patients who are resistant to one mood stabiliser on to cocktails of up to six or seven mood stabilisers, on the basis that someone has apparently always responded to the one of the many combinations that are possible (Sheehan 2000). This is difficult to endorse. In the case of rapidly cycling mood disorders, an earlier consideration of ECT is probably a better option. Many of these other drugs interfere with a variety of vitamins such as folate, or essential minerals such as zinc, potentially setting up a situation where a decent response is unlikely to be obtained. While it is clear that these newer drugs have something to offer, their proper place has not yet been established, and there is the possibility that patients are being brought down this path when, for many, more effective options such as lithium and ECT are available.

All of these agents have withdrawal syndromes associated with their use. Dose reduction therefore must be gradual. Convulsions and a range of other problems have been produced by over-rapid cessation.

References

Abou-Saleh MT (1987) The dosage regimen. In: Johnson FN, ed. Depression and mania: modern lithium treatment, pp 99–104. Oxford: IRL Press.

Angst J (1985) Switch from depression to mania – a record study over decades between 1920 and 1982. Psychopathology 18: 140–154.

Balfour JA, Bryson HM (1994) Valproic acid. A review of its pharmacology and therapeutic potential in indications other than epilepsy. CNS Drugs 2: 144–173.

Beaumont G, Healy D (1993) The place of clomipramine in psychopharmacology. Journal of Psychopharmacology 7: 383–393.

Blaska B (1990) The myriad medication mistakes in psychiatry: a consumer's view. Hospital and Community Psychiatry 41: 993–998.

British Association for Psychopharmacology Consensus Statement (1993) Guidelines on treating depressive illness with antidepressants. Journal of Psychopharmacology 7: 19–23.

Carlsson A, Healy D (1996) The impact of the basic sciences on neuropsychopharmacology and clinical psychopharmacology. In: Healy D, ed. The psychopharmacologists, pp 51–80. London: Chapman & Hall.

Comité Lyonnais pour la Research et Therapie en Psychiatrie (2000) The birth of psychopharmacotherapy: explorations in a new world, 1952–1968. In: Healy D, ed. The psychopharmacologists, vol 3, pp 1–54. London: Arnold.

Creaney W, Murray I, Healy D (1991) Antidepressant induced suicidal ideation. Human Psychopharmacology 6: 329–332.

Cunningham-Owens DG (1999) A guide to the extrapyramidal side-effects of antipsychotic drugs. Cambridge: Cambridge University Press.

Donovan S, Clayton A, Beeharry M et al (2000) Deliberate self-harm and antidepressant drugs. Investigation of a possible link. British Journal of Psychiatry 177: 551–556.

Fink M (2000) Electroshock: Restoring the Brain. New York: Oxford University Press.

Frasure-Smith N, Lesperance F, Talajic M (1993) Depression following myocardial infarction: impact on 6-month survival. Journal of American Medical Association 270: 1819–1825.

Glenmullen J (2000) Prozac backlash. New York: Simon & Schuster.

Goodwin G (1994) Recurrence of manic-depression after lithium withdrawal. British Journal of Psychiatry 164: 149–152.

Greil W, Ludwig-Mayerhofer W, Erazo N et al (1997) Lithium versus carbamazepine in the maintenance treatment of bipolar disorders – a randomised study. Journal of Affective Disorders 43: 151–161.

Healy D (1990) The suspended revolution. Psychiatry and psychotherapy re-examined. London: Faber & Faber.

Healy D (1991) The marketing of 5HT: depression or anxiety? British Journal of Psychiatry 158: 737–742.

Healy D (1993) Images of trauma. London: Faber & Faber.

Healy D (1994) The fluoxetine and suicide controversy. CNS Drugs 1: 223–231.

Healy D (1997) The Antidepressant Era. Cambridge, MA: Harvard University Press.

Healy D (2000) Antidepressant induced suicidality. Primary Care Psychiatry 6: 23–28.

Healy D, Savage M (1998) Reserpine exhumed. British Journal of Psychiatry 172: 376–378.

Healy D, Williams JMG (1989) Moods, misattributions and mania. Psychiatric Developments 7: 49–70.

Hoehn-Saric R, Lipsey JR, McLeod DR (1990) Apathy and indifference in patients on fluvoxamine and fluoxetine. Journal of Clinical Psychopharmacology 10: 343–345.

Jick SS, Dean AD, Jick H (1995) Antidepressants and suicide. British Medical Journal 310: 215–218.

Johnson FN (1984) The history of lithium. Basingstoke, UK: Macmillan.

Johnson FN (1987) Depression and mania: Modern lithium treatment. Oxford: IRL Press.

Kuhn R (1990) Artistic imagination and the discovery of antidepressants. Journal of Psychopharmacology 4: 127–130.

Lejoyeux M, Ades J, Rouillon F (1994) Serotonin syndrome: incidence, symptoms and treatment. CNS Drugs 2: 132–146.

O'Hanlon JF (1995) Minimising the risk of traffic accidents due to psychoactive drugs. Primary Care Psychiatry 1: 77–85.

Okuma T (2000) The discovery of the psychotropic effects of carbamazepine. In: Healy D, ed. The psychopharmacologists, Vol 3, pp 259–280. London: Arnold.

Pichot P (1996) The Birth of the Bipolar Disorder. European Psychiatry 10: 1–10.

Rosenbaum JF, Fava M, Hoog SL, Ashcroft RC, Krebs W (1998) Selective serotonin reuptake inhibitor discontinuation syndrome: a randomised clinical study. Biological Psychiatry 44: 77–87.

Sachdev P (1996) Akathisia. Cambridge: Cambridge University Press.

Sandler M (1990) Monoamine oxidase inhibitors in depression: History and mythology. Journal of Psychopharmacology 4: 136–139.

Schou M (1992) Phases in the development of lithium treatment in psychiatry. In: Samson F, Adelman G, eds. The neurosciences: paths of discovery, vol II, pp 149–166. Boston, MA: Birkhauser.

Sheehan D (2000) Angles on panic. In: Healy D, ed. The psychopharmacologists, vol 3, pp 479–504. London: Arnold.

Small JG, Klapper HH, Kellams JG (1988) Electroconvulsive treatment compared to lithium in the management of manic states. Archives of General Psychiatry 45: 727–732.

Sternbach H (1991) The serotonin syndrome. American Journal of Psychiatry 148: 705–713.

Taylor D (1999) Truth withdrawal. OpenMind September.

Williams JMG (1990) The psychological management of depression. Beckenham, UK: Croom Helm.

Use of psychostimulants

SECTION CONTENTS

8

The history of the psychostimulants

INTRODUCTION

Unlike other sections of this book which are about the management of clinical conditions, this section is about the use of a group of drugs. This is not the only feature that is unusual about this section. It is the only new section in this edition and, furthermore, it is new despite the group of drugs concerned being an older group of drugs than either the antipsychotics or antidepressants. Clearly there must have been something unusual about the psychostimulants in recent years to warrant such an approach. There has been: the explosive increase in their use for attention-deficit hyperactivity disorder (ADHD). But this is not all the section will deal with. There is a rich history underlying the various uses of the psychostimulants.

DIFFERING REACTIONS TO STIMULANTS

Stimulants such as arsenic, strychnine and coca (later cocaine) have been used for over a century in the treatment of nervous problems. In a famous natural experiment, a flood in Pavlov's laboratory in Leningrad in 1924, which nearly drowned his experimental dogs, left many of them nervous. Even though the shock in each case was the same, the reactions of the dogs was quite different, with some becoming severely disabled and others less so. Also different was their response to treatments: some were helped by sedatives and others by stimulants. This raises the possibility that quite different drugs could be effective for the same condition, depending on the constitutional type (the personality) of the individual (Healy 2001).

These ideas were later elaborated into a sophisticated theory of personality by Hans Eysenck, who distinguished between introverts and extroverts. According to Eysenck, introverts handle their fears internally and in so doing predispose themselves to phobic and obsessional disorders, as well as neurotic anxiety. Extroverts handle their difficulties in the interpersonal space, so that they become problems both for themselves and others. In so doing they predispose themselves to hysteria and psychopathy. These dimensions of introversion and extroversion were, for Eysenck, biological realities. In support of this he pointed to a differential sensitivity between introverts and extroverts to the effects of stimulants and sedatives. Answers on the Eysenck Personality Questionnaire, can, in fact, predict how much anaesthetic will be needed to put someone to sleep for surgery: introverts need much more than extroverts. Similarly, extroverts are much more sensitive to the effects of stimulants, which can have apparently paradoxical effects on them.

AMPHETAMINES

The amphetamine series of molecules, one of which was later given the street name Ecstasy, were first made in the decades preceding World War One. It took some years for chemists to appreciate their stimulant properties. Exploring these further led to the discovery of dexamphetamine (Dexedrine) in 1935, an amphetamine with much more marked stimulant properties than other amphetamines. This quickly swept away the use of other stimulants. Dexamphetamine was tried out in a range of conditions and found to be helpful. These included narcolepsy, anxiety disorders and a condition that has since come to be called attention-deficit hyperactivity disorder (ADHD) (Bradley 1937, Healy 2001).

In 1937, Charles Bradley reported on the beneficial effects of benzedrine on a series of disturbed children in care in the following terms: 'to see a single dose of benzedrine produce a greater improvement in school performance than the combined efforts of a capable staff working in a most favorable setting, would have been all but demoralizing to the teachers had not the improvement been so gratifying from a practical viewpoint' (p 584).

Reporting effects like this in a group of acting-out children opens up the possibility that what Bradley had found was what Pavlov before him and Eysenck after found: the different effects of stimulants on extroverts compared with introverts. However, the field developed in a different direction, towards categorical disease entities rather than dimensional drug effects. The discovery of the effects of amphetamine in disturbed children led on to the notion of minimal brain dysfunction, and then to hyperactivity syndrome, conditions that were thought might be linked to food allergies or other such problems. In 1954, another stimulant appeared: methylphenidate (Ritalin). (Methylphenidate is now also available as Equasym.) This was put into clinical trials for the same group of children Bradley had looked at, and was also found to be effective.

ADHD AND RITALIN

In 1980, with the creation of DSM-III, hyperactivity disorders and minimal brain dysfunction disorders merged to become attention-deficit hyperactivity disorder (ADHD) (Klein 2000, Rapoport 2000) and Ritalin, which had been available for 25 years before that, exploded into popular consciousness.

Initially, these results from America were discounted in Europe. In America, the first explanations were in terms of something clearly being wrong with the brains of hyperactive children, so that drugs that abolished appetite, interfered with sleep and stimulated normal children produced the opposite effects in these 'hyperactive' children. Then, Judy Rapoport demonstrated that similar effects could be shown in normal children, which introduced the notion that there was a paediatric response to these drugs that differed from the responses of adults (Klein 2000, Rapoport 2000). This idea has also since been discarded, leaving us with the options of either ADHD on one side, a brain disorder corrected by psychostimulants, or something akin to extroversion on the other side, a constitutional predisposition that many people have which makes them more sensitive to the calming effects of stimulants than introverts are. There is a third option outlined in the next chapter, which is that the effects of psychostimulants depend in part on the baseline activity rates of the person or animal taking them, leading to slowing down effects against a background of high activity rates and a stimulant effect against a background of low activity rates.

There are a number of extraordinary features of the current scene. One is that a taboo has been breached: the taboo of giving psychotropic drugs to children. Children, especially in North America, are being given cocktails of psychotropic drugs on a vast scale. A second point is the lack of pharmacological distinction between the drugs being used – Ritalin and Dexedrine – and a number of banned or controlled agents such as cocaine and speed. On the one hand, we can look at a group of drugs and see them as harmless, and then look back a moment later and see a major threat to society (DeGrandpre 1998).

In Section 10, I cover some of the mechanisms that I believe are responsible for producing this situation.

9

Psychostimulants and their uses

ADHD/EXTROVERSION

As outlined in Chapter 8, the 1990s saw an explosion in the use of psychostimulants, mainly for attention-deficit hyperactivity disorder (ADHD). This began in the United States, but the trend has now extended to Europe. It began with the use of stimulants for children, and has now extended to their use for adults also. There is little doubt, based on the clinical trial evidence, that stimulants can produce dramatic behavioural changes in some children (Healy & Nutt 1997). The benefits are so great in some cases that there can be little doubt but that the child's life is transformed and they are enabled to get on with socialising and other developmental tasks. In other cases, while the superficial effects may be clear, surprisingly there is much less evidence that these benefits actually translate into improved school performance or better socialisation.

There are grounds, therefore, for handling the prescription of psychostimulants to children, adolescents or even adults with ADHD/extraversion with caution. The effects should be monitored with some care to ensure that there are clear superficial benefits, and ideally indicators of deeper improvements.

Having made this point, an equal but opposite one also needs to be made: that refusing to prescribe on the basis that behavioural approaches are in some way ethically preferable is difficult to defend given the significant improvements for the individual and their families that can be produced by the judicious prescription of stimulants.

Table 9.1 Commonly used psychostimulants

Generic drug name	UK trade name	US trade name
dexamphetamine	Dexedrine	Dexedrine
methylphenidate	Ritalin/Equasym	Ritalin
pemoline	Cylert	Cylert

Psychostimulants (Table 9.1) are given in slowly increasing doses, dexamphetamine and methylphenidate in doses from 5 to 60 mg and other stimulants in the equivalent dose range. These medications have a short half-life and therefore often have to be given in twice or thrice daily doses. Slow-release preparations are available in some countries, including North America.

User Issues

SIDE EFFECTS AND INTERACTIONS

There are two main sets of side effects to psychostimulants. One is an increasing anxiety, leading to a paranoid state developing over the course of a few days or weeks. This is quite rare in clinical doses. More commonly these agents may lead to a hyperactive state, where an individual has too much motor energy and drive. The energy is relatively unfocused, so that, rather than getting lots of useful things done, the person is left pacing up and down restlessly. They also may be unable to sleep properly. Side effects such as this should lead to a discontinuation of treatment. Related to these effects may be an increase in nervousness, palpitations, increased irritability and aggression, and an increased number of tics. In toxic doses, all of these may be much more pronounced.

There may also be loss of appetite and either weight loss or, in the case of children, a reduced rate of growth. This delay in growth may be overcome by a drug holiday, for instance during the school holiday.

Stimulants potentially interact with MAOIs and some antihypertensives.

PSYCHOSTIMULANTS IN ANXIETY AND DEPRESSION

The psychostimulants were traditionally distinguished from the antidepressants on the basis that they supposedly had little effect on depression. However, the depression on which they had little effect in the 1940s and 1950s was the hospitalised melancholic or patient with endogenous depression. These depressions paradoxically responded to the more sedative tricyclic antidepressants.

In fact, however, through the 1950s, 1960s and 1970s, psychostimulants were used regularly for community depressions – tired all the time states – as well as anxiety disorders. In fact, the first placebo-controlled clinical trial in medicine involved the use of dexamphetamine in depression and schizophrenia; this demonstrated that dexamphetamine helped patients with depression but not those with schizophrenia (Dub & Lurie 1939). There is, indeed, considerable evidence that stimulants are just as good as selective serotonin reuptake inhibitors (SSRIs) for community nervousness in general (Chiarello & Cole 1987). In fact, the SSRIs have never been shown to be effective for melancholic depressions of the kind that responded to the first antidepressants, suggesting that if they had been introduced in the 1950s or 1960s they would never have ended up being called antidepressants.

In addition to use as antidepressants, stimulants are used as adjunctive therapies with other antidepressants.

The doses and side effects used for depression are the same as those for ADHD.

PSYCHOSTIMULANTS IN SCHIZOPHRENIA

In any consideration of the dopamine hypothesis of schizophrenia, one of the arguments invariably put forward is that psychostimulant drugs, in particular the amphetamines, can lead to mental disorder, characterised by prominent paranoid feelings and a stereotyped thought disorder. This state has similarities with some schizophrenic states. As the psychostimulants increase brain dopamine levels or neurotransmission and the antipsychotics block dopamine neurotransmission, the thinking has been that schizophrenia must therefore involve increased dopamine functioning and, accordingly, giving a stimulant to someone with schizophrenia would not be a good idea.

However, the picture in real life is considerably more ambiguous. In the first place there is a substantial amount of evidence that up to one-third of individuals with 'schizophrenia' actually do well on stimulants (Lieberman et al 1987).

Second, there are good grounds for suggesting that not all individuals who are labelled as having schizophrenia, or who get antipsychotics, actually have schizophrenia. There is some evidence that a proportion of individuals have an attention deficit disorder (Bellak et al 1987). Some patients who have suffered from hyperactivity in childhood may present with a psychotic disorder later in life, at which point they are likely to be given antipsychotics. But because psychostimulants are an appropriate treatment for hyperactivity, antipsychotics, which do just the opposite to psychostimulants, are likely to make the condition worse.

Third, the collapse of the dopamine hypothesis of schizophrenia removes much of the worry that hindered the use of psychostimulants in psychotic states. This hypothesis made it all but impossible to prescribed psychostimulants to people with psychosis, even when clinically there were clear benefits.

Aside from the beneficial therapeutic effects that psychostimulants might have for some psychoses, there are compelling reasons to believe that they will ameliorate a number of antipsychotic side effects (Bowers & Swigar 1988, Huckle & Thomas 1991). In practice, while amphetamines may lead to psychotic breakdowns and admissions, this is usually linked to high dosage and chronic use. Most mental health staff, however, will know of other individuals who are taking amphetamines, while also taking antipsychotics. The orthodox view is that the antipsychotics may be preventing amphetamine use from leading to a psychosis, but very often it looks as though the alternative view applies: amphetamine use may be helpfully reversing some of the less helpful features of neuroleptic therapy.

The literature in this area is scant, but in recent years I have been using psychostimulants in some cases to reverse antipsychotic-induced side effects. It seems possible, in many cases, to combine a stimulant with an antipsychotic, so that the helpful effect of the antipsychotic is maintained but a troublesome side effect is ameliorated. This is easier to understand post-clozapine, if neuroleptics are understood in terms of a filter and their effectiveness, in part, depends on their blocking a number of receptor systems; in this case the reversal of blockade in one system may not prove immediately catastrophic.

For example, antipsychotic-induced demotivation can be helped by a combination of lowering the dose of the antipsychotic and adding a psychostimulant. Weight gain on olanzapine, clozapine or other antipsychotics may also be counteracted by stimulants. Antipsychotic-induced increases in levels of the hormone prolactin, which lead to menstrual irregularities, increased breast size and the production of milk, even in men, may respond to a stimulant or a dopamine agonist such as bromocriptine. Motor side effects, which are unresponsive to the usual antidotes, may also respond well.

In general, it seems probable that psychostimulants are most likely to be of benefit to people who appear to be more sensitive than average to the dopamine-blocking effects of antipsychotics. There appears to be a small subgroup of such individuals (probably 5–10% of us) for whom antipsychotics, even in relatively low doses, produce marked motor side effects and/or demotivation, so much so that the taking of these drugs may be quite distressing, and in the long run possibly harmful to mental health.

NARCOLEPSY

This disorder, which involves falling asleep abruptly (see Section 5), responds well to low doses of psychostimulants. Recently, a new drug, modafinil (Provigil) has been released for the management of narcolepsy. Its makers claim that it has the alerting properties of dexamphetamine without the euphoriant properties or the activity-increasing effects. It is not yet clear how closely modafinil resembles other psychostimulants, or whether it might have benefits in other nervous states or reduce the side effects of antipsychotics in the way that other stimulants do.

OTHER USES OF PSYCHOSTIMULANTS

There is a place for the psychostimulants in a range of brain disorders from Alzheimer disease and other dementias, especially subcortical dementias, to head injuries and Parkinson disease. In subcortical dementias and following head injury, the benefits may stem from a simple speeding up of cognitive functions. In the case of Alzheimer disease and other cortical dementias, the benefits seem more like the effects in ADHD – excessive activity is 'paradoxically' inhibited.

This paradoxical inhibition of excess activity even extends to mania. A number of clinicians have given dexamphetamine or other psychostimulants to manic patients and have found that it calms them down – temporarily. This links into a neglected line of work on psychostimulants by Robbins and colleagues, which emphasises the fact that the results observed may depend in part on the baseline level of activity of the person to whom they are given (Robbins & Sahakian 1979).

References

Bellak L, Kay SR, Opler LA (1987) Attention deficit disorder psychosis as a diagnostic category. Psychiatric Developments 5: 239–263.

Bowers MB, Swigar ME (1988) Psychotic patients who become worse on neuroleptics. Journal of Clinical Psychopharmacology 8: 417–421.

Bradley C (1937) The behavior of children receiving benzedrine. American Journal of Psychiatry 94: 577–585.

Chiarello RJ, Cole JO (1987) The use of psychostimulants in general psychiatry. Archives of General Psychiatry 44: 286–295.

DeGrandpre R (1998) Ritalin nation. New York: Oxford University Press.

Dub LM, Lurie L (1939) Use of benzedrine in the depressed phase of the psychotic state. Ohio State Medical Journal 35: 39–45.

Healy D (2001) The rise of psychopharmacology. Cambridge, MA: Harvard University Press.

Healy D, Nutt D (1997) British Association for Psychopharmacology Consensus on Childhood and Learning Disabilities – Psychopharmacology. Journal of Psychopharmacology 11: 291–294.

Huckle PL, Thomas R (1991) Pemoline and neuroleptic induced side effects. Irish Journal of Psychological Medicine 8: 174.

Klein R (2000) Children and psychopharmacology. In: Healy D, ed. The psychopharmacologists, vol 3, pp 309–332. London: Arnold.

Lieberman JA, Kane JM, Alvir J (1987) Provocative tests with psychostimulant drugs. Psychopharmacology 91: 415–433.

Rapoport J (2000) Phenomenology, psychopharmacotherapy and child psychiatry. In: Healy D, ed. The psychopharmacologists, vol 3, pp 333–356. London: Arnold.

Robbins TW, Sahakian BJ (1979) 'Paradoxical' effects of psychomotor stimulant drugs in hyperactive children form the standpoint of behavioural pharmacology. Neuropharmacology 18: 931–950.

Management of anxiety

The anxiety disorders

DRUGS USED IN ANXIETY

Six groups of drugs are used to manage anxiety, as shown in Box 10.1.

Box 10.1 Groups of drugs used to treat anxiety

- The antipsychotics particularly chlorpromazine, haloperidol, flupentixol and thioridazine. These are considered in Section 1.

- The antidepressants including the tricyclic antidepressants, the MAOIs and the SSRIs. These are dealt with in Section 2.

- Minor tranquillisers of the benzodiazepine type. These are covered in Chapter 11.

- Drugs active on the serotonin system, which are discussed in Chapter 12.

- Beta-blockers such as propranolol, which is considered in Chapter 13.

- Psychostimulants. These have historically been used extensively for nervousness, but are not in favour for this purpose now (see Section 3).

TYPES OF ANXIETY

To understand how any of these drugs may be useful it is necessary to understand the various types of anxiety. The term anxiety covers four sets of experiences, one or other of which may be more prominent in any individual case.

There may be mental anxiety, which roughly translates as worry or a mental preoccupation with things that might go wrong. This may also include intrusive ideas or thoughts or impulses, which are of a distressing nature. This form of anxiety may be present without much in the way of physical symptoms such as increased muscular tension or increased heart rate or sweating or shaking of the hands.

The second form is physical tension, which basically consists of a tensing up and knotting of the various muscles around the body. This most probably results from a constant suppression of action. When we get emotional or worried, we review or think about possible things to do to sort our problems out. Thinking about things commonly produces a state of preparing muscles for the intended action – tensing them up and getting them ready to swing into action. All we do is think about things, and we don't actually do anything, the result is that our muscles get tensed up without that tension being discharged. It may go on to become chronic, if an individual gets into the habit of being physically tense. Physical relaxation exercises work for anxiety by acting principally on this component of the anxiety spectrum.

The third aspect to anxiety is a set of physical symptoms, which include increased heart rate and increased intensity of the heart beat so that the person becomes aware of their heart thumping in their chest. These are called palpitations. Other symptoms include a shake in the hand, sweating from the palms, the back of the neck, the forehead, etc., feeling weak and faint and liable to keel over, feeling butterflies in the pit of the stomach and sometimes frank nausea, as well as a loosening of the bowels which may lead to diarrhoea. There is usually also a tendency to breathe more shallowly and quickly. This hyperventilation can, in turn, produce a set of symptoms such as tingling feelings in the hands and legs, pins and needles, a feeling of being light-headed and even visual disturbances.

Related to the symptoms produced by hyperventilation there is a fourth form of anxiety that has been increasingly recognised in recent years, called dissociative anxiety. The cardinal features of this are:

- Depersonalisation – a feeling of being somehow detached or removed from oneself or as though one's body is not operating normally (see Ch. 5).
- Derealisation – an impression that the world somehow seems unreal, flat, or as though everything is happening on a stage (see Ch. 5).
- Experiences of leaving one's body and somehow looking back at oneself. These out-of-body experiences probably relate closely to depersonalisation and derealisation.
- Hallucinations – usually of the auditory type, although visual hallucinations are possible.

- Recurrent waves of emotion or recurrent short-lived black moods.
- Episodic feelings of being totally numb either mentally or physically, even to the point where one can cut oneself and not feel any pain.
- Amnesia for past events – whether the happenings of the day or episodes in one's past life.

OCCASIONS OF ANXIETY

In addition to the types of anxiety mentioned above, there are a number of different situations in which anxiety arises and according to which it is categorised and treatment given.

Stage fright

This is the kind of anxiety that everyone gets when faced with an interview or having to speak before a crowd or having to perform in some way for others. The typical manifestations of stage fright are increased muscular tension, sweating, butterflies, a tremor in the hand and palpitations, as well as a feeling perhaps of being unreal or out of touch. In other words, some aspects of all of the forms of anxiety mentioned above may be experienced. Stage fright can often be helped by either minor tranquillisers or beta-blockers.

The basis for a response to these drugs appears to lie in part in an interruption of the feedback from increased heart rate or muscular tension to the mental state. Typically, when we get anxious, we are worried about something and our heart rate increases, our hands shake and we begin to perspire. These in turn lead us to be more anxious. If these signs of anxiety are blocked, we appear to assume that we are less anxious and as a result we do become less anxious. In other words, we can trick ourselves into thinking that we are not as anxious as we actually may be by blocking the usual signs of anxiety. This is a legitimate manoeuvre and is undoubtedly what human beings have been doing for millennia, mostly hitherto by using alcohol to abolish the manifestations of anxiety – giving us Dutch courage.

There are two potential problems with this procedure, however. One is that it is normal to feel anxious before a performance of any kind and, indeed, a certain amount of anxiety probably contributes to a good performance and helps us to perform at a level higher than we would otherwise do. People who are too relaxed and at ease may lose a certain amount of 'edge'. One pitfall, therefore, is that over-zealous tranquillisation may impair performance.

A further pitfall lies in starting the treatment of anxiety too early. In the case of a concert, a speech or an interview, treatments should be used only on the day of the performance or, at the most, to include the night before. Danger arises when performances come close together and an individual is self-medicating for too long before each performance, so that they slide into a routine of constant medication. This may produce dependence in the case of drugs such as alcohol or benzodiazepines.

Another problem is that, while it is probably legitimate to use drugs of this sort in an appropriate way, if they are found effective, there is an inevitable tendency to rely on the drugs rather than to develop the skills to help manage activities such as interviews, speaking in public or playing snooker. This presents a dilemma in that a judicious use of anxiolytics to combat stage fright may enable the person to go on stage and perform more readily and thereby potentially become more accustomed to performing in front of others and, as a consequence, less anxious about this. In other words anxiolytic drugs can lead gradually, if used properly, to their own discontinuation.

Neurotic anxiety

We all become acutely anxious on occasions. If the anxiety is intense or long lasting, or if it catches us at a vulnerable time, there is a tendency for it to organise itself into a neurosis. A neurosis is a relatively long-lasting and self-perpetuating maladaptation to anxiety.

For example, someone who has a shock while out shopping may perhaps be left nervous. They may then subsequently, when they come to go shopping next, find that they are apprehensive about going out. If they do not go out to the shops, perhaps by getting one of their children or a neighbour to go instead, the likelihood is that a certain nervousness about going shopping will become established. Not going shopping in order to avoid becoming anxious about shopping leads progressively to an inability to go shopping, and to even more anxiety when one has to face up to what it is that one has been avoiding. Such problems can be self-perpetuating.

Sometimes the difficulty may clear up spontaneously. Many neuroses also respond very well to behaviour therapies, which act on much the same principle as telling someone who has just fallen off a horse to get up and ride again as quickly as possible. Blocking avoidance responses and exposing oneself to the thing that one is afraid of are the basic behavioural methods for handling neurosis. They work extremely well and are, broadly speaking, the optimal therapy for phobic and obsessive–compulsive neuroses (Marks 1978).

However, there are other treatments and anxiolytics that are commonly used for various neuroses. To understand their place we will first lay out the different kinds of neuroses and then indicate where and why drug treatments may also be employed.

FORMS OF ANXIETY

Phobic neurosis

There are both general and specific phobias. A general phobia of going out is termed agoraphobia. The specific phobias involve phobias of a particular thing such as a fear of spiders, snakes, or thunder and lightning.

Exposure therapy is the treatment of choice for a phobic disorder uncomplicated by a depressive illness. Antidepressants are also often used for agoraphobia, although they are rarely, if ever, used for the more specific phobias. One rationale for using antidepressants in these conditions is that many people who are agoraphobic will also have a concomitant depressive disorder; if this is tackled the neurosis may clear up. However, in addition to the clearing up of a depressive disorder, the SSRIs and MAOI antidepressants appear to be independently anxiolytic and there is some evidence that treatment with these drugs may be of some benefit to those who are phobically anxious but not depressed. Whether treatment in such a group should ever rely solely on drug treatment without including a behavioural input also is a matter of some dispute.

Panic disorder

Panic disorder is a state that can come on either in company, out of doors, or indoors at home alone. The experience of panic usually seems intensely physical to the affected individual. They become aware of their heart thumping and hands shaking. They may have feelings of nausea, and feel weak and short of breath. They may also have feelings of impending doom. Panic disorders typically come out of the blue. These feelings may lead secondarily to a phobia of going shopping if, for example, the first panic attack happens in the supermarket – afflicted individuals are then often understandably nervous about going to supermarkets again (Klein & Healy 1996).

There have been vigorous attempts to market a number of antidepressants and anxiolytics, particularly the minor tranquilliser alprazolam, for panic disorder (see Section 10). Most of the antidepressants – the tricyclics, the MAOIs and, more recently, the SSRIs – have been tested in clinical trials for panic disorder and have been shown to have a certain amount of usefulness.

Exposure therapy is used widely to manage panic disorder, as well as a recently developed variation of cognitive therapy (McNally 1990). Briefly, the behavioural and cognitive approaches propose that people who panic experience the symptoms of anxiety such as increased heart rate, breathlessness, feelings of weakness and palpitations, and interpret these in terms of an imminent stroke or loss of control or heart attack or outburst of some sort. They then take evasive action to avoid such things. Typically, a person who fears a heart attack will, for example, sit down – just as any reasonable person who actually thought they were having a heart attack would do. This sitting down and taking things easier, however, perpetuates the problem. Treatment aims to get the person to do the opposite to what they have been doing and to try to get hold of the thoughts that come to their mind during episodes of panic, so they can recognise what is happening. Over and above this, the cognitive approaches further emphasise the thinking style of affected individuals.

Social phobia

Three forms of social phobia are described. The first is a specific form that involves having to perform in front of others – a degree of stage fright sufficient to lead to avoidance. Second, a generalised form of social phobia involves avoidance of most occasions of interaction with others. This may range from avoidance of shopping because of difficulties in asking for things, to avoiding the bank teller and using automated tellers instead, to crossing the street when aware of the approach of anyone who might want to stop and engage in conversation. The difficulty with this phobia is extreme self-consciousness: affected individuals are constantly evaluating themselves and feeling that they are boring. Finally, there is a condition termed 'avoidant personality disorder', which, as the name implies, is a state where an individual's freedom to act is heavily constrained by their interpersonal difficulties. In its extreme form, individuals with this condition may become housebound. There is a high incidence of alcohol abuse and co-occurrence with other phobic disorders, panic disorder and depression.

Until recently, social phobia was all but unrecognised in the West, although it is commonly diagnosed in the East. The condition is still likely to be viewed by sufferers and others as a form of shyness, in other words not as something that would lead to the seeking of medical help. Accordingly, it neither presents in primary care nor is detected by primary care physicians, despite estimates that up to 3% of the population may be affected (Healy 1995). There are a number of programmes in place to increase recognition, as the condition may lead those affected to be unable to sustain a relationship or to hold down employment.

Clinical trials have recently shown that the MAOIs and SSRIs may bring about some improvement in the condition, and may do so for individuals with severer forms of the disorder, even in the absence of any obvious depressive disorder. In contrast, beta-blockers or benzodiazepines appear to be of limited usefulness. A number of behavioural and cognitive strategies are also emerging and, as with the phobic disorders, it would seem that the best management in future will probably involve an appropriate combination of pharmacotherapy and behavioural approaches.

Obsessive–compulsive disorder (OCD)

Three fairly dissimilar behaviours may be subsumed under this title. First is a general indecisiveness and inability to take action. Another is an obsessional and ritualised checking on things, such as whether one's hands are clean or whether one has locked the back door, turned off the gas – things we all do but which may be done in OCD to an extraordinary degree and disabling extent (Rapoport 1990). The third is having images or urges present themselves to one's mind that it is feared will be given into. Examples include images of oneself shouting out obscenities in public or impulses to pick up a knife and skewer one's children. The fear that such imagery or impulses may generate can be extreme.

In recent years, there have been many claims that antidepressants with serotonin reuptake inhibiting properties can be useful for individuals with OCD.

The drug for which most research has been done and for which most claims have been made has been clomipramine (Anafranil) (Beaumont & Healy 1996). However, there is now clinical trial evidence that each of the SSRIs may be useful in OCD. However, if there is agreement that these drugs may be of some usefulness, there is less agreement about what exactly it is that they do. Are they anxiolytic in some way or antidepressant? And just how useful are they? This will be developed in Chapter 12.

As with the other neuroses, one good reason for using an antidepressant in OCD is that there will often be an underlying depressive disorder, the stress of which has precipitated the full-blown neurosis. Resolution of the underlying depression may bring about an improvement of the neurosis or make the person more accessible to a behavioural programme. This, however, might be expected to be true for any antidepressant and not just for antidepressants with serotonin reuptake inhibiting properties.

Is the usefulness of the SSRIs in OCD, then, down to some anxiolytic effect of 5HT reuptake inhibition, or are these drugs in some way specifically anti-obsessional (Healy 1991)? In favour of the idea that the SSRIs help because they are non-specifically anxiolytic is the fact that these drugs also seem to be useful in panic disorder, social phobia and other anxiety states. This raises the question of whether any other anxiolytics may also be useful for obsessive–compulsive disorders. The simple answer to this is that we do not know. No proper clinical trials have been done on any other agents. It seems unlikely that beta-blockers or benzodiazepines would be particularly useful as there are no prominent physical symptoms of anxiety in OCD.

However, there is often a marked degree of agitation and, on this basis, one might imagine that antipsychotics would be useful. Before the recent vogue for using SSRIs, antipsychotics were used quite widely and successfully for some people with OCD. The recent literature suggests that the antipsychotics may be particularly useful when the clinical picture contains tics or other features of Tourette disorder.

The main form of treatment for OCD is behavioural management, for both the ritualistic type of OCD and the intrusive imagery and impulse type of OCD. Behaviour therapy is much less successful, it would seem, for OCD characterised almost solely by indecisiveness or slowness. The principle behind a behavioural approach in these disorders is to expose the sufferer to the thing that is frightening them the most and to block, at least temporarily, their avoidance of what they have been avoiding. This forces the individual to encounter the stimulus to their fears and to habituate to it. Such an approach may produce a brief spell of intense anxiety, but it appears to be an effective way of breaking obsessive compulsive cycles of behaviour.

Hysterical or dissociative disorders

At one time, hysteria was the commonest diagnosis in medical circles for patients who had any kind of trouble with their nerves or psychological disorder of any sort. It has fallen out of favour for a variety of reasons. It remains the case, however, that there are a number of patients who have classical hysterical neuroses, where they seemingly become paralysed in a leg or an arm, for instance, or go blind in an eye without there being any apparent physical basis for the problem. Ordinarily this will be triggered by some sort of psychological shock or ongoing stress.

While there are unquestionably a number of such cases that happen without the affected individual also being depressed, it is common to find at least mild degrees of hysteria in many patients who are depressed. The reverse is also true, in that it is quite rare to find people who have hysteria who are not depressed. Very often, effective treatment of an underlying depression will help to clear up a hysterical neurosis. One of the mechanisms by which patients who are depressed become hysterical is something like the following. People who are depressed may have clear problems concentrating or in trying to remember things. Given that being anxious about remembering may itself interfere with being able to remember, someone who is both depressed and anxious may conclude that their memory problems indicate a possible Alzheimer disease or something similar and, if prone to extroversion, they may start behaving accordingly. Both depression and anxiety produce a range of other physical and psychological symptoms that may crystallise out in a similar fashion.

Today, there is a certain swing back towards a diagnosis of hysteria, but the condition is called a dissociative disorder rather than hysteria (Healy 1993). Simply put, dissociation means that psychological functioning is in some way split by pressure or stress. For example, the idea of how to use your arm is cut off from the actual arm itself so that, while there may be nothing wrong with your arm, you may not be able to use it – it may effectively be paralysed. Under strain or stress, people may often be cut off from memories of things that happened in the past, even so profoundly cut off as to be unable to remember their own name or how they got to where they are. This is not uncommon in people before interviews or exams.

At the turn of the century, Sigmund Freud, Pierre Janet and others argued that hysteria more often than not arose in response to trauma. Many of the features of hysteria as they described it then correspond well with what is now termed post-traumatic stress disorder (PTSD). PTSD officially came into being in 1980. It is a condition that comes on after trauma – whether rape, physical violence, sustained mental torture or disasters of one sort or another. These are thought to precipitate a dissociation or split within the individual, so that they are in part cut off from what happened to them. Their feelings or experiences subsequently are of recurrent intrusive images of what has happened or awarenesses of something that they may be afraid might have happened to them but which they cannot clearly remember, or uncertainties regarding things they feel they ought to have done during the traumatic episode, such as struggle more in the course of a rape. These alternate with episodes of numbness, blankness and amnesia. There may be a pervasive feeling of unreality and a generalised anxiety, with an increased liability to be startled.

There is, at present, no effective pharmacological treatment for this disorder. If caught soon after the initial trauma, tranquillisation with benzodiazepines or barbiturates may help. Quite commonly people who have a PTSD also develop a depressive disorder at points during the course of their post-traumatic state. Antidepressants in this case may be helpful for the depressive component to the picture. SSRIs also appear to be helpful, even in the absence of depression, because of their anxiolytic effects, although at present the evidence is more convincing for their usefulness in women than in men.

PTSD has only recently been recognised, and a number of attempts have been made to try to produce techniques to manage the recurrent intrusive images and episodes of emotion that happen in this disorder. Such developments are at present at an early stage. At present, the condition seems more likely to resolve (at least temporarily) if the subject can actively engage in doing new things and getting on with life.

When the condition has become chronic, it is common to find that sufferers resort to alcohol or minor tranquillisers to numb the distress they feel. While these may work very effectively in the short term, and may even in the short term assist in the resolution of the disorder, neither works well in the long term. Where the disorder is long lasting, and characterised by recurrent intrusive memories and flashbacks or nightmares, there is some evidence that drugs active on the 5HT system may help (see Ch. 12).

There is a variation of PTSD called a borderline disorder or borderline personality organisation. Present research suggests that this condition results from chronic trauma during childhood, which leads to recurrent dissociative experiences and later unstable interpersonal relationships and self-injurious episodes. One hundred years ago this condition would also have been called hysteria. In recent years, individuals with this disorder have been more likely to be diagnosed as having schizophrenia.

Antidepressants may sometimes be of use in these states. On other occasions, they may aggravate the depersonalisation and derealisation to which such individuals are prone. Antipsychotics may help to reduce the impulsive behaviour, such as self-mutilation, that often goes with the condition. However, benzodiazepines appear to be the most reliable means of bringing to an end the acute episodes of dissociation or extreme agitation that accompany this disorder.

Health anxiety or hypochondriasis

There seems to be a widespread tendency to rename conditions when an older name conjures up pejorative associations. Often the renaming appears to lose something of the resonance of the older term. Recently, the condition of hypochondriasis has been subject to this process and has become health anxiety instead. But, in contrast to some other renamings, the term health anxiety far more clearly indicates what this condition is all about.

As has been pointed out, both depression and anxiety may give rise to a range of physical sensations, some of which may be extremely uncomfortable and may give the impression that there is something physically wrong. Consulting a textbook for the sensations of weakness and tingling feelings that may come about as a result of anxiety, in particular after hyperventilation, would be quite likely to lead many of us to give ourselves a diagnosis of something like multiple sclerosis, for example.

It may be very difficult to shift an individual from such a diagnosis, as symptoms of multiple sclerosis are non-specific and often, if it is an ongoing anxiety, it may well appear that the physical sensations being experienced map fairly well on to the diagnosis worked out from a textbook. Besides which, the medical profession has a certain reputation for not telling patients when they have got something seriously wrong with them such as cancer, schizophrenia or multiple sclerosis. Accordingly, the fact that your doctor does not confirm the diagnosis you have come to yourself may, for many people, not be very reassuring.

A number of other factors may play a part in the generation of a health neurosis. One is that attention to a physical complaint is all too likely either to aggravate that complaint or at least to give it a salience that then becomes difficult to ignore. Such attention may have a defensive quality to it. When any of us are anxious or under stress, one defence mechanism for coping with the problem we are faced with is what is termed a displacement reaction. This is what happens when, for example, we have to study for an exam or write an awkward letter, and somehow it seems there are a whole range of other things that seem easier to do – tidying the pens in the holder, clearing out the drawer in the desk, etc. In the same way, displacement on to what might appear to be a physical problem requiring attention may be a means of not facing something more stressful. Prolonged displacement on to the supposed physical problem may lead to an ongoing awareness of that aspect of health functioning long after the original stressor has been resolved.

An unhelpful focus on aspects of health is more likely in someone who has particular ideas about their health. Thus, someone who believes that their bowels must move at least once per day, and that there are serious consequences for their health if they do not, may get very preoccupied by the constipation that often goes with depression. In Section 5 I will argue that, in many respects, chronic insomnia can be viewed as a form of health anxiety. Fixed ideas about health, such as the need to move the bowels daily or for a regular 8 hours' sleep, tend to run in families.

Far from being a mild disorder, health anxiety will often lead to repeated visits to general practitioners, alternative therapists and a range of 'other healers'. The disorder can become extreme, with an individual becoming paralysed by their fear of interfering with the physical condition they are afraid they may have. They may even, for example, get to the state of urgently calling in the police to bring them to hospital as they are sure something terrible is happening. Repeated physical investigations rarely yield anything of note. The complaints of ill-health are often incessant so that other family members, as well as general practitioners and others, become either very irritated or very concerned.

At present a number of cognitive therapy strategies for health anxiety are being developed (Warwick & Salkovskis 1990) which resemble those in use for panic disorder (both conditions, it can be noted, involve a misinterpretation of physical symptoms). Behaviour therapies have not been as effective as in obsessive or phobic disorders. A general anxiety management strategy may help, particularly if there is any evidence that some of the symptoms come on after episodes of hyperventilation.

On the basis that health anxieties often become established in someone who is depressed, treatment with an antidepressant is common if there is any hint that the individual concerned has an underlying depressive disorder. The hope is that treating the depression will lead to a resolution of the neurosis.

Generalised anxiety disorder (GAD)

This is what used, rather more simply, to be called anxiety (Smail 1984). It involves unrealistic or excessive anxiety and apprehensive expectation about two or more life circumstances, such as worry about possible misfortune to one's child (who is in no danger) and worry about finances (for no good reason), for 6 months or longer. During this time, a person must be bothered by these concerns for more days than not. The condition may affect children and adolescents, taking the form of anxiety and worry about academic, athletic and social performance. When the person is anxious, there should be signs of motor tension, of autonomic hyperactivity and of increased vigilance and arousal.

The symptoms of motor tension include: trembling, twitching or feeling shaky; muscle tension and aches or soreness; restlessness; and easy fatigability. Those of autonomic hyperactivity include: shortness of breath or smothering sensations; palpitations or accelerated heart rate, sweating, or cold clammy hands, dry mouth, dizziness or light-headedness; nausea, diarrhoea or other abdominal distress; hot flashes or chills; frequent urination; and trouble swallowing or a 'lump in the throat'. The symptoms of increased vigilance and arousal include: feeling keyed up or on edge; exaggerated startle response; difficulty concentrating or finding one's mind going blank because of anxiety; trouble falling asleep; and irritability.

In diagnosing the disorder, other disorders that are frequently associated with generalised anxiety need to be ruled out. Thus, the diagnosis is not made if the worry and anxiety are present only when the person is depressed. In practice there is considerable overlap between GAD and the other neuroses, both with regard to symptomatology and the fact that many individuals may present with what appears like a phobic neurosis one year, GAD the next, and perhaps OCD the following year. If one of the worries is about health, then distinguishing GAD from health anxiety may be very difficult.

But, broadly speaking, GAD refers to the large number of anxious states, in which individuals appear globally or diffusely anxious, in which there has been no crystallising of the anxiety into a clear phobic or obsessive state, or preoccupation with health as the sole focus of concerns. For these reasons, it may be difficult to see a point of entry for cognitive or behavioural strategies. GAD, therefore, is the anxiety state for which general practitioners and others have tended to resort to the use of minor tranquillisers and for which they have been blamed for an inappropriate tranquillisation of distress. They are now being encouraged to use antidepressants, particularly the SSRIs, on the basis that these drugs do not produce dependence, are anxiolytic and that behind a GAD there may often be a depressive disorder.

The typical picture of a GAD is of a person who has multiple problems on their plate and who is, in many respects, legitimately anxious. The problem lies in the maladaptive or habitual nature of the anxiety, or in its severity. Very often the problems may be relatively intractable and 'out of sympathy' a doctor will prescribe something to try to calm the person down or to take the edge off their distress. This may lead, when the pills fail to work, to an increased level of prescription or to the addition of yet other drugs into the cocktail. The person in question has their distress dulled – but often at a cost.

When not disablingly severe, GAD is the form of anxiety that lends itself most readily to interpretative approaches. These may include an identification of the real stresses that the individual may be under, such as an unsatisfying marriage, isolation in a suburban housing estate or in a tower block cut off from other family members, or pressures at work stemming perhaps from a downturn in the general state of the economy. The identification of such stresses and the institution of appropriate anxiety management strategies may be all that is needed to bring about considerable change.

THE NOTION OF AN ANXIOLYTIC

The first treatments for nerves were generally sedating and were termed sedatives. There was no notion that there was anything else to do with nervous problems other than sedate the affected person. The first breach in this way of thinking came with the use of stimulants for nervous problems, although the change implied was noticed by very few at the time.

In 1955, Frank Berger launched meprobamate, the first non-barbiturate sedative. In the course of developing this drug, which had pronounced muscle relaxant properties, Berger became convinced that it would ultimately be possible to produce a drug for nervous problems that was not sedative – a drug that might, in the case of meprobamate, work by producing muscle relaxation.

In order to distinguish his new drug from the older sedatives, Berger stumbled on the term tranquilliser, which had been coined by Yonkman of Ciba the previous year to describe the effects of the first neuroleptics, reserpine and chlorpromazine. Meprobamate and the generation of benzodiazepine drugs that followed it were accordingly termed tranquillisers – or minor tranquillisers, to distinguish them from the major tranquillisers such as chlorpromazine.

The benzodiazepine dependence crisis of the 1980s made the term tranquilliser as much of a problem as the term sedative had been before it. In the course of the next decade, pharmaceutical companies will bring a new generation of agents for nervous problems on stream. These will in all likelihood be termed anxiolytics, a term that, for the moment, does not have the connotations of a tranquilliser.

11

Benzodiazepine anxiolytics

INTRODUCTION

To attempt to write an impartial account of the benzodiazepines (Table 11.1) is all but impossible (Hindmarch et al 1990). When they were first introduced, these drugs were seen as being of major benefit. They were widely regarded as extremely safe and obviously effective. They were popular with physicians, consumers and the pharmaceutical industry. More recently the benzo-diazepines have been described as one of the greatest menaces to society in peacetime. They have been seen as the epitome of the psychotropic drug

Table 11.1 Commonly used benzodiazepine anxiolytics

Generic drug name	UK trade names	US trade names
diazepam	Valium/Diazemuls/Stesolid/Valclair	Valium
chlordiazepoxide	Librium	Librium
lorazepam	Ativan	Ativan
bromazepam	Lexotan	Lexotan
oxazepam	Serenid	Serax
alprazolam	Xanax	Xanax
clobazam	Frisium	Frisium
medazepam	Nobrium	Nobrium
clorazepate	Tranxene	Tranxene
clonazepam	Rivotril	Klonopin

juggernaut whose prescription must be curbed at all costs. It has been claimed that coming off them is harder than coming off heroin. There have been a variety of television and radio programmes highlighting the dangers of benzodiazepines and the horrors of dependence.

But, strangely, benzodiazepine dependence is perhaps the only case of drug dependence in which the dependent person is viewed with sympathy. He or she is portrayed as a victim of forces beyond their control rather than as author of their own destiny (Bury & Gabe 1990). This suggests that the benzodiazepines mark a point where consumers took up arms against the medicopharmaceutical complex, rather than simply against the dangers of this particular group of drugs.

The other half of the argument, which is still put forward by medical practitioners and the pharmaceutical industry, is that these drugs remain remarkably safe, that reports of dependence and withdrawal reactions are exaggerated in the extreme, and that withdrawal phenomena are probably more linked to the personality of the sufferer than to the pharmacology of the drugs.

These opposing views have become so polarised over the past few years that it is difficult to write an account of the benzodiazepines that will not alienate someone. The position taken here will be that the benzodiazepines are far safer for most people than they are currently perceived to be but that there is a subgroup of individuals who, through no fault of their own, will encounter serious difficulties with them. The benzodiazepines have provided something of a stick with which to beat the pharmaceutical industry. Perhaps the wrong stick has been chosen, but the choosing of these things is rarely a calculated matter: it is much more likely to result from a combination of accidental factors interacting with the spirit of the times.

When the benzodiazepines came on the market in 1960, the available alternatives were the barbiturates or the first neuroleptics (antipsychotics). There were serious drawbacks to the barbiturates: excessive sedation, a high risk of dependence and substantial fatalities in overdose. The antipsychotics, while not afflicted with these problems, have their own drawbacks, as outlined in

Section 1, and their prescription is seen by many as inappropriate for milder or neurotic disorders.

The benzodiazepines, in contrast, had none of the side effects of the antipsychotics. Compared with the barbiturates, they appeared to produce a relatively mild sedation, to be free of the risk of physical dependence and, most of all, to be very safe in overdose. They became increasingly popular and widely prescribed. A wide-scale chemical tranquillisation of anxiety ensued.

We now recoil from what happened during the 1960s and 1970s. There is evidence that many patients do as well with brief counselling from general practitioners as they do on benzodiazepines, and that they are as happy with such counselling. General practitioners, today, often squirm in the face of such findings, but it should be mentioned that before the large-scale prescription of benzodiazepines there was a great deal of chemical management of neurotic and anxiety disorders. Before the mid-1960s this involved the use of barbiturates and a significant number of deaths were consequent on this use.

Furthermore, the chemical tranquillisation of anxiety appears to be something that both the medical profession and we, the drug takers, engaged in even before the establishment of the modern pharmaceutical industry. In the last century, opium was used widely in a variety of preparations. These were bought in large quantities over the counter and were used widely, sometimes explicitly to sedate cranky children. The demand for tranquillisation was, and still is, often clearly consumer led. Hence it may be somewhat naive to ascribe the dark side of the benzodiazepine story solely to the pharmaceutical industry following the siren call of the profit motive oblivious to any greater good.

Quite apart from barbiturates and opiates, it should also be pointed out that human beings have relied extensively on alcohol for millennia to tranquillise anxiety and provide sedation. By any standards alcohol must be seen as a far more dangerous compound than the benzodiazepines and yet society's concern regarding it seems much less than its anxiety about the benzodiazepines.

MECHANISM OF ACTION OF THE BENZODIAZEPINES

We know more about how benzodiazepines work than we do about almost any other psychotropic drug. Attempts to unravel the mechanism of action of benzodiazepines have, furthermore, in recent years led to significant advances in psychopharmacology generally.

The first development in our understanding of the benzodiazepines came with the discovery that a compound called γ-aminobutyric acid (GABA) is one of the most plentiful neurotransmitters in the brain – much commoner than serotonin or noradrenaline. It is the brain's principal inhibitory neurotransmitter. Benzodiazepines bind to and modulate GABA receptors. They neither block messages through the GABA system nor create artificial messages, but rather modulate normal functioning. There are three types of BZ receptor,

BZ_1, BZ_2 and BZ_3, mediating sedative, myorelaxant and anxiolytic effects respectively.

It has emerged that there are a number of natural compounds within the brain that bind to the same sites on the GABA receptor as the benzodiazepines. The implication of this is that there are a set of natural compounds in the brain performing much the same function that benzodiazepines perform. The best candidates for these natural compounds at present seem to be a group of compounds called the β-carbolines.

One surprising finding has been that β-carbolines may both alleviate anxiety and produce relaxation just as benzodiazepines do, but also that other β-carbolines may cause anxiety, tension and convulsions. This finding has led to significant changes in our understanding of how neurotransmitters and receptors work naturally. It had previously been thought that neurotransmitters act on receptors and that drugs may either mimic this action or antagonise it. It now seems clear that some compounds within the brain may produce opposite actions at the same receptor site. Where actions on benzodiazepine receptors are concerned, we can now produce compounds that relieve anxiety, compounds that increase anxiety, and compounds that block both of these effects. These three types of compounds differ, but all act at the same receptor site.

Another interesting feature of the benzodiazepines is that the benzodiazepine receptor appears to have emerged only in higher animals. The other neurotransmitters that have been discussed in this book, such as noradrenaline, dopamine and serotonin, are all found in single-celled or quite simple organisms. Benzodiazepine receptors, in contrast, are confined mostly to cortical areas of the brain and have emerged only in, relatively speaking, higher animals; they also occur naturally in certain plant species.

CLASSES OF BENZODIAZEPINES

By convention the benzodiazepines are divided up according to their half-life – the length of time it takes for the amount of the drug in the blood to decrease to half its initial level after a standard dose. There was a great deal of interest in this concept during the 1970s, as it was thought that producing a benzodiazepine with a short half-life might overcome problems such as hangover sedation that were apparent with some of the earlier compounds, such as diazepam. The half-life of some of the earlier compounds was so long that taking the pills regularly meant that a first pill had not washed out of the system by the time a second was taken, and so on. This led to a steady accumulation of the drug, which in the elderly was a particular problem. However, even in the case of the supposedly shorter-acting compounds, it should be kept in mind that, while the duration of action depends on the chemical make-up of the compound, it also depends on how much of the drug is given: a large amount of a short-acting compound may act for a long time (see Box 11.1).

Box 11.1 Benzodiazepines classified by duration of action

Long	Intermediate	Short	Ultra-short
chlordiazepoxide	flunitrazepam	alprazolam	midazolam
clorazepate	nitrazepam	lorazepam	triazolam
diazepam	lormetazepam		
	oxazepam		

CLINICAL USES FOR BENZODIAZEPINES

Benzodiazepines give a relaxing warm glow, like alcohol. There is a sense of muscular release and a soothing feeling which most people who take them describe as being positively pleasant. In one sense they are one of the twentieth century's greatest inventions. After 2000 years of trying to improve on alcohol, they represent success. They can be used for the same purposes as alcohol: for general relaxation purposes, as antianxiety agents for acute crises such as interviews or whatever, and they are just generally pleasant in the way alcohol is. Furthermore they are free of many of the drawbacks of alcohol, as they do not cause liver, heart, joint or gut problems, or the generalised brain cell loss that alcohol causes. They do not cause weight gain, or throwing up after one too many; they are much cheaper than alcohol and, above all, are much safer in overdose than alcohol.

Anxiolysis

To say that benzodiazepines are anxiolytic seems rather superfluous. They are, but they are by no means universally anxiolytic. They are of benefit in anxiety states that have a significant muscular tension or dissociative component to them. The anxiolytic effect of benzodiazepines appears to resemble most the effects of alcohol. The anxiolysis differs clearly from the 'anxiolytic' effect of the antipsychotics, which work best in distraught and agitated rather than in anxious states. Benzodiazepine anxiolysis also differs from the anxiolysis brought about by beta-blockers, which work best in states characterised by increased heart rate, palpitations, butterflies in the stomach and other shakes of the hand. It also differs from the serenic effect produced by SSRIs and other compounds acting on the serotonin system (see Ch. 12).

The above description of the anxiolytic effects of benzodiazepines is only approximate. Greater precision is not possible at present, which seems remarkable given that so many benzodiazepines have been prescribed and taken in the past 30 years. One might expect that there would be a better appreciation of just what kind of anxiolysis they bring about. This is a major indictment of the way we develop drugs at present.

Anticonvulsant

In addition to being anxiolytic, the benzodiazepines are generally anticonvulsant. They are not used widely for epilepsy because phenytoin, carbamazepine, valproate and others are more effective anticonvulsants. In states of intractable epilepsy, however, the benzodiazepines may often be used in conjunction with these other compounds. One benzodiazepine in particular, clobazam, is used more widely in epilepsy as it provides the anticonvulsant effects of a benzodiazepine without producing the sedation associated with most benzodiazepines. In status epilepticus, intravenous diazepam is the drug of first choice. Another benzodiazepine, clonazepam, is also used for the management of epilepsy, restless leg syndrome, myoclonic jerks and a range of other neuropsychiatric indications.

Sedation

Benzodiazepines are sedative in much the same way as barbiturates, although somewhat less so. The sedation produced, however, varies from individual to individual and from benzodiazepine to benzodiazepine. With regular ingestion of benzodiazepines, tolerance to these sedative effects develops quite quickly. In addition, as mentioned above, there is little or no sedation associated with clobazam. The sedative effects of benzodiazepines provide the basis for their use as hypnotics (see Section 5). While the use of benzodiazepines as anxiolytics has fallen off dramatically in the past 10 years, their use as hypnotics has not. They are prescribed for sleeping purposes as regularly now as they were 10 years ago.

Muscle relaxants

Benzodiazepines are also effective muscular relaxants and are used for this purpose in patients with spasticity, dystonia and multiple sclerosis. A proportion of their anxiolytic effect may stem from this action, although there also appears to be an independent central anxiolytic effect.

Amnesia

The benzodiazepines can produce an amnesia that resembles the effect of alcohol on memory. Essentially, they impair the registration and subsequent recall of events that take place after they have been taken. This seems to be most marked for short-acting agents such as lorazepam, midazolam and triazolam. It is also more marked when the drugs are given intravenously. For this reason short-acting benzodiazepines are given before operations in order to produce amnesia regarding the events of surgery. Something like this effect may also be partly responsible for the complaints of people who took benzodiazepines during the years their children were growing up, that the past seems indistinct, hazy or blotted out to some extent.

The effects of benzodiazepines on memory are at present the subject of much investigation, as they provide a window on the study of memory. In general, it has been believed that drugs that improve memory do so by being stimulants of some sort, while drugs that sedate generally impair memory. This appeared to apply to the benzodiazepines, until recently, when it became clear that many benzodiazepines, particularly when they enter the brain quickly, as after intravenous injection, produce striking memory deficits for periods after the sedative effects have worn off. Another odd thing about these findings was that amnesia was being produced less by the action of a drug on some receptor but rather as a consequence of the rate of binding to the receptor.

Abreaction

Paradoxically, the benzodiazepines may also be used for abreaction. Abreaction is a technique used to recover buried memories, often following trauma. It involves getting individuals to remember scenes from their past life in great detail. In the course of such remembering, it is hoped that hints about or glimpses of the significant event or trauma will be recovered. Abreaction can be conducted without pharmacological intervention of any sort, but commonly the relaxation produced by a tranquilliser helps and mystique is introduced into the process by hints that remembering is being assisted by a truth drug. A simplistic rationale is that relaxation permits memories that are suppressed to re-emerge into consciousness.

This rationale is obviously simplistic given that benzodiazepines are, if anything, amnestic rather than memory enhancing. A partial reconciliation of the amnestic effects of benzodiazepines and barbiturates, and their role in bringing back buried memories, lies in the fact that the amnesia induced by these compounds is for events that happen after they have been taken, rather than for events that may have happened in the past. It is, for example, reasonable to work for an oral examination for weeks and then take a benzodiazepine the night before or morning of the oral without the homework done being wiped out. What is more likely to happen is that memory for the actual oral exam itself may be hazy but performance should not be affected.

Alcohol withdrawal

The benzodiazepines are the standard first line of treatment for alcohol withdrawal. The early institution of a comprehensive benzodiazepine regimen for such individuals has all but abolished the rigours of alcohol withdrawal, and prevents individuals going into delirium tremens on withdrawal. Before the benzodiazepines this was a condition with a high level of fatalities. The benzodiazepines can then be tailed off over the course of a week or two.

Catatonia and neuroleptic malignant syndrome

In recent years the benzodiazepines have become the favoured first-line treatment for both catatonic signs or syndromes and for neuroleptic malignant syndrome (see Ch. 2). Lorazepam is used most often, in doses of up to 16 mg per day, but diazepam or other benzodiazepines in high doses are equally likely to be effective.

Mania

Benzodiazepines are regularly prescribed in mania, particularly in North America. There seems to be no clear theoretical rationale, but it may be that the high incidence of catatonic features in bipolar disorders leads to a noticeable benefit and that this perceptible benefit underpins the practice.

Rapid tranquillisation

Concern has developed in recent years about deaths that have occurred during the course of the rapid tranquillisation of disturbed or violent behaviour with antipsychotics. The intramuscular use of agents such as chlorpromazine has been particularly implicated, but there is no clear evidence that chlorpromazine is uniquely responsible. The concerns, however, have prompted a fresh look at regimens for rapid tranquillisation and a consensus is emerging that benzodiazepines have a place. The agent most commonly used at present is lorazepam (0.5–2.0 mg) because of its short duration of action and lower likelihood to accumulate. It can also be given orally, or by intramuscular or intravenous routes, in contrast to diazepam. Emerging regimens involve the use of lorazepam alone or in combination with an antipsychotic (Pilowsky et al 1992).

The primary hazard in the use of benzodiazepines for rapid tranquillisation is respiratory depression. If this occurs, it can be reversed by flumazenil (Anexate), which can be given continuously (200 µg intravenously, up to 600 mg) or administered in a glucose or saline solution.

 User Issues

SIDE EFFECTS OF BENZODIAZEPINES

Sedation

Sedation is a feature of all benzodiazepines except clobazam. This may be put to use for hypnotic purposes. However, it can also impair normal daily functioning. It was to avoid such effects that the intermediate and short-acting benzodiazepines were synthesised. The impairment of daily functioning that can occur with tranquillisers such as diazepam or with sleeping pills such as nitrazepam are comparable to the effects produced by alcohol. These compounds also impair reflex reactions and car-handling ability. Surprisingly, however, given current concerns with alcohol and driving, there are no legal proscriptions against driving under the influence of benzodiazepines (see below).

The sedative effects of benzodiazepines depend heavily on the state of arousal of the individual concerned. For a subject who has never had

continued

benzodiazepines before, 5–10 mg of diazepam may be heavily sedating. For an individual who has had a modest amount of benzodiazepines in the past, taking 5–10 mg of diazepam may produce a noticeable but not undue sedative effect. The same individual going to have a tooth extraction, to an interview or engaging in some anxiety-provoking procedure may be able to take 30–40 mg immediately before their ordeal without significant sedative effects. Up to 100 mg of diazepam may be necessary in some agitated states to produce noticeable sedation.

Rebound anxiety

In some cases benzodiazepine intake may cause as much anxiety as it alleviates. This effect is similar to an effect produced by alcohol. Individuals with marked anxiety problems, such as phobias, often turn to alcohol to help them cope with situations they know will provoke anxiety. While it may help in the short term, becoming alcohol dependent leads to withdrawal anxiety as the alcohol wears off. Similarly, intake of benzodiazepines, particularly of the shorter-acting benzodiazepines, may lead in susceptible individuals to an early development of withdrawal based rebound anxiety. (See Rebound insomnia in Section 5).

Amnesia

The amnestic effects of benzodiazepines have been the basis for many complaints regarding their use. However, these amnestic effects can also be put to good use, before operation for instance, as well as for dental procedures, endoscopy or other procedures, which involve the passage of tubes or instruments into the body for investigative purposes.

Concerns surrounding procedures such as these led to the first clear recognition of the amnestic effects of benzodiazepines. Patients undergoing dental procedures and endoscopy claimed that they had been taken advantage of (Hindmarch et al 1990, Wheatley 1990). The investigation of these claims led to the recognition of a complicated picture. There was usually a clear relationship between events that had occurred and the complaint made. For example, in the case of dental procedures and endoscopy it was claimed that oral sex had taken place. Similarly, in procedures involving an individual having to squeeze a hand in order to pump up their vein before a blood sample was taken, it was claimed that the patient had been forced to masturbate the other person. In some cases accusations have been upheld; in others the judgement has been that the drowsy state the subject was in made them more suggestible.

Ordinarily, the amnestic effects of benzodiazepines are not noticed. Every so often, however, people taking benzodiazepines find that something dramatic happens. For example, a colleague of mine after flying home from abroad and taking a short-acting benzodiazepine on the flight to promote sleep, went to his parents' house immediately after getting off the plane. He met his sister in the drive and talked with her at length. The following day, when he met her again, he had no recollection of their encounter the previous day.

The benzodiazepines produce an anterograde amnesia – events that occur after taking them may not be registered fully. This effect is similar to the anterograde amnesia produced by anticholinergic compounds and by alcohol. Benzodiazepines may interact with both the anticholinergics and alcohol to make amnesia even more likely. The effects are comparable in many respects to the blackouts that some people have on alcohol, which can occur after having had only one or two units of alcohol. Conversations that have taken place after this modest amount of alcohol may not be recalled the next day.

Dissociation

Occasionally the benzodiazepines may produce dissociative reactions. The most commonly described reactions are states of hyperactivity. It is often thought that these involve disinhibition – that the benzodiazepines have inhibited some inhibitory pathway on the brain. This seems unlikely. What seems more likely is that, just as alcohol may in certain individuals produce quite marked dissociative reactions characterised by profound amnesia and explosive behaviour following the intake of sometimes less than a pint of beer, so also the benzodiazepines in certain individuals who are particularly sensitive to their effects may produce markedly excitable and overactive or explosive behaviour. Benzodiazepines have also been reported to produce depersonalisation, derealisation and hallucinatory experiences. The frequency of these is unknown.

Depersonalisation, derealisation and dissociative experiences are most commonly a feature of anxiety. When they occur in this context, a benzodiazepine is the most reliable treatment.

 User Issues

BENZODIAZEPINES AND DRIVING

Psychiatric illnesses of all sorts slightly increase the risks of a road traffic accident (RTA). However, this includes the effects of dementia; at present it is not possible to calculate the mean effect of any one illness, such as anxiety or depression. Neither has work been done to differentiate between the RTAs stemming from untreated illness and those that stem from individuals on treatment but in a better frame of mind. It would seem highly likely that antidepressants, particularly tricyclics, benzodiazepines or other agents with sedative properties, may also contribute to RTAs, although the risks posed by such agents are much less than those posed by alcohol.

Section 4 of the 1988 Road Traffic Act makes it a criminal offence for a person to drive under the influence of drugs, prescribed or otherwise. Present recommendations from the Royal College of Psychiatrists (1993) suggest that driving licences should not be issued to or renewed for individuals who regularly take psychotropic regimens that would hamper their ability to drive safely. There are a number of problems here, one of which is the fact that there can be considerable interindividual variability in terms of how disabling a compound or regimen may be. Another concerns the locus of responsibility should an accident happen. At present the climate is shaping up that mental health professionals are best advised to warn subjects taking benzodiazepines, other sedatives or antidepressants of the potential risks, of the need for them to avoid driving if they are experiencing difficulties and to record that they have issued such advice. In the case of individuals who drive large goods vehicles or passenger-carrying vehicles, the problems are clearly of a much more serious order and merit careful consideration. This is one of those situations where, in certain circumstances, the professional duties of confidentiality may be outweighed by other considerations and it may be necessary to report an individual to the appropriate driving licence authority.

BENZODIAZEPINE DEPENDENCE AND WITHDRAWAL

The significance of benzodiazepine dependence will be considered further in Section 8. This chapter overviews the clinical management of possible problems.

While there do appear to be a significant number of people who have problems with withdrawal from benzodiazepines, these are only a small proportion of the overall numbers of people who have had benzodiazepines. It would seem, therefore, that the dependence potential of the benzodiazepines cannot be as serious as it is often now claimed to be, if so many people could have been prescribed these drugs so often over the course of 20 years and not had significant problems.

On the other hand, the medical response to this issue has been to write off the problem as stemming solely from individuals who either have a personality problem or who are experiencing a recrudescence of the initial anxiety, which their benzodiazepines had suppressed successfully for a considerable period of time. This recourse to personality is unwarranted given the current state of the evidence.

The recent developments in our understanding of how benzodiazepines work, outlined above, are beginning to shed some light on the question of why some individuals develop problems on these drugs. The nature of the benzodiazepine receptor and the dual action of endogenous compounds, such as the β-carbolines on it, opens up the possibility that one cause of problems following benzodiazepines may be that the receptors on which they work have been blocked for so long by these compounds that they become hypersensitive to the effects of the natural compounds in the brain that cause anxiety, insomnia, muscular tension and convulsions. Discontinuing drug treatment then leaves a hypersensitive receptor being bombarded by anxiogenic compounds.

This appears, however, not to be the whole story. The degree to which the BZ receptors shift to a state of being sensitive to the natural compounds acting to produce anxiety in the brain is almost certainly genetically determined. There will therefore be a range of liabilities to shift. This range is, in turn, likely to cause some people to become more sensitive to withdrawal of these compounds and to become sensitive at a quicker rate than others. Experimental findings and clinical experience bear this out.

If a large number of people are given the same benzodiazepine for the same period of time, different people will show differential rates at which rebound anxiety and rebound insomnia develops. It is almost certainly the case, therefore, that quite apart from personality there will be a physiological propensity to having difficulties with benzodiazepines. Current research suggests that 20–25% of us are at risk of having marked sensitivity to BZ withdrawal.

The corollary of this is that, for the remaining 75%, benzodiazepines are safer than current alarms would suggest. Indeed, for a proportion of us there may be quite minimal risks associated with taking them, unless very large amounts are taken chronically.

Apart from physiological factors in the takers of benzodiazepines, there appear to be pharmacological factors to do with the drugs themselves which may produce sensitivity to withdrawal. It increasingly appears that benzodiazepine compounds that have a short half-life and that enter the brain rapidly are more likely to produce marked effects on withdrawal. Such compounds include alprazolam and lorazepam. The irony here is that the short-acting compounds were produced in the first instance in order to avoid the prolonged sedation that may be associated with benzodiazepines with a longer half-life such as diazepam or chlordiazepoxide. Thus, there are good grounds for suggesting that, while personality may be a factor in benzodiazepine dependence, there are also significant physiological and pharmacological inputs to dependence, independent of the personality of the individual.

Symptoms of benzodiazepine withdrawal

Box 11.2 lists the symptoms that have been claimed as features of the withdrawal syndrome associated with benzodiazepines – and equally dismissed by sceptical medical practitioners as manifestations of a recrudescence of anxiety.

Withdrawal is most likely to occur if a person is taking a high dose of a short-acting benzodiazepine that is tapered abruptly. It also seems somewhat

---

Box 11.2 Symptoms associated with benzodiazepine withdrawal

- Increased anxiety with all its physical symptoms
- Poor sleep
- Unsteady gait
- Numbness
- Muscle pains
- Feeling of things moving, as though on a boat
- Aggressive feelings
- Depression
- Weakness and tiredness
- Flu-like symptoms
- Hallucinations
- Paranoid ideas
- Seizures
- Confusion
- Depersonalisation or derealisation
- Craving
- Restlessness
- Nausea, abnormal taste and gastrointestinal cramps

more likely if the individual was highly anxious before being put on benzo-diazepines and if they have a previous history of neurosis, although this latter is controversial. Current recommendations are that an individual should consider themselves hooked or at serious risk if they cannot stop benzo-diazepines for 2–3 days, whenever called upon to do so.

At present it is also recommended that benzodiazepines should not be prescribed for longer than 4 weeks. After that, prescribers should review the issues rather than simply repeat the prescription. As a result of these restrictions and replacement by the SSRIs, doctors are now prescribing benzo-diazepines infrequently as a first-line treatment for anxiety, and most pre-scriptions are being issued to individuals who have been long-term takers.

Along with recent horror stories of medical negligence in creating physical dependence on benzodiazepines has gone a set of stories, less widely publi-cised, of doctors who, reacting with therapeutic calvinism to the current cli-mate, have withdrawn all benzodiazepines from all their patients regardless. This is often highly inappropriate, particularly in the case of individuals aged 60 years and upwards who have been on the drugs for 10 years or more with little or no ill effect.

Withdrawal strategies

There is a recognised strategy for withdrawal management. If an individual has difficulty in withdrawing from a short-acting benzodiazepine, they should be switched to a compound with a long half-life, such as diazepam, as this is less likely to give rise to rebound phenomena.

Using the long half-life strategy, the usual regimen is to taper over 6 weeks or so, reducing one-quarter of the dose in the first week, one-quarter in the second week and one-eighth in each of the subsequent 4 weeks. The last dose level or two may need to be drawn out longer in some cases.

There have been attempts to find a compound that would attenuate benzo-diazepine withdrawal. To date, none seems particularly effective. Clonidine, carbamazepine, antidepressants and beta-blockers have been used, but with no convincing effects. The benzodiazepine antagonist, flumazenil, can both push individuals into withdrawal and dramatically shorten the length of time for which withdrawal is liable to last, but is not used clinically for this purpose.

There is some dispute as to how long the withdrawal syndrome lasts in those most severely affected. For most individuals it appears to be effectively over in a matter of weeks, but for some there have been claims of symptoms recurring for months or up to a year.

Psychological management of withdrawal

While it is clear that dependence is not a matter of some neurotic flaw in the personality of the affected individual, an individual's psychology may play a part in the ease or otherwise with which they can withdraw from benzo-diazepines. People given benzodiazepines are very often anxious and prone to phobias. A phobia of withdrawal is accordingly something that can be predicted in certain individuals and, where it occurs, it can be managed psychologically as any other phobia might be managed.

There have now been a number of trials showing that a package involving education about the nature of panic and anxiety, training in slow diaphragmatic breathing, correction of maladaptive thinking about anxiety and repeated exposure to feared bodily sensations can make a significant difference for such individuals (Albany et al 1997, Barlow & Craske 1989).

12

Anxiolysis and the serotonin system

INTRODUCTION

The 1990s were the decade of the neurotransmitter serotonin (otherwise called 5-hydroxytryptamine; 5HT). This was first isolated in the intestine in 1933 and called enteramine. It was rediscovered in blood vessels in 1947 and found to cause them to constrict, which led to it being called serotonin. In 1949, it was established that the chemical structure of serotonin was 5-hydroxytryptamine, or 5HT for short. Both names, 5HT and serotonin, have remained in use. The name serotonin survives partly because Smithkline Beecham stumbled on the marketing appeal of the acronym SSRI (selective serotonin reuptake inhibitor) for paroxetine.

Shortly before serotonin was discovered in the brain, lysergic acid diethyl-amide (LSD) had been discovered and it had been recognised that there were structural similarities between serotonin and LSD. This led, at the beginning of the psychopharmacological era, to great interest in the role that brain serotonin might play in mental illness (Carlsson & Healy 1996, Healy, 1991, 1997). However, serotonin more or less disappeared from view for over 20 years. One important reason for this was the emergence in 1965 of the catecholamine hypothesis for depression. This led to a focusing of research on the catechol-amine system and a virtual ignoring of the serotonin system.

One consequence was that an association between serotonin and anxiety developed. The reason for this was in part as follows. By the early 1970s, it seemed that dopamine was the 'psychosis' neurotransmitter, noradrenaline the 'mood' neurotransmitter and acetylcholine the 'dementia' neurotransmitter (see Section 6). This left serotonin without an accompanying psychiatric disorder, and one disorder with which it might be associated was anxiety.

While this parcelling out of disorders appears simplistic, there has always been some evidence to support it. We noted in Chapters 3 & 10 that the SSRIs appear to be in some way anxiolytic. Clomipramine, fluoxetine and fluvoxamine are useful for phobic and obsessional states as well as depression. This applies to all antidepressants with serotonin reuptake inhibiting properties and far less so to those antidepressants that do not inhibit serotonin reuptake.

With the development of the SSRIs, there was increasing interest in the serotonin system. This led during the 1980s to a sustained effort to characterise the receptors that serotonin acts on and to develop drugs specific to each of these.

SEROTONERGIC RECEPTORS AND DRUGS

Drugs acting on serotonergic (S) receptors divide into agonists (acting on a receptor) and antagonists (blocking the receptor) (Table 12.1).

S_1 receptors

Buspirone, an S_1 agonist, was launched under the trade name Buspar in 1985 in the USA, and in 1988 in the UK, and marketed as an anxiolytic. Given the degree of concern there had been about the use of benzodiazepines in the treatment of anxiety, it seemed a safe bet that a non-benzodiazepine anxiolytic, an anxiolytic that did not produce dependence, would sweep the market. Buspirone did not do this.

There seem to be three reasons why not. First, buspirone does not give the same pleasant feeling that the benzodiazepines produce, and consumers accordingly did not 'go for it'. Another is that it does not work immediately.

Table 12.1 Serotonergic system drugs

	Agonist	Antagonist
S_{1a}	buspirone flesinoxan gepirone	spiperone propranolol
S_{2a}	D-LSD	ketanserin mianserin trazodone nefazodone all antipsychotics
S_{2b}	mCPP	ritanserin mianserin mirtazapine
S_3		ondansetron

It takes anything from 2 to 4 weeks for effects to appear, which is not much help in many forms of acute anxiety. Finally, the reaction to claims that it is not dependence producing have been: 'Oh yes, we've heard that one before where anxiolytics are concerned and look what happened...'.

In the treatment of anxiety, buspirone is used in doses from 5 mg three times a day to 30–60 mg daily for severely anxious individuals. The most prominent side effects are headache, nausea and dizziness. Nervousness/akathisia has also been reported, as have stiffness (dystonia) and/or odd movements (dyskinesias). This is a mild version of the side-effect profile of the antipsychotics, and very similar to the side effects of the SSRIs. Such effects seem more likely to occur when drugs active on the serotonin system, such as the SSRIs or S_1 agonists, are combined with antipsychotics. The use of drugs active on the serotonin system in combination with a variety of other psychotropics also may lead to the development of a 'serotonin syndrome' (see Ch. 5). This appears to be a mild version of neuroleptic malignant syndrome (see Ch. 2).

Since the introduction of buspirone, a number of drugs that are more specific for the S_1 receptor have been developed, including gepirone and flesinoxan. These compounds all show efficacy in screening tests for anxiolytic compounds. In general, they appear to have a significantly different profile to the benzodiazepines, being inactive in the screening tests used to detect benzodiazepine-type anxiolysis. However, in contrast to buspirone, flesinoxan and gepirone, if marketed, are likely to be produced as antidepressants and, in fact, buspirone itself is now being remarketed as an antidepressant. Why?

There is some clinical trial evidence in support of this strategy but the real reason appears to be because the drug treatment of anxiety has such a bad name, in the wake of the benzodiazepines, that the very word anxiolytic has become a problem. General practitioners and others are much happier handing out antidepressants, which they feel certain are not habit forming. This process is assisted by current education campaigns to bring home to general practitioners how often they miss the diagnosis of depression and how much misery they could alleviate if they got it right.

There is, in fact, little basis to distinguish between S_1 agonists and SSRIs. If the SSRIs work, it must be through one of the serotonergic receptors, and most people's guess as to the most likely receptor is the S_1 receptor. S_1 agonists are arguably cleaned-up SSRIs – there is less serotonin around to act indiscriminately on a range of other receptors. Just like the SSRIs, S_1 agonists take 2–4 weeks to take effect. This is quite unlike benzodiazepine anxiolytics and much more like an 'antidepressant'. Are the S_1 agonists then antidepressants? Or are the SSRIs anxiolytics that are effective in milder depressions? Is the marketing of both of these groups of drugs (Healy 1991) as antidepressants a clever or perhaps even a cynical marketing exercise?

This returns us to the question of what do the SSRIs do; see Chapter 4. The SSRIs are beneficial in milder depressions, obsessive–compulsive disorder (OCD), panic disorder, social phobia, generalised anxiety disorder and post-traumatic stress disorder. The easiest way to explain this broad effectiveness is to argue that SSRIs have some common serenic effect across these conditions. There is, in fact, good physiological evidence to indicate that SSRIs damp down fight-or-flight anxiety systems in the brain, making the individual less responsive to either internal or external signals of threat. Clinically it is very clear that when SSRIs work they make the taker more mellow, more docile and more serene or sanguine. In some cases they do this to a greater extent than is desired, leading to complaints of emotional blunting or numbness. An action such as this would explain why SSRIs are of benefit in a broad range of anxious states and beneficial only in anxious or primary care depressions and not in hospital or melancholic depressions.

Migraine

Before leaving the S_1 receptor, some mention can be made of the triptans, of which the first launched was sumatriptan, even though these are neither antidepressant nor anxiolytic. These drugs are used for the treatment of migraine. Serotonin is released into the bloodstream during a migraine attack. The traditional treatments for migraine hitherto have been compounds derived from the fungus, ergot, such as dihydroergotamine, which acts weakly on most serotonin receptors as well as on many non-serotonin receptors.

By acting on the S_1 receptor on arteries leading to the brain, sumatriptan appears to constrict cerebral arteries and thereby prevent the alternating constriction and dilatation of arteries that gives rise to the throbbing headache of migraine. By extension, most drugs active on the serotonin system, including the SSRIs, have some potential either to alleviate or to aggravate migrainous attacks.

S_2 receptors

It is now clear that LSD, mescaline and related hallucinogens produce their effects by binding to the S_2 receptor. These effects can be blocked in animals by ketanserin, an S_2 antagonist. Perhaps surprisingly, however, neither ketanserin nor any other pure S_2 antagonists appear to be of much use in the treatment of psychotic conditions.

The issue is complex in that all current neuroleptics, in addition to having common actions on dopamine D_2 receptors, also block S_2 receptors. It remains possible, therefore, that the tranquillising as opposed to the 'strait-jacketing' effects of neuroleptics may be as much related to their actions on the serotonin system as to those on the dopamine system. And, as noted in Chapter 2, clozapine, the antipsychotic that acts most potently on the S_2 receptor, is particularly useful in treatment-resistant psychoses, this is attributed to a serenic aspect of its actions.

The presence on the list of S_2 antagonists of mianserin, mirtazapine, nefazodone and trazodone, which have all been marketed as antidepressants, is also of interest. Mianserin, mirtazapine and trazodone also have significant effects on adrenergic receptors, but this is much less so with nefazodone. A compound related to trazodone, mCPP, which is an agonist for the S_{2b} receptor, is potently anxiogenic. Also of interest is that trazodone and cyproheptadine and nefazodone, which are S_2 antagonists, have aphrodisiac properties (see Section 7).

It seems likely that S_2 antagonism produces two further effects. One is weight gain. The weight-gaining properties of antipsychotics such as chlorpromazine and clozapine, which act more potently at the S_2 receptor, may stem from this source. Similarly mianserin is particularly likely to cause weight gain. A further effect is sedation. Compared with other antipsychotics, clozapine and chlorpromazine are sedative. Trazodone and mianserin, which are S_2 antagonists, are also among the most sedative antidepressants.

It remains somewhat unclear, however, just what role pure S_2 drugs have. While ketanserin and ritanserin are relatively pure antagonists, clinical trials have not revealed them to be particularly good anxiolytics, antidepressants or antipsychotics. One possibility is that they may be useful in the management of the dissociative symptoms of anxiety such as derealisation or depersonalisation – symptoms that may be provoked by LSD.

S_3 receptors

It was initially thought that there were only S_1 and S_2 type serotonergic receptors, with drugs such as buspirone binding to the S_1 type, and LSD or ketanserin binding to the S_2. It now seems that there may be S_3, S_4, S_5 and other serotonergic receptors. At present the picture is most clear in the case of the S_3 receptor.

It initially appeared that S_3 antagonists might be effective in schizophrenia. This led to the development of a number of compounds such as ondansetron and granisetron, which may have some anxiolytic rather than 'antipsychotic' effects. This anxiolytic profile differs from that of both benzodiazepines and S_1 agonists, although the precise differences are not clear at present. There is also some evidence from animal studies that both S_3 and S_2 antagonists enhance cognitive function (see Section 6).

At present, ondansetron (Zofran) and granisetron (Kytril) are marketed for nausea, such as is caused by cancer chemotherapy, for example. Before this, the drugs used for this purpose were dopamine antagonists, closely related to the antipsychotics (see Ch. 1). This points to a close relation between the dopamine and serotonin systems.

SEROTONIN AND ANXIOLYSIS

It seems clear that there is a role for compounds acting on the serotonin system in anxiety states. What is involved?

It appears that there is a substantial overlap between the serotonin and dopamine systems. Both S_3 and D_2 antagonists are antiemetic. Antipsychotics,

SSRIs and S_1 agonists all produce akathisia and dyskinesias. More directly it has been shown that S_3 antagonists modulate dopamine release in the brain. One possibility, therefore, is that many of these compounds that are active on the serotonin system are, as it were, atypical neuroleptics. That is, they produce the benefits of an antipsychotic without the same side effects.

Of note here are the reports of a possible benefit of clomipramine and SSRIs in OCD (see Ch. 10), which suggest that these agents help by producing a state of indifference to intrusive thoughts and imagery. In Chapter 1, it was argued that the beneficial effects of neuroleptics also consist of an induction of a state of psychic indifference, although one that appears to come on far more rapidly than that induced by clomipramine or SSRIs.

There are data that argue against similarities between the two sets of compounds. Some patients can have both groups of drugs at the same time and distinguish between the 'indifference' caused by each. Furthermore, where antipsychotics help in schizophrenic disorders, SSRIs and tricyclics with clear actions on the serotonin system will often lead to a decompensation if not given concurrently with an antipsychotic.

Nevertheless, there is sufficient overlap here to ask whether drugs that are active on the serotonin system produce much the same type of anxiolysis as antipsychotics, albeit with a slower onset. There is a good case here for saying that the best scientific way forward with this question would be to enlist the takers of these various drugs to attempt to determine whether the effects of antipsychotics and the effects of drugs active on the serotonin system are similar. If not similar, in what way do they differ? This, however, is not the way in which the modern pharmaceutical industry works (see Section 10). Uncontrolled observations by users or clinicians are not welcome. From the industry's point of view, any recognition of similarities of this type would not help the marketing process, which works better in distinguishing difference and gearing up strategies around these differences.

Quite apart from the interaction between the serotonin and dopamine systems, there is another possible interaction between the serotonin system and the GABA system on which benzodiazepines work. Thus, it may be that benzodiazepines in part exert their anxiolytic action through effects on the serotonin system. While this is theoretically possible, it seems that the benzodiazepines and the drugs active on the serotonin system bring about very different kinds of anxiolysis.

It is difficult to be more specific than this because, as is the case with so many other drugs that have effects on behaviour, we know a lot about what brain receptors the various anxiolytics work on and a lot about the kind of patients that can be managed with these drugs and how quickly they respond, but very little about what the drugs actually do to those who take them. We know little about what it feels like to have them and exactly what aspects of anxiety respond to particular anxiolytics. We know a lot about where drugs go in the brain, but very little about how they work.

This is surprising because, on the face of it, these should be the easiest of all data to collect. It reflects the fact that we simply have not been in the habit of sitting down and listening to the reports of those who take the pills. In part, it seems to me, this is because we appear to assume that taking pills for a psychiatric disorder of any sort must render the taker unfit to make objective observations. This is an unfortunate – and indeed dangerous – assumption.

Beta-blockers and anxiety

INTRODUCTION

In recent years, with concern over benzodiazepine use, there has been interest in the use of beta-blockers in the treatment of anxiety. The principal drugs in this group used psychiatrically are shown in Table 13.1.

Beta-blockers are used mainly in the treatment of hypertension, angina and cardiac arrhythmias. The rationale for their use in psychiatry is that they block the peripheral manifestations of anxiety, such as increased heart rate or shaking in the hands. Signs such as these are the cues we all use to judge how anxious we are. When these effects of anxiety are controlled, it seems that two sets of feedback loops may be interrupted. Part of getting anxious involves getting anxious at signs that one is getting anxious, such as increased heart rate and shaky hands. These manifestations of anxiety can lead to worries in their own right, for example the concert performer who may worry about both the audience and the effects of a shaky hand on the violin bow. Similarly public speakers may have their nervousness faced with an audience augmented by nervousness about the effects of a tremulous voice or a dry mouth on the act of speaking itself. Controlling effects such as heart rate, voice timbre and

Table 13.1 Beta-blockers used psychiatrically		
Generic drug name	**UK trade name**	**US trade name**
propranolol	Inderal/Beta-Prograne	Inderal
atenolol	Tenormin	Tenormin

hand steadiness, therefore, can interrupt one feedback loop by taking away one set of stimuli to further anxiety. It can also interrupt another and ease the central anxiety by, as it were, removing the cues by which we all judge just how anxious we are.

PERFORMANCE-RELATED ANXIETY

The role of beta-blockers in the management of anxiety has been highlighted by musicians experiencing stage fright, who find that by using them they are able to cope with being on stage and to give more assured performances than they would otherwise have been able to give. Up to a third of orchestral musicians have been reported to use beta-blockers in order to steady their hands or control palpitations. There is a somewhat more notorious use for beta-blockers by snooker players, who have been using them supposedly for medical conditions, but who in actual fact may have been using them to reduce the amount of shake in their cue arm, allowing them to hit the ball more surely (Wheatley 1990).

As little as 10 mg of propranolol per day may be all that is needed to block the manifestations of stage fright of this type. Doses greater than 40 mg are rarely needed.

GENERALISED ANXIETY DISORDER (GAD)

With increasing concern about the use of benzodiazepines for anxiety, general practitioners have in recent years taken to prescribing beta-blockers for many of their more diffusely anxious patients. The rationale for this is tenuous. In the case of stage fright there is a very clear rationale and treatment is tied to specific situations. This is not possible with GAD and, as a consequence, much larger doses of beta-blockers have tended to be used and for longer periods of time.

The standard dose for propranolol used for GAD has been 20 mg four times a day, or 80 mg of longer-acting preparations such as Inderal LA (long acting). There have been trials on four beta-blockers for GAD: propranolol, oxprenolol, sotalol and practolol. Practolol has since been withdrawn from widespread use. Sotalol and oxprenolol had no clear anxiolytic effects. Propranolol, however, came out as being significantly anxiolytic, without causing the sedative effects found with benzodiazepines. It brings about significant improvement in palpitations, sweating, diarrhoea and tremor.

There are a number of other beta-blockers such as labetalol, metoprolol, timolol, pindolol, nadolol and atenolol, but these have not been investigated systematically for anxiolytic effects. The fact that propranolol is particularly effective raises, however, a further possibility in that propranolol has prominent effects on the serotonin system (see Ch. 12). Given that other beta-blockers are not particularly effective in GAD, it seems quite possible that it is propranolol's effect on the serotonin system that is helpful. If this is the case, then a more specific serotonergic drug probably should be used instead, as propranolol and other beta-blockers may cause significant rebound anxiety on discontinuation.

PANIC ATTACKS: A PUZZLE?

The use of beta-blockers can generally be considered in individuals who have anxiety states characterised by prominent peripheral manifestations of anxiety – increased heart rate, etc. Surprisingly, however, there are no reports of these drugs being beneficial in panic attacks which are characterised by physical symptoms of disabling intensity.

TREMOR

The beta-blockers are also of use for lithium-induced tremor (see Ch. 6) and for a number of neuroleptic-induced dyskinesias (see Ch. 3).

AKATHISIA AND RESTLESSNESS

Propranolol, but not other beta-blockers, may also be of benefit in states of akathisia unresponsive to anticholinergic compounds (see Chs 2 & 5). It also seems to be of some benefit in SSRI-induced akathisia or dyskinesia.

 User Issues

SIDE EFFECTS OF BETA-BLOCKERS

◆ All beta-blockers can cause shortness of breath. They should therefore be used with caution in anyone who has a history of wheezing or asthma.
◆ Beta-blockers can also cause reduced circulation of blood to the extremities. In cold weather this may lead to painful and cold fingers. Such painful and cold fingers, of course, may in their own right interfere with performances requiring dexterity, such as playing music.
◆ Beta-blockers also reduce the circulation of blood to muscles, and on this basis may need to be used with caution for performance-related anxiety. They may be unhelpful for singers and dancers – unhelpful to singers because they may cause wheezing or shortness of breath, and unhelpful to dancers or athletes generally because they reduce blood flow to muscles that may be needed for use. They may also inhibit performance by dropping blood pressure, leading to fainting.
◆ Some individuals have difficulties with sleep and have nightmares on beta-blockers, especially propranolol. The reason for this is uncertain.
◆ Tiredness and lassitude are sometimes reported. This may be allied to a clear feeling of muscle weakness on exertion. There is no clear sedative effect of these compounds, however, and no indication that they interfere with ability to drive, for instance.

continued

- Poor concentration and memory disturbances have also been reported. Propranolol does seem to reduce short-term memory span, even in healthy control subjects. This is different to the effects of benzodiazepines on memory, which involve not being able to recall things afterwards. Beta-blockers involve not being able to take in as much as usual at any one time.
- Hallucinations. In common with many other centrally acting compounds, the beta-blockers seem capable of producing dissociative effects, including hallucinations and confusion.
- In high doses beta-blockers may cause nausea and vomiting, diarrhoea, dry eyes and skin rashes, but such doses should never be needed for the control of anxiety.
- Beta-blockers may interact with other drugs used for heart disease or hypertension, including clonidine and calcium channel blockers such as verapamil.

References

Barlow DH, Craske MG (1989) Mastery of your anxiety and panic. Albany, NY: Graywind.

Beaumont G, Healy D (1996) The place of clomipramine in psychopharmacology. In: Healy D, ed. The psychopharmacologists, pp 309–328. London: Chapman & Hall.

Bury M, Gabe J (1990) A sociological view of tranquilliser dependence: challenges and responses. In: Hindmarch I, Beaumont G, Brandon S, Leonard BE, eds. Benzodiazepines: current concepts, pp 211–226. Chichester, UK: John Wiley.

Carlsson A, Healy D (1996) Early brain research in psychopharmacology: the impact on basic and clinical neuroscience. In: Healy D, ed. The psychopharmacologists, pp 51–80. London: Chapman & Hall.

Healy D (1991) The marketing of 5HT: depression or anxiety? British Journal of Psychiatry 158: 737–742.

Healy D (1993) Images of trauma: from hysteria to post-traumatic stress disorder. London: Faber & Faber.

Healy D (1995) Social phobia in primary care. Primary Care Psychiatry 1: 31–38.

Healy D (1997) The antidepressant era. Cambridge, MA: Harvard University Press.

Hindmarch I, Beaumont G, Brandon S, Leonard BE (1990) Benzodiazepines: Current Concepts. Chichester, UK: John Wiley.

Klein DF, Healy D (1996) Reaction patterns to psychotropic drugs and the discovery of panic disorder. In: Healy D, ed. The psychopharmacologists, pp 329–351. London: Chapman & Hall.

McNally RJ (1990) Psychological approaches to panic disorder. Psychological Bulletin 108: 403–419.

Marks IM (1978) Living with fear. London: McGraw-Hill.

Pilowsky L, Ring H, Shine P J, Battersby M, Lader M (1992) Rapid tranquillisation. British Journal of Psychiatry 160: 831–835.

Rapoport J (1990) The boy who couldn't stop washing. London, Fontana.

Royal College of Psychiatrists (1993) Psychiatric standards of fitness to drive large goods vehicles and passenger carrying vehicles. Psychiatric Bulletin 17: 631–632.

Smail D (1984) Illusion and reality: the meaning of anxiety. London: Dent.

Spiegel DA, Bruce TJ (1997) Benzodiazepines and exposure-based cognitive behavior therapies for panic disorder: conclusions from combined treatment trials. American Journal of Psychiatry 154: 773–781.

Toates F (1990) Obsessional thoughts and behaviour. Wellingborough, UK: Thorsons.

Warwick HMC, Salkovskis PM (1990) Hypochondriasis in cognitive therapy in clinical practice. In: Scott J, Williams JMG, Beck AT, eds. An illustrative casebook, pp 78–102. London: Routledge.

Wheatley D (1990) The anxiolytic jungle; where next? Chichester, UK: John Wiley.

Management of sleep disorders and insomnia

SECTION CONTENTS

Sleep disorders and insomnia

INTRODUCTION

This chapter focuses on both sleep disorders and insomnia. Strictly speaking, insomnia is a complaint rather than a condition. The management of insomnia is not the management of people who have sleeplessness. Rather it is the management of people who complain about sleeplessness. In fact, the sleep of those who complain about insomnia differs little from that of those who do not complain. In both groups there are a number of people who have little sleep or apparently poor-quality sleep. In both groups there are individuals who appear on objective tests, such as sleep electroencephalography, to have excellent sleep. Surveys suggest that about one in five individuals in the general population feel their sleep is not as satisfying as it should be.

The management of this state of affairs will therefore be complex. There is a fault-line down this section between the management of sleeplessness and sleep disorders and the management of insomnia. In some instances a simple pharmacological management of sleeplessness will be appropriate. In others an entirely psychological management of a complaint may be called for. In many others a judicious use of both pharmacological and psychological approaches is required.

THE SLEEP DISORDERS

An initial complaint of insomnia may refer to a number of different things, as shown in Box 14.1.

A range of physical problems causing coughs, itches, pain, restlessness, frequency of urination and breathlessness can contribute to sleep disturbances.

Box 14.1 Aspects of insomnia

◆ An inability to get to sleep

◆ An inability to stay asleep

◆ Waking too early

◆ Unsatisfying sleep

◆ Tiredness during the day, which individuals assume is caused by inadequate sleep the previous night

These may include cancer, infection, trapped nerves, depression, drug reactions and many others. These conditions need diagnosis and the proper treatment for whatever condition is revealed.

One condition deserves special notice: obstructive sleep apnoea. This is commonest in middle-aged men who may be overweight but who, in particular, have large necks. In a serious form, it may affect up to 3% of men. It involves the airway collapsing on inspiration during sleep. It typically happens when sleeping at night lying on the back. Collapse of the airway leads to breathing stopping until the respiratory drive becomes so intense that the airway is forced open – usually with a loud snort. The effort is so intense that the individual usually has their sleep disturbed, leading to poor-quality sleep and hence to tiredness the next day. The snort is so dramatic and loud that bed partners are often woken. The diagnosis is therefore often made by interviewing the sleeping partner, who complains about snoring. They will usually have noticed that their partner often appears to stop breathing for anything from 10 to 60 seconds. The significance of this condition is that poor sleep and fatigue the next day may lead to requests for something to improve sleep – but treatment with hypnotics may be fatal. The condition can be treated successfully with continuous positive airways pressure (CPAP).

There are two other notable but relatively rare conditions, which are partly physical and partly social: advanced sleep-phase insomnia and delayed sleep-phase insomnia. In advanced sleep-phase insomnia individuals fall asleep too early in the evening and wake too early, while in delayed sleep-phase insomnia, they fall asleep too late and are then unable to get up the next day. These disorders stem from the functioning of the circadian clock. Essentially we all tend constitutionally to be either 'larks' (waking early and at our best early in the day) or 'owls' (at our best later in the day or in the evening). Advanced and delayed sleep-phase disorders are exaggerations of these tendencies that may require specialist help to set right.

In brief, the management of delayed sleep-phase insomnia involves getting the individual to go to bed even later by 3–4 h, every night for five to seven nights until their sleep-onset time has come all the way back to normal. The rationale behind this – as anyone who enjoys a sleep in at the weekend knows – is that it is easier for the circadian clock to drift backwards rather than for it to be advanced. This behavioural strategy is more likely to be successful than any efforts to medicate the person to sleep at the correct time (Espie 1991, Waterhouse et al 1990).

The parasomnias

Alongside these sleep disorders, there are a group of disturbances called the parasomnias. These involve disturbance of arousal–sleep maintenance mechanisms that lead to behaviours associated with (para) sleep. The most common parasomnias are the motor parasomnias, which include sleep walking, bruxism (tooth grinding), night terrors and restless leg syndrome. These different conditions run in families. The behaviours usually have their onset in association with the deeper stages of non-rapid eye movement (non-REM) sleep. Therefore, they typically start around 2 h after the onset of sleep, unlike sleep apnoea, which leads to disturbances immediately after falling asleep.

Restless leg syndrome may appear first as a distinctly unsettling pre-sleep impatience or twitchiness of the legs. This is a familial condition, which can be treated successfully with clonazepam.

Narcolepsy

As with the parasomnias, narcolepsy involves a disturbance of arousal mechanisms, but where the parasomnias involve the production of behaviour even in someone who is deeply asleep, narcolepsy involves an abrupt onset of sleep in an individual who is wide awake. This starts usually around the age of 19–20 years. The primary feature of the condition involves falling asleep in company.

Linked into narcolepsy is a spectrum of other problems including catalepsy, sleep paralysis and hypnogogic hallucinations. Catalepsy refers to episodes of what seems like a temporary paralysis of the mouth, limbs and sometimes even of the whole body. This can appear unprovoked but it is often triggered by strong emotion. On laughing or crying, the individual may suddenly collapse. The problem can be triggered by a wide variety of drugs. If troublesome, this symptom, which may occur without narcolepsy, often responds to a selective serotonin reuptake inhibitor (SSRI).

Sleep paralysis refers to waking up to find oneself unable to move – even to speak. The condition usually lasts for only a few minutes, but may be sufficiently alarming to lead people to make a 'buried will' out of fear of mistakenly being thought to be dead and ending up being buried alive. Finally individuals with narcolepsy may have intense visual or auditory hallucinations on falling asleep or waking up. These may sometimes lead to a referral to a psychiatrist with a query as to whether the condition might not be an early schizophrenia.

The treatment of narcolepsy is with psychostimulants (see Ch. 9). The most commonly used drugs are methylphenidate, dexamphetamine or the anti-parkinsonian drug selegiline, which breaks down in the body to produce methamphetamine.

INSOMNIA

Aside from the transient causes of sleep disturbance such as jet lag, shift work or the physical causes of sleeplessness, poor sleep and/or a complaint of poor sleep most commonly arise:

- as a consequence of an emotional shock
- as part of an anxiety state
- spontaneously
- initially either spontaneously or after a shock or as part of an anxiety state, but subsequently become a matter of habitual inability to get asleep properly and increasing frustration or anxiety at this inability
- as a symptom of depression (see Ch. 4). Depression typically causes early morning wakening with an inability to fall asleep again. It may also cause repeated awakening during the night. The treatment in this case is an antidepressant. In depression, the usual benzodiazepine hypnotics may be relatively ineffective. Depression should be thought of in any chronic sleep problem, and early morning wakening should be taken as indicative of depression, until proven otherwise.

The proper management of a complaint of insomnia will eliminate any possible physical causes of poor sleep as well as recognise and treat any depressive disorder or anxiety state. However, there will still be a group of individuals who complain of poor sleep. This group is particularly likely to expect drug treatment to solve the problem, but the role of pharmacotherapy here is as uncertain as it is in the management of anxiety states such as hypochondriasis.

The great problem here is that current evidence suggests that many people in this group have sleep that is no worse than that of the rest of the population. Complainers are often slightly older, in which case the complaint will be justified to the extent that sleep depth does decline with age and naps during the day may lead to less than the former 6–8 h of sleep at night. The problem remains, however, that others who are ageing do not complain.

In the non-complaining population there are individuals who, for no apparent reason at some point during their lives, find themselves unable to sleep for more than only 2–3 h. This may be highly distressing as they are left wandering around the house while everyone else is sleeping peacefully. Often the only remedial treatment that can be undertaken in such cases is to minimise the frustration that the problem causes, for example by finding something constructive to do.

In the case of complainers, the problem seems in many respects similar to that of health anxiety (see Ch. 10), with a specific focus on sleep. As in health anxiety, individuals become concerned about a symptom, which is made worse by noticing it. The problem may start during a period of stress, which in its own right will cause sleep quality to fall off. All of us faced with stress have a tendency to focus away from the stressor and on to something else; this is called displacement. Focusing on sleep (or stomach problems, for instance) means that individuals end up thinking or feeling that everything would be okay, if only their sleep (or their bowels) were okay. This is likely to become a chronic rather than just a passing problem, if the individual has a history of sleep problems or a family history of sleep problems, or very fixed ideas about sleep.

Unhelpful ideas about sleep may include the idea that it is necessary to get 8 h sleep a night or else health will suffer. This is similar to the idea that it is necessary to have a bowel motion every day. Temporary constipation is clearly going to be far more worrying to people who have fixed ideas about regular bowel motions, and such ideas in turn are more likely in someone who comes from a home where there were such ideas or where there were bowel problems of one sort or another.

Another unhelpful idea is the notion that sleep is something that should be under conscious control. There is a paradox here in that we all, to some extent, have the illusion that we control our sleep, but attempts to sort out sleeplessness by re-exerting control are likely to fail.

Studies suggest that the complaint of insomnia may cover a number of different conditions that are important to distinguish as the treatment for each differs (see Ch. 15) (Coyle & Watts 1991):

◆ For some people, the primary concern is with the after-effects of poor sleep on how they are likely to concentrate and operate in general the next day.

◆ For others, the concern is with the problem of falling asleep. These people have a sleep-related performance anxiety.

◆ For yet others the problem seems to be one of finding their mind more active just as soon as their head hits the pillow, and this activity then interferes with sleep.

◆ A fourth group has difficulty in staying asleep. They wake up and are bothered by their awakenings more than others and in a way that interferes with being able to get back to sleep. We all awake more often during the night than we suspect, but it seems that we are in the main unaware of such episodes or even amnesic for them.

◆ Finally there is a group that is simply dissatisfied with the quality of their sleep.

One further problem that needs to be mentioned is the question of perception. Individuals with insomnia appear to overestimate the amount of time it takes them to fall asleep and the frequency with which they wake up during the night. Hypnotics may in fact make this perceptual difficulty worse (Schneider-Helmert 1988). It seems that individuals on sleeping pills underestimate the time it takes them to fall asleep and have amnesia for their awakenings during the night. This, of course, compounds the problem of how adequate or inadequate sleep is perceived to be on withdrawal of sleeping pills. On withdrawal there appears to a rebound overestimate of how long it takes to fall asleep and a hyper-awareness of any awakenings that occur during the night.

Non-pharmacological management of insomnia

There are a number of steps that can be taken in the management of insomnia before a resort is made to hypnotics.

CAFFEINE

A first step is to eliminate all caffeine-containing drinks, such as tea, coffee and colas, even if taking tea or coffee late in the evening has not been the cause of the problem. (See routine below.)

ENVIRONMENTAL FACTORS

It is important to ensure quiet surrounds. This is a particular problem for shiftworkers, especially where the shiftworker wants to burn the candle at both ends, or resents having to be on shiftwork. There are further shiftwork-related difficulties; see Body awareness below.

RELAXATION

Relaxation exercises, particularly progressive muscular relaxation, are useful in their own right but they are not particularly sleep inducing in the short term. They also require considerable patience and regular practice to master, as a great part of how they work depends on building up associations between relaxation and sleep. With regular practice, subjects find they drift off half way through their exercises. Cassette tapes or relaxation programmes promising sleep, however, rarely mention the fact that considerable hard work and patience is required. The failure of these methods to deliver, in the short term, leads many subjects to feel frustrated and to abandon what is a useful skill.

BODY AWARENESS

There is a regular cycle, operative in all of us called the basic rest–activity cycle (Waterhouse et al 1990). This produces alternating peaks and troughs in arousal and activity at regular intervals. This rhythm can be seen most clearly in infants, who wake and sleep on a 3–4-h cycle. In later life this cycle continues so that we have our mid-morning sags and mid-afternoon dips. The same cycle also underlies the stages of sleep. In normal sleep we progress regularly through a series of stages of sleep called stages 1, 2, 3 and 4 of non-REM sleep and then REM sleep. In this process we sink deeper into sleep and come back to the surface before sinking again, several times during the night.

What often happens in insomnia is that an individual goes to bed and finds that they seem to become more awake as they lie there. This is no illusion. It is a correct perception of what is happening. But what may also be happening is that, owing to difficulties in getting to sleep, the person has waited until they are exhausted and gone to bed, thinking that they have thereby given themselves the best chance for falling asleep. In fact, they are just about to 'turn the corner' and head into an upswing in the arousal curve, which will make it very difficult to fall asleep. What is needed in such instances is for the individual to get out of bed before becoming too worked up about not being able to drift off. They should go downstairs, have a small snack or hot milk drink, read the newspaper or listen to something soothing and wait until they feel the first hints of a downward swing. What they should not do is to wait until fatigue sets in.

A regular sleeping pattern makes this easier to achieve, because the rest–activity cycle switches around to track cues from the environment indicating likely sleep-onset times and rising times. Switching typically takes several days to a week or two depending on how great the change is from the former routine. The resolution of jet lag is based on just such switching. Our sleep rhythms are tied in to important processes such as the temperature rhythm. Normally as we fall asleep, our body clock programmes a drop in temperature, and falling asleep is associated with this. As body temperature rises in the early morning, there is an associated gearing up of a range of physiological functions in preparation for the day ahead. These, in part, are what lead to our waking up. It becomes increasingly difficult to get off to sleep in the face of this rise, and this underlies the particular problems that shiftworkers, who have to sleep during the day, may have.

The significance of this is that, with practice, it is possible to learn to read our bodily cues quite accurately. A complication of the treatment of insomnia with alcohol or drugs is that these agents will mask the bodily cues we might be better off in the longer term learning to read. Having said all this, on occasion our lifestyles get out of kilter with our basic rest–activity cycles, at which times the inappropriate alerting effects of the rest–activity cycle can be usefully over-ridden by alcohol or hypnotics. This should be necessary only on a short-term basis, as the cycle realigns itself to a new routine.

STIMULUS–CONTROL TREATMENTS

This approach grew out of learning theory, which believes that behaviour is determined or at least shaped by associations. According to this, treatment should aim to build up associations between behaviours and sleep and to reduce behaviours associated with being awake. This leads to advice such as never to do work in the bedroom, remove the television from the bedroom, or not to read in bed. Do nothing except sleep. (Leaving sexual activities in is not seen as a problem, although in theory it should be.) This approach may often be helpful, although there are good grounds to believe that learning theory has little or nothing to do with automatic behaviours such as sleep or sex. Another explanation why this approach works may simply be that it gives some people the impression of control and this is sufficient to allay their anxiety and permit sleep.

ROUTINES

A number of the above techniques interface with the issue of the generation or maintenance of routines. Routines are probably the single most potent contributors to sleep. This becomes clear in the case of individuals who routinely drink a cup of strong black coffee just before going to bed and who, far from having problems falling asleep on it, would have much greater problems if they were denied their coffee. In this case coffee has become part of the bedtime routine. In the case of many people on continuous treatment with a hypnotic, it is quite certain that the pills have stopped working physiologically and are now working because they have been incorporated in a successful routine. It is worth noting that essentially the same pills may be used during the day for anxiolytic purposes, but in these circumstances people do not fall asleep with them.

PARADOXICAL INTENTION

This involves telling the individual to try to stay awake as long as possible. This may be particularly useful in those who have a performance anxiety where sleep is concerned. This technique picks up on the paradox inherent in sleep, which is that we have the impression we control it but actually have very little control one way or the other. This leads to a range of paradoxes. For example, giving good advice, such as don't take your worries to bed, is likely to be unhelpful, as it will only lead to the individual worrying about not worrying. This is an instance of the pink elephant principle, whereby telling someone to avoid thinking about pink elephants causes them immediately to think of pink elephants and of almost nothing but pink elephants.

FORWARD PLANNING

This technique advocates spending some time during the evening in reviewing the day and settling or at least noting worries. These may be reviewed and then symbolically filed or binned. The method appears to work, especially for people who have difficulties falling asleep. This technique is one that most cultures seem to have discovered. The Guatemalan Indians for instance used Troubledolls for the purpose – hanging a separate worry on each of a number of dolls – and the German philosopher Immanuel Kant did something very similar.

USE OF MANTRAS AND YOGIC BREATHING EXERCISES

A technique common to many transcendental meditation exercises involves the creation of a personal mantra. This is a word or set of words, which are chanted or thought about. Alternatively a breathing technique may be used. There are good grounds in current psychological theory to believe that such approaches induce sleep (Levey et al 1991). In brief, these approaches, which are variations of the age-old remedy of counting sheep, act to suppress the intrusion into consciousness of thoughts that might be alerting. Current evidence suggests that this type of procedure works best when the problem is one of waking up during the night with subsequent difficulties in getting back to sleep. Just as with relaxation exercises, transcendental meditation and yoga techniques are deceptively simple. Their mastery, however, requires weeks or even months of regular practice. They will not provide a quick fix for insomnia.

16

Hypnotics

INTRODUCTION

What is the place for hypnotics in this scheme of things? Basically they are in the same place that alcohol has occupied for centuries. Most of us, every so often, if we are anxious, worked up or have a lot of things on our mind, will have resorted to alcohol to knock ourselves out. It does this effectively on an episodic basis. There are drawbacks to regular alcohol, however. One is that it produces a rebound insomnia: it knocks you out but also wakes you up several hours later as the effects wear off. It may also wake you up to pass urine or because of dehydration.

Hypnotics do roughly the same thing, with similar benefits and side effects. Judiciously used, they are wonderful. Taken in the early stages of a problem they may abort the later development of habitual or anxiety-based insomnia. Taken too regularly or chronically, they may produce their own problems.

The place for the hypnotics lies in the management of sleeplessness rather than in the management of insomnia. Where there is genuine sleeplessness stemming from jet lag or an underlying physical condition or problems with falling asleep in what may be uncomfortable circumstances or situations of stress, a hypnotic may be of benefit. The presumption in these cases is that there is a transient sleeplessness, which is being managed until normality returns. Where a chronic physical condition regularly compromises sleep,

Table 16.1 Common hypnotics

Generic drug name	UK trade name	US trade name
nitrazepam	Mogadon	
flurazepam	Dalmane	
temazepam	Normison	
loprazolam	Dormonoct	
lormetazepam	Noctamid	
triazolam	–	Halcion
zolpidem	Stilnoct	Ambiens
zopiclone	Zimovane	

hypnotics can be used chronically without causing dependence or other problems. The management of acute or chronic sleeplessness is important as, although the sedative effects of hypnotics may pose risks to driving for example, the fatigue consequent on sleeplessness is at least as hazardous, if not more so. A great number of road and industrial accidents stem from this source. Too often the management of sleeplessness is seen as a rather trivial issue.

The hypnotics in current use include a number of benzodiazepine and related compounds (Table 16.1), which act at different sites on the γ-amino-butyric acid (GABA) receptor. These bind to a 'benzodiazepine' receptor on the GABA receptor and thereby modulate the action of GABA. At present, distinctions are drawn between benzodiazepine BZ_1, BZ_2 and BZ_3 receptors within this family. The BZ_1 receptor is thought to be responsible primarily for sedative effects, the BZ_2 for myorelaxant and anticonvulsant effects, and BZ_3 for anxiolytic effects. The older benzodiazepines bind to all three types and are, therefore, sedative, anxiolytic, muscle relaxant and anticonvulsant. It is claimed that newer agents such as zolpidem bind primarily to the BZ_1 site and are accordingly primarily hypnotic.

COMMON HYPNOTICS

Any of the benzodiazepines listed in Chapter 11, such as diazepam, may be used in additional to the hypnotics given in Table 16.1.

Benzodiazepine hypnotics

The benzodiazepine hypnotics are essentially the same as the benzodiazepine anxiolytics. Calling one compound an anxiolytic and another a hypnotic is a marketing convenience, although a compound is likely to have greater potential as a hypnotic if it penetrates the brain quickly. It was this that underlay the success of temazepam gels. The same compound in tablet form is simply not as effective a hypnotic.

Zopiclone

This is technically a cyclopyrrolone. It was initially marketed as a non-benzodiazepine hypnotic that gave more natural sleep, was free of hangover effects and would not produce dependence. It binds, however, to BZ_1 receptors, which makes it effectively a benzodiazepine. It can produce hangover effects and dependence – and no hypnotic gives natural sleep.

It has a short half-life, however, which means that in older individuals, for instance, who are slower to excrete hypnotic drugs from their system, zopiclone and zolpidem are the only hypnotics that are not likely to accumulate. For this reason, these drugs may be better than some longer-acting benzodiazepine hypnotics for this age group. Among the side effects reported with zopiclone are a metallic taste, heartburn and a lightening of sleep on withdrawal.

Zolpidem

This agent is an imidazopyridine, which binds preferentially to BZ_1 receptors. Claims that zolpidem leads to more natural sleep and less dependence, rebound insomnia, or some of the other problems associated with benzodiazepine hypnotics, need to be treated with scepticism. Whether it does or not is uncertain. Side effects include drowsiness, fatigue, depression, falls and amnesia.

 User Issues

SIDE EFFECTS OF HYPNOTIC DRUGS

The side effects of the hypnotics resemble those of benzodiazepine tranquillisers, outlined in Chapter 11, with the following additional problems.

Tolerance

Within 2–4 weeks of continuous use, tolerance is likely to develop to hypnotics. This means that they will not be as sedating after this length of treatment and little further sedative benefit will be gained by continuing with them. Nevertheless, continuing with a hypnotic beyond 2–4 weeks may be helpful for two reasons. First, although no longer as sedative, the same drug may continue to be anxiolytic, and this may help. Second, and as mentioned in the last chapter, the psychological effect of getting into the habit of falling asleep on these drugs may also help to promote sleep even after the sedative effect of the drug has worn off.

Rebound insomnia

This effect probably relates to the development of tolerance, as instanced by the example of taking coffee before going to bed. Once the habit is created of sleeping on hypnotics, their absence may make sleep difficult, until new habits are established. Rebound insomnia may be demonstrated within 2 weeks of continuous hypnotic ingestion. In practice, what this means is that individuals who stop a sleeping pill may lie awake for several nights afterwards, which of course confirms their worst fears – that they need the pills.

Broken sleep

Just as with alcohol, modern hypnotics induce sleep but may also cause a wakening from sleep as their effects wear off. This is particularly likely to be the case with the shorter acting compounds: temazepam, lormetazepam, zolpidem and zopiclone.

Hangover

Hypnotics with shorter half-lives were synthesised in order to avoid the hangover effects produced in some individuals by older benzodiazepines, such as nitrazepam or flurazepam. This was a state of muzziness, with slowing of cognitive functioning and impairment of reaction times, the morning after the night before. In occasional individuals, this can last for most of the next day. This problem usually reduces in severity as tolerance develops. In controlled clinical trials, the shorter-acting compounds appeared to eliminate this problem. However, in real life, they may also cause a similar problem if people resort to having another short-acting sleeping pill on waking up at 3 or 4 am.

Often, sometimes for the benefit of carers, the dose of a hypnotic will be pushed up in an elderly individual, in which case traces of the drug will begin to build up in the system just as if the subject had been put on a compound with a longer half-life. If the original dose fails to work – and in the elderly the dose should be lower than for younger subjects – management strategies should involve recourse to means other than increasing the dose.

Inappropriate sedation

Packages of hypnotics usually state that driving or operating machinery after taking a hypnotic may be hazardous. In practice, if the individual does not feel unduly affected, they are likely to take a risk and drive or work. It is difficult to calculate what the effects on the economy might be if everyone on any psychotropic drug were to refrain from driving or operating machinery. The problem is that some people will be more impaired than they are aware of, and there is an increasing body of evidence that a significant number of road traffic accidents happen to individuals who are taking psychotropic medication (although at present much less than are caused by alcohol).

Other

All the other side effects of benzodiazepines listed in Chapter 11 apply to these hypnotics. Amnesia is less of a problem, as the person sleeps it off. This does not apply if the pill is taken during the day. When taken in large amounts either intravenously or orally, one of the notable side effects of temazepam abuse has been a profound amnesia. Abusers who present at clinics often appear to have no recollection of visits they may have made to the same clinic several days before.

In contrast to amnesia, dissociation may be a greater problem when these compounds are used as hypnotics, precisely because the confused overactivity that results may be more at odds with the tranquil sleep that is being sought than it would have been with anxiety if the pills had been given during the day. Dissociation is more likely with the elderly but, as with antidepressants or neuroleptics, a range of problems – from confusion to hallucinations – is possible.

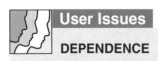

DEPENDENCE

The use of the benzodiazepines as hypnotics raises the issue of possible dependence – an issue that clouds the use of zolpidem and zopiclone. In part, however, the risks of dependence with modern hypnotics stem not just from the pills themselves but from the marketing process that distinguishes hypnotics from benzodiazepine anxiolytics. When the benzodiazepines were used more widely as anxiolytics, it was common to find individuals on a benzodiazepine anxiolytic, such as lorazepam or diazepam, by day and a benzodiazepine hypnotic at night. Such combinations promote a more rapid production of tolerance, a greater likelihood of dependence, and a more general scrambling or overriding of the body prompts that might otherwise be used to come to grips with both insomnia and anxiety. In the past decade the prescription of benzodiazepine anxiolytics has dropped substantially, and this makes it much less likely that the more recently introduced hypnotics will be implicated in the widespread production of dependence – although not necessarily because they are intrinsically less dependence producing.

Where individuals have been taking hypnotics for years, there is no good argument for forcing them to discontinue. There is substantial evidence that for a great number of subjects, chronic hypnotic intake, provided there is no concurrent daytime use of benzodiazepines, does not cause significant physical dependence or withdrawal. This is because taken once at night, rather than regularly over the 24-h period, the drug may not build up in the system to any great extent. At the correct dose, there may be little more harm in taking hypnotics for such individuals than in taking Ovaltine or a nightcap. The harm is more likely to come from the levels to which the dose of the drug has been pushed by prescribers than from the intrinsic properties of the drug. At high doses, these hypnotics cause sedation the next day, confusion, amnesia and possibly ataxia.

Despite the relative safety of these compounds, the current climate is such that guidelines for the use of hypnotics now suggest limiting their use to a regimen of something like 10 pills per month (Lader & Healy 1992). Many takers are likely to find increasing pressure on them to stop their continuous use of these compounds. Where discontinuation is indicated or desired, a regimen like that for the withdrawal of benzodiazepine anxiolytics is indicated (see Ch. 11), with supplementary education about sleep hygiene and the misperceptions the person is likely to experience on halting a hypnotic after some months or years of intake.

Sedatives

Before the benzodiazepines, both anxiety and sleep problems were treated with sedatives. The emergence of the benzodiazepines led to distinctions between anxiolysis and sedation, and to the discovery of the idea of an anxiolytic. It also led to distinctions between sedatives and hypnotics. The concerns about the overprescription of benzodiazepines in the 1980s led some prescribers to look at alternative agents. This meant either a return to older sedatives, such as the barbiturates or chloral agents, or the use of anti-depressants or antipsychotics with a sedative profile. There are a number of problems with either of these options.

CHLORAL COMPOUNDS

Chloral compounds (Table 17.1) were first produced in 1869 (Healy 2001). Their sedative effects were quickly recognised. A number of factors militated against their widespread use. One was the difficulty in making them in other than foul-tasting liquid formats. The subsequent discovery of the barbiturates around 1900 led to a decline in their use.

The chloral compounds are now produced in tablet and liquid form. They are popular with some prescribers as they do not appear to give the buzz

Table 17.1 Chloral compounds

Generic drug name	UK trade name
chloral hydrate	Noctec/Welldorm elixir
chloral betaine	Welldorm tablets
triclofos sodium	–

sometimes got from benzodiazepines and are, therefore, considered by some less likely to be abused. For this reason they are used in some hospitals as the sedative of choice for illicit drug users. They are also popular with hospital pharmacies in that they cost pennies rather than pounds. A chloral prescription may cost the pharmacy as little as 5 p per week.

Chloral compounds may, however, cause dependence, as well as gastric irritation, heartburn and rashes. They are hazardous in overdose. These compounds are contraindicated where there is a coexisting disorder of almost any sort – cardiac, renal or gastric.

The trend to prescribe any hypnotic other than a benzodiazepine, owing to the fear of creating dependence, ignores the fact that the benzodiazepines came to prominence because they were much safer than older compounds. In particular, they are less likely to cause problems such as heartburn. In recent years it has become increasingly common to find people taking chloral hypnotics, who have also been put on ranitidine (Zantac), cimetidine (Tagamet) or omeprazole (Losec) for heartburn or ulcers. These are more expensive than most new psychiatric drugs and have side effects of their own.

BARBITURATES AND RELATED COMPOUNDS

The first barbiturate compounds were produced in the 1860s, but the discovery of their useful sedative properties stems from 1900. They were the first group of psychotropic drugs to be marketed systematically. Since then, there have been a great number of barbiturate compounds. They are widely used in anaesthesia and for the control of epilepsy, with far fewer complications than their fearsome reputation in psychiatry might suggest. Until the mid-1960s the barbiturates and related compounds, such as glutethimide, were the standard hypnotics (Table 17.2). Concern about their dependence-producing potential, their dangers in overdose, and the fact that these drugs interacted with a large number of other psychiatric drugs led to their abandonment with the emergence of the benzodiazepines. But, essentially, the barbiturates and benzodiazepines both work on the same GABA receptor complex.

It is rare to find any barbiturate prescribed now as a hypnotic. Barbiturates have some use as general sedatives in states of acute agitation. They combine

Table 17.2 Barbiturates and related drugs

Generic drug name	UK trade name
amylobarbitone	Amytal/Sodium Amytal
butobarbitone	Soneryl
quinalbarbitone sodium	Seconal Sodium
quinalbarbitone–amylobarbitone	Tuinal
glutethimide	Doriden

well with antipsychotics in the short term, allowing lower doses of each to be used. They may also be used for abreactive purposes.

CHLORMETHIAZOLE

Marketed as Heminevrin, this is one of the most widely used hypnotics. It is also used in alcohol withdrawal. It seems to be either loved or hated. It is liked by prescribers in that it works and does not produce hangover effects because of its short half-life. This makes it suitable in the elderly, for whom it is particularly marketed and used. It is also popular with consumers because for a considerable proportion of takers its effects are distinctly pleasant, giving it a greater street value than benzodiazepines, for instance.

Chlormethiazole is disliked by many psychopharmacologists because it is a drug that defies conventional classification. It is distrusted by some prescribers, because it is over-liked and has a high dependence potential. In terms of side effects, it can also produce nasal congestion, nasal irritation and heartburn.

SEDATIVE ANTIDEPRESSANTS AND ANTIPSYCHOTICS

Given current levels of concern about both benzodiazepines and barbiturates, as well as hypnotics and anxiolytics in general, a number of clinicians prefer to prescribe a sedative antidepressant (such as trimipramine, trazodone, mianserin or mirtazapine) or an antipsychotic (such as chlorpromazine or thioridazine). Although these may work, if handled properly, it is almost certainly better to prescribe a conventional hypnotic.

Antidepressants, and in particular the older more sedative ones, can be fatal in overdose and they produce more in the line of side effects (see Ch. 4). The sedative antipsychotics are only sedative for some and they, too, produce side effects, a number of which may be very worrying if the person affected is unaware of what to expect. If prescriptions of such compounds are made without the taker being briefed as to the possible emergence of tardive dyskinesia or other problems, one imagines that prescribers would be on very shaky grounds.

Against that, there is a certain logic to the prescription of these agents. A common feature of all the agents used is S_2 antagonism. The serotonin system is involved in the generation of what is termed slow-wave sleep, and drugs that act on S_2 receptors can increase the amount of slow-wave sleep. In some cases this will happen without any obvious sedation. In other patients, because of other effects of these drugs, there may be clear sedation. There may be some place for such agents in chronic sleep disorders but they have little use in the management of acute sleeplessness. In the case of electroencephalographic evidence of deficient stage 4 or stage 3 sleep, the picture may be quite different and such compounds may be quite appropriate.

ANTIHISTAMINES

A number of antihistamines, especially promethazine (Phenergan/Avomine) and trimeprazine (Vallergan), are also used as sedatives, mainly for children. They often 'work', although their use arguably should be discouraged for this purpose as they may have marked hangover effects on the child's behaviour the next day, which may potentially lead to accidents and/or poor performance at school.

References

Coyle K, Watts FN (1991) The factorial structure of sleep dissatisfaction. Behaviour Research and Therapy 29: 513–520.

Espie C (1991) The psychological treatment of insomnia. Chichester, UK: John Wiley.

Healy D (2001) The Creation of Psychopharmacology. Cambridge, MA: Harvard University Press.

Lader M, Healy D, Beaumont G et al (1992) The medical management of insomnia in general practice. Royal Society of Medicine Round Table Series no. 28. London: Royal Society of Medicine Publications.

Levey AB, Aldaz JA, Watts FN, Coyle K (1991) Articulatory suppression and the treatment of insomnia. Behaviour Research and Therapy 29: 85–89.

Schneider-Helmert D (1988) Why low-dose benzodiazepine-dependent insomniacs can't escape their sleeping pills. Acta Psychiatrica Scandinavia 78: 706–711.

Waterhouse JM, Minors DS, Waterhouse ME (1990) Your body clock: how to live with it, not against it. Oxford: Oxford University Press.

Management of cognitive impairment

SECTION CONTENTS

18

Cognitive enhancement and the dementias

INTRODUCTION

The 1990s saw the first systematic attempts to enhance cognitive perform-ance, whether in normal subjects of all ages or in individuals who suffered from either strokes or a dementing process. Cognitive enhancement refers to the action of a drug that in some way improves cognitive performance, with memory being the performance most commonly looked at. An older term for this group of drugs was the nootropics.

The initial goal in this field has been to find drugs to treat dementia. More recently efforts have broadened out to include, on the one hand, drugs that might limit the consequences of having a stroke or might be more generally neuroprotective and, on the other hand, drugs that might enhance age-associated decline in memory. It is quite probable that drugs that are cogni-tively enhancing will not in any meaningful way treat or reverse any of the dementing processes. Conversely agents that bring a dementing process to a halt are unlikely otherwise to be cognitive enhancers. There is accordingly a fault-line down the middle of this section, with the treatment of dementia on the one side and on the other cognitive enhancement, which is increasingly forming a separate, if related, field of endeavour.

In part, at least, for pharmacoeconomic reasons, many of the larger pharma-ceutical companies have in recent years been moving out of the antidepres-sant, neuroleptic and anxiolytic fields and into the area of neuroprotection and cognitive enhancement (Waldmeier 1996). It is worth bearing in mind, however, as with all other agents considered in this book, that any treatments that come out of such research programmes should be looked at closely by all of those involved in their clinical use because there is no such thing as a drug working on the brain that affects only one set of behaviours. The example of the antidepressants and sexual functioning is worth bearing in mind here (see Section 7). It is not inconceivable that a new generation of neuroprotective agents will be as useful in the management of schizophrenia as they may be for dementia. The people best placed to discover this will be drug takers and those closely involved in their care, such as nursing staff.

THE DEMENTIAS

Part of the problem in finding drugs that may be effective for dementia is that our ideas about what constitutes dementia have been undergoing radical change in recent years. It had been traditional to distinguish between Alzheimer's dementia, or senile dementia of the Alzheimer's type (SDAT), and multi-infarct dementia (MID), which is theoretically caused by stroke. These are usually small strokes, which insidiously pick off brain tissue to the point where an individual's cognitive function is compromised.

Stage 1

It was originally thought that MID accounted for more than 60% of the dementias. Accordingly, early attempts to treat the dementias concentrated on the multi-infarct dementias. The initial hypothesis was that these multiple small strokes were being caused by hardening of the arteries, sometimes called arteriosclerosis and sometimes atherosclerosis (although these terms refer to two different disorders), which impaired blood supply to the brain. The logical treatment, therefore, was to attempt to dilate the blood vessels. This led to the use of a number of vasodilating drugs such as hydralazine. It is now quite rare for such drugs to be used for this purpose. Arguably, if anything, such treatment may have made the condition somewhat worse in that vasodilators can reduce blood pressure, leaving the brain less perfused with blood.

Stage 2

More recent attempts to treat the dementias have proceeded on the basis that Alzheimer's disease is the commonest form of dementia. For many years, the term Alzheimer's dementia was reserved for dementias that came on before the age of 65 years (for this reason, it was also called presenile dementia). It was conceded that there was another dementia that was like Alzheimer's dementia, which appeared to come on after the age of 65 years, called senile dementia. Distinctions on the basis of age have collapsed and all dementias of the Alzheimer type are now called senile dementia of the Alzheimer type (SDAT). The amalgamation of these two groups led to an awareness that Alzheimer-type dementia is the commonest form of dementia.

In terms of treatment, the focus has been on possible dysfunction of cholinergic pathways in the brain. There are both historical and clinical reasons for this focus. Historically, in the 1960s, there were only four known neuro-transmitters: noradrenaline, serotonin, dopamine and acetylcholine (ACh). Noradrenaline became linked to depression and mood disorders. Dopamine was known to be involved in Parkinson's disease but, through the antipsychotics, it also became linked to schizophrenia. Serotonin was for the most part associated with either depression or anxiety. This left ACh without a function. It seemed convenient to parcel it out to the dementias.

There was, in addition, some clinical evidence in favour of an association between the cholinergic system and dementia. Part of the reason for this claim is that drugs with anticholinergic effects have been noted as potentially causing amnesia or confusion (see Ch. 3).

Stage 3

More recently, a number of other dementias have been described. One is senile dementia of the Lewy body type (SDLT) (McKeith et al 1995). This is a mixed cortical and subcortical dementia, more likely to show motor abnormalities than Alzheimer's disease, and to be characterised by prominent visual hallucinations or confusion. It appears to be related to Parkinson's disease, in that the Lewy bodies of SDLT are inclusion bodies that are also found in the brain cells of patients with Parkinson's disease. Unlike SDAT, which tends to begin insidiously and progress relentlessly, although slowly, SDLT may present dramatically and follow an episodic course. The first presentation may be episodic confusion. At times the person may seem almost delirious but, on later testing, may perform almost normally. The confusional episodes and disturbed behaviour that go with them may lead to the use of a neuroleptic in the management. This can be particularly hazardous, as in Lewy body dementia neuroleptics may lead to a dramatic worsening of the clinical picture. Owing probably to its relationship to Parkinson's disease, patients with SDLT are more likely to have extrapyramidal symptoms even without neuroleptics. Faints and falls are common with SDLT.

A distinction has also been drawn between cortical and subcortical dementias. The cortex of the brain is the area responsible for higher cognitive functions such as speaking, reading, planning and executing actions. In the cortical dementias, memory is usually the function most noticeably affected, but sufferers also have problems with planning even simple functions such as dressing, reading, drawing or any complex tasks. Alzheimer's disease and MID are cortical dementias. There are also subcortical parts to the brain. These are common to humans and other mammals. They involve a number of what are termed midbrain and brainstem structures. When these are affected, the results may be a slowing of mental activity rather than its destruction (see below).

Current estimates about the relative proportion of the various dementias are:

◆ Alzheimer's dementia (SDAT) is now thought to comprise more than 40% of the dementias.

- The contribution of MID has shrunk to somewhere around 20% of the dementias.
- SDLT may account for 10–20% of the dementias.
- Frontal lobe dementia comprises 5–10% of the dementias. This condition used to be called Pick's disease. As the name suggests, the frontal lobes of the brain are particularly affected. This leads to a clinical presentation in which disinhibited, silly or odd behaviour rather than memory difficulties are the first things that are noticed.
- Subcortical dementia. All of the above disorders are cortical dementias; they affect the cortex of the brain. The subcortical areas of the brain may be affected by strokes and other diseases, such as Parkinson's disease, Huntingdon's disease, Wilson's disease, tumours, infections and trauma. If affected, the net result may be a profound slowing of cognitive functioning rather than an outright loss. Answering even simple questions, however, may be so slow that the questioner may assume that the affected individual has a profound memory problem, indicating SDAT or some such disorder. The importance of distinguishing this group of dementias from the others is that treatment may make a considerable difference to the picture.

19

Cognitive enhancement and neuroprotection

INTRODUCTION

There is no good evidence that damage to the cholinergic pathway is the central deficit in Alzheimer's dementia. Indeed, it has recently become clear that a number of other neurotransmitters are affected in both Alzheimer's disease and other cortical dementias. It is also clear that, because of the interactions between various neurotransmitter systems, it is almost impossible to manipulate one neurotransmitter without affecting the others.

In addition, current research suggests that many cortical dementias involve cell-protective mechanisms that have been thrown out of gear. Normally, there is a range of mechanisms within cells aimed at neutralising toxins of various sorts. These frequently involve the binding of a protein to the toxin, which labels it so that the cell's own degradative processes destroy the offending agent. In the dementias, such mechanisms appear to have been stimulated to the point where large amounts of the cell-protective proteins are produced – to the point that they themselves poison the cell. Whether the stimulus to this production is genetic, viral, toxic (as in aluminium), or some combination of these and other factors, is uncertain. It may even represent a feature of normal ageing, with some people programmed to age quicker than others. The treatment options are to find compounds that will either switch off the process or else compensate for it.

For the most part, the aim of current treatments remains largely one of giving a boost to the cholinergic system. The rationale here is not to cure the dementia but rather to stimulate cognitive function. Early efforts to do this clinically included the following:

◆ Choline. This is a precursor of the neurotransmitter acetylcholine (ACh). The rationale has been that, by increasing supplies of choline in the body, the brain might synthesise more ACh. Initial studies reported some success, but this has not been confirmed. Choline is also present in the essential fatty acid lecithin. For this reason, lecithin supplements have also been given in dementia, but with little benefit.

◆ Piracetam/oxiracetam/aniracetam/pramiracetam. In animal studies these drugs release ACh within the brain. They appear to be mildly stimulant in humans, but relatively ineffective in dementing conditions. It has been claimed that combining them with lecithin and an anticholinesterase does give some benefit.

◆ Cholinesterase inhibitors. These compounds block the breakdown of ACh. The first drug of this type was physostigmine. Some reports suggest that this drug may bring about improvements in some subjects with SDAT on some tests of performance. However, physostigmine has an extremely short half-life, and doses that bring about improved performances in one person produce deterioration in others.

◆ Tetrahydroaminoacridine (THA) (tacrine). This is a longer-acting anticholinesterase agent, which has seemed to be of benefit in some studies. The findings overall have not been sufficiently robust to persuade large numbers of clinicians that a significant breakthrough has been made, although they have been sufficient for the drug to be licensed in the USA for dementia. There are suggestions that this type of compound may be of greater benefit in SDLT than in other dementias. If so, however, it is worth noting that compounds such as tacrine also block potassium channels, and any therapeutic benefit may stem from such sources. The most significant problem with THA and related compounds has been liver toxicity.

◆ Angiotensin-converting enzyme inhibitors (ACE inhibitors). The best-known ACE inhibitors, captopril, enalapril and lisinopril, are used in the treatment of hypertension and cardiac failure. They also bring about a release of acetylcholine in the brain. The marketing of ACE inhibitors for blood pressure heavily emphasises the fact that these drugs not only lower blood pressure but seem to provide some sort of 'zest for life'. There appears to be a poorly worked out stimulant quality or mild cognitive-enhancing quality to these compounds. In studies with aged rats, the ACE inhibitors appeared to be able to improve performance in a range of behavioural tasks back to the level of performance shown by young rats. It is too early yet to say, whether these will be of significant benefit in the dementing disorders. A number of open studies at present have suggested that the drugs may be helpful, but exactly how helpful, and for which of the many forms of dementia, remains to be determined.

MANAGEMENT OF SDAT AND SDLT: SECOND-GENERATION AGENTS

A second generation of agents acting on the cholinergic system has proven somewhat more successful than these earlier attempts, but the use of these agents has been controversial because of their cost. Critics claim that the clinical trials provide barely perceptible benefits in dementing disorders, and that the widespread and indiscriminate use of such agents, given the modest benefits set against the high costs, would be crippling financially.

The modest clinical trial effects, however, may stem from two sources. One possibility is that these drugs are debatably effective. The other possibility is that they work reasonably well in some patients but not at all in others; adding up scores in a group therefore underestimates the benefits that can be obtained in some patients. In dementia, clinical experience appears to support the latter option. There is no reason to believe, however, that the cognitive-stimulating effects such drugs produce will be of benefit only in clear dementia. There is a potential for patients with difficulty following head injury to respond, as well as the cognitive decline found in many other states.

Donepezil (Aricept)

The claims are that this cholinesterase inhibitor given in 5- or 10-mg doses can produce cognitive benefits in patients with mild to moderate dementia, that it sustains functional ability, and delays the emergence of behavioural symptoms. (Similar claims have been made for rivastigmine and galantamine.)

User Issues

SIDE EFFECTS OF DONEPEZIL

The commonest side effects are diarrhoea, muscle cramps, fatigue, nausea and insomnia. There is a potential to slow the heart so patients with cardiac conditions should be monitored. Another possibility is that treatment may provoke confusion or other neuropsychiatric disturbances. At present, there is little established about the possible interaction of this drug with others that elderly patients are likely to be taking.

Overdosage, whether because of some interaction or for another reason, produces nausea, vomiting, diarrhoea, confusion, convulsions, and cardiac and respiratory depression. This can be treated with atropine.

Rivastigmine (Exelon)

This, another cholinesterase inhibitor, is used in doses of 3–12 mg per day. It has a similar profile of side effects and precautions as donepezil.

Galantamine (Reminyl)

Galantamine is also a cholinesterase inhibitor, used in doses of 16–32 mg per day, again with a similar profile of side effects and precautions as donepezil and rivastigmine.

MANAGEMENT OF MULTI-INFARCT DEMENTIA

It is now believed that the brain damage caused by strokes can be managed to some extent. The greatest destruction of brain tissue does not happen when the stroke begins, but rather happens anything over the course of several hours to 1–2 days later. The initial stroke often affects only a very small group of nerves, but these release a neurotransmitter called glutamate. Glutamate increases the permeability of adjacent nerve cells, which absorb both sodium and chloride, causing water also to enter the cell, and this leads the cell to swell and burst.

This process does not happen if there is a low level of calcium in the medium surrounding the cells. Furthermore, the absorption of sodium and chloride also leads to a greater than usual entry of calcium into the cell, and this causes the activation of a number of enzymes which break down proteins and fats within the cell. If this entry can be blocked, the chances for cell survival are greatly increased. In essence, therefore, the toxicity of a stroke appears in a large part to be a question of calcium toxicity.

Efforts are currently, therefore, focusing on trying to prevent calcium entry into nerve cells in the period immediately after the onset of the stroke. This can be done in two ways. One is to block a group of receptors called N-methyl-D-aspartate (NMDA) receptors, which are one of the receptors on which glutamate acts and which form one of the principal means of calcium entry (Rothman & Olney 1987). NMDA receptors can be blocked by anaesthetic agents such as ketamine, dextorphan and a variety of barbiturate-related compounds. The other is to block voltage-operated calcium channels, with calcium channel blockers, such as verapamil, nifedipine and diltiazem.

MANAGEMENT OF SUBCORTICAL DEMENTIAS

The subcortical dementias are the most treatable of the dementias. Sometimes, if the precise nature of the disturbance can be diagnosed, the condition can be cured entirely; this is the case for benign subcortical tumours and hydrocephalus. If an underlying disorder cannot be identified and corrected, treatment with psychostimulants, such as dexamphetamine or pemoline, or cholinomimetics, such as the ACE inhibitors, is worth trying and is more likely to yield improvements than in the case of the cortical dementias.

NEUROPROTECTION

The initial focus of interest in neuroprotection centred on Parkinson's disease and stemmed from several discoveries. One was that a severe Parkinson's disease-like state could be precipitated by the designer drug MPTP. This is oxidised in the brain to MPP by monoamine oxidase B (MAO-B), which destroys the substantia nigra cells containing dopamine. This raised the possibility that MAO-B inhibitors, such as deprenyl (also given the generic name selegiline; trade names Eldepryl/Zelapar), might protect against the toxicity of MPTP and perhaps also that of some unknown toxin that is responsible for the naturally occurring form of Parkinson's disease. A large study comparing deprenyl with other treatments (the DATATOP study; see Knoll 2000) suggested that it did slow the progression of the disease.

Whether deprenyl helps by this means or some other is less clear. There is some evidence now to suggest that deprenyl and related compounds can inhibit apoptosis. Apoptosis is the term for a recently discovered process of programmed cell death, a process that seems to be activated in cells in response to a variety of stimuli, one of which appears to be toxin overload.

Another possibility is that deprenyl might work by reducing the production of what are called free radicals. These are derivatives of oxygen, which, if they arise within the body, may inhibit a range of enzymes, the polymerisation of proteins and the reading of DNA. The oxidation of dopamine by MAO can in certain circumstances increase free radical production and there is some evidence of such processes at work in Parkinson's disease. Deprenyl can block a number of the enzymatic processes that might lead to increases in the levels of free radicals. Antioxidants, such as tocopherol or vitamin C, are often promoted in health food shops as the natural way to reduce free radicals but, while these agents may reduce free radical formation in parts of the body, it is not clear that they get into the parts of the brain necessary for effective action in the degenerative disorders (Mizuno et al 1994).

However, much more intriguingly, it appears that deprenyl, in addition to acting on MAO, also acts on a series of other monoamine mechanisms responsible for the release of noradrenaline, dopamine and serotonin. In laboratory animal experiments there is a considerable amount of evidence that boosting the release of amine neurotransmitters through these monoamine release-enhancing mechanisms promotes longevity. The argument put forward by Josef Knoll, the discoverer of both deprenyl and monoamine release-enhancing mechanisms, is that the functioning of monoamine systems is intrinsically bound up with longevity and pushing these systems to a higher level of physiological functioning can prevent the appearance of disorders associated with senescence. As with any other physiological system, he argues, variation between individuals is to be expected, so that some age quickly and some more slowly. On this argument, Parkinson's and Alzheimer's diseases are simply evidence for the early ageing that would be expected in some people; the trick is not so much to treat a discrete disease as to postpone ageing (Knoll 2000).

The dose of deprenyl required to achieve these effects, according to Knoll, is only 1 mg per day, compared with the 10-mg dose usually employed for monoamine inhibition. A range of new agents aimed at stimulating mono-amine release mechanisms that have no effects on MAO are at present being developed by Knoll and his collaborators.

COGNITIVE ENHANCEMENT AND THE POLITICS OF DIAGNOSIS

At present, in addition to finding potential drugs that might be useful for the various forms of dementia, manufacturers have their eyes on what may be an even larger market. As mentioned, there are two ways to tackle the problem of dementia. One is to find a drug that would reverse the illness. The other is to find compounds that might enhance cognitive function. The rationale behind the latter approach is that, if the function of remaining brain tissues can be maximised, then the quality of life of individuals who have dementia will be improved.

However, this has led to an appreciation of a much larger issue: if drugs can be found that have these benefits for individuals with Alzheimer's disease, why not give them to the population at large? Awareness of this possibility has led to a proposal that there is a condition called age-associated memory impairment (AAMI).

AAMI is a state that is proposed to affect a great number of us once we get over the age of 50 years (McEntee & Crook 1990). Many individuals over the age of 50 complain of changes in their memory, but formal testing with the usual tests for dementing disorders rarely picks up anything of note. At present, therefore, it is not clear just what exactly AAMI consists of, except that it is thought of as being part of normal ageing rather than as being related to dementia. The notion has developed, however, that there is such a condition and that cognitive enhancers may help it. In general, in younger populations it has been difficult to demonstrate that any drugs enhance cognitive function. Any results that have been positive have tended to come from older populations.

This seemingly minor point raises an issue about the politics of diagnosis. In general, cognitive-enhancing agents when used in animal populations offer benefits to less able or aged animals compared with younger more able animals.

In our society, discrimination on the basis of sex, age, race or religion is unlawful, but discrimination on the basis of intelligence remains legitimate. Clever children go to college and are subsidised to do so. They end up with the better-paying and more prestigious jobs because of this advantage. This advantage, however, stands to be eroded by cognitive enhancers, unless, for instance, the use of these drugs is confined to diseases such as AAMI (Ray 1998). The political influence of current prescription-only arrangements and disease models to channel developments in particular directions can be seen clearly in the case of the possible restriction of cognitive-enhancing drugs to AAMI.

SMART DRUGS

Despite this, there has been a widespread interest at ground level in the idea of using cognitive enhancers. This has led to the notion of 'smart drugs' (Dean & Morgenthaler 1990). In the USA, in particular, it is now common for many individuals to take a wide range of compounds in an attempt to boost their cognitive performance and give themselves a competitive edge.

The compounds most commonly used are:

◆ Nootropics such as piracetam, oxiracetam, aniracetam, pramiracetam and pyroglutamate (see above).

◆ ACh precursors such as choline, lecithin and acetylcarnitine (see above).

◆ Stimulants such as caffeine, pemoline, ginseng or gingko bibloka.

◆ Hydergine – derived from ergot, a fungus that grows on rye. It is closely related to LSD. Claims have been made that hydergine protects brain cells from damage by free radicals, increases blood supply to the brain, enhances brain cell metabolism, and increases intelligence, memory, learning and recall. Some of the above metabolic effects may be true, but whether hydergine has consistent effects on any mental abilities is not yet clear. What is clear is that it is not a treatment for dementia. Nevertheless, it is used widely in the USA, often in combination with nootropics such as piracetam, with users claiming that they feel much more alert, attentive and lively on these regimens. Cynics might say that, given the amounts of money spent, it would be unlikely that takers would claim anything other than clear benefits.

◆ Phenytoin (Dilantin/Epanutin). This drug is one of the standard treatments for epileptic convulsions. More recently, it has had advocates who claim that, in lower doses than those used for epilepsy, phenytoin may enhance cognitive function. At present, the evidence remains anecdotal. Richard Nixon was perhaps the most famous user of phenytoin for this purpose.

◆ Vasopressin. This is a hormone secreted by the pituitary gland, also called antidiuretic hormone, which, as its name implies, has a role in maintaining the fluid balance of the body. It does seem to have a role in memory formation, but the precise nature of this is still unclear. Vasopressin is used widely as a smart drug at the moment, usually by inhalation in the form of a nasal spray.

Users typically claim to feel much more alert and attentive within seconds of taking it.

♦ Vitamins. Vitamins are used increasingly for smart drug purposes or as cerebroprotectants. Among those most commonly used are the B vitamins, B_1 (thiamine), B_3 (niacin), B_5 (pantothenic acid), B_6 (pyridoxine) and B_{12} (cyanocobalamin). Also used for this purpose are vitamins C and E. It is true that deficiencies of any of these compounds may cause nervous tissue damage and affect psychological performance, but there is no evidence that increasing levels of these vitamins beyond the normal enhances cognitive functioning beyond the norm.

♦ Hormones. The stress hormone cortisol leads to brain cell loss when levels are raised chronically. One of the body's antidotes to cortisol is dihydro-epiandosterone (DHEA). This enjoys considerable sales over the counter in North America as an anti-ageing agent. Another such agent is melatonin.

The smart drugs issue at present involves health food preparations, over-the-counter preparations, and drugs for which there is little clear clinical use, being pressed into service. Individuals who are enthusiastic about cognitive enhancement are possibly spending several hundred, if not several thousand, pounds per year on these preparations. Whether they do anything at all, either to protect the brain from insult or actually to improve performance, is at present unproven. The suggestion from AAMI research is that, if these compounds do anything, it will be for older individuals who do not have dementing processes rather than for those who have begun to dement or for those under the age of 50 seeking some competitive edge.

References

Dean W, Morgenthaler J (1990) Smart drugs and nutrients. Santa Cruz, CA: B & J Publications.

Kafka MS (1995) Sexual impulsivity. In: Hollander E, Stein D, eds. Obsessive–compulsive spectrum disorders, pp 201–228. Chichester, UK: John Wiley.

Knoll J (2000) The psychopharmacology of life and death. In: Healy D, ed. The psychopharmacologists, vol 3, pp 81–110. London: Arnold.

Kolodny RC, Masters WH, Johnson VE (1979) Textbook of sexual medicine. Boston, MA: Little Brown.

McEntee WJ, Crook TH (1990) Age-associated memory impairment: a role for catecholamines. Neurology 40: 526–530.

McKeith IG, Galasko D, Wilcock GK, Byrne EJ (1995) Lewy body dementia – diagnosis and treatment. British Journal of Psychiatry 167: 708–717.

Mizuno Y, Mori H, Kondo T (1994) Potential of neuroprotective therapy in Parkinson's disease. CNS Drugs 1: 45–56.

Ray O (1998) A psychologist in American neuropsychopharmacology. In: Healy D, ed. The psychopharmacologists, vol 2, pp 435–454. London: Arnold.

Rothman SM, Olney JW (1987) Excitatotoxicity and the NMDA receptor. Trends in Neuroscience 10: 299–302.

Waldmeier P (1996) From mental illness to neurodegeneration. In: Healy D, ed. The psychopharmacologists, pp 565–586. London: Chapman & Hall.

Management of sexual difficulties

SECTION CONTENTS

The range of sexual difficulties

POTENCY

The sexual problem in men most likely to lead to a seeking of medical assistance is impotence. This refers to an inability to achieve or sustain an erection. Impotence may derive from either an organic or a psychogenic source (Kolodny et al 1979).

The organic causes of impotence stem from problems with either the nervous supply to the blood vessels of the penis (neurogenic causes) or the blood vessels themselves (vasculogenic causes). The commonest vasculogenic causes involve blockage of the blood vessels by atherosclerosis, consequent on or associated with excessive smoking, or disorders that destroy the smooth muscle walls of the penile blood vessels, such as diabetes.

The commonest neurogenic causes stem from diseases such as multiple sclerosis or diabetes that lead to damage to the nervous supply to the sexual organs, or following trauma to the spine or directly to the nerves serving the sexual organs. There are two neural pathways involved in mediating the erectile response and either can be damaged separately. One is the parasympathetic nervous system, which runs from the end of the spinal column and mediates reflex erectile responses, such as when the penis rubs up against material, etc. It also mediates the spontaneous erections that happen throughout the day and night in a rhythmic manner.

There is another pathway, which is part of the sympathetic system. This has been seen as a more 'psychogenic' pathway, which leads to erections at the sight of erotic material, for example.

A number of illnesses or disorders may cause problems. There are local diseases of the penis, such as Peyronie's disease, which involves excessive curvature of the penis (few penises are entirely straight when erect). Diseases that affect the whole body, such as liver or kidney disease, may also affect sexual functioning through an accumulation of toxic metabolites or other effects.

EJACULATION AND ORGASM

In the male, climax usually involves an ejaculation. The extremes of pleasure – orgasm – are usually associated with this function. Ejaculation and orgasm, however, need not be tied together. There are a number of common problems affecting ejaculation and orgasm, but there is a separate set of problems that can also affect orgasm, indicating that these two functions are not identical. In the female, orgasm is not tied to an obvious ejaculatory event and the differences between the two functions are more clear-cut.

Ejaculation depends on the production of seminal fluid from the prostate gland and the mobilisation of semen from the testes. Seminal fluid is produced before ejaculation and may be noticeable on the tip of the penis during arousal, when it appears to add to the sensitivity of the penis and to facilitate intromission.

Ejaculation involves a complexly organised set of events in which the bladder neck must be closed off, seminal fluid produced and passed down the urethra to mix with semen coming from the testes, and the lot discharged by a coordinated 'Mexican wave' of muscle movements. At any point along this chain of events, a quite minor imbalance or disruption may compromise the whole operation.

Problems with ejaculation may involve premature, delayed or retrograde ejaculation. Premature ejaculation involves consistent ejaculation too early in sexual activity, often before intromission is achieved or else within an unsatisfyingly short time of entry.

Delayed or retarded ejaculation involves an inability to ejaculate within a reasonable period of time, so that no release is achieved. With time, this makes for tension and frustration.

Retrograde ejaculation involves the bulk of the seminal discharge passing back into the bladder rather than out into the vagina. The individual has the experience of ejaculating but not the results. Afterwards, when it comes to passing water, the urine may be cloudier than usual because of the seminal fluid it contains.

Quite apart from the achievement of ejaculation, which is what is commonly thought of as orgasm, most people will be aware of a certain quality to their orgasms, which varies, so that some may be more pleasurable than others. This quality of orgasm may be affected by drugs so that, although ejaculation takes place, it may not be the pleasurable thing it once was.

LIBIDO

A third aspect of sexual functioning is libido. This refers to the degree of interest in sexual stimuli and activities – in lay terms, feeling randy or sex drive.

As with erections and orgasms, libido appears to have several components. There are the diurnal and seasonal surges of interest that appear to have no specific trigger. They come on in much the way that hunger does, as though something builds up gradually and then needs discharge. And there is the specific increase in sexual interest and preoccupation with sexually related imagery, etc., that develops on exposure to erotic stimuli.

SEXUAL ORIENTATION, OBJECTS AND PRACTICES

This refers to the subject matter that an individual finds erotic. This ordinarily refers to members of the opposite sex. In some cases it will involve members of the same sex. To some extent, this issue does not depend on whether a person is homosexual or heterosexual in their practices, but rather what the nature of their fantasies is when they fantasise about sex. If these consistently involve members of the same sex, even though the person's usual sexual partner is of the opposite sex, then there are elements of a homosexual orientation.

This latter distinction points to the fact that a great range of individuals and materials may be used as sexual objects. Sexual intercourse or relief, for example, may be obtained with animals. The fact that this is so does not indicate that an individual is necessarily zoo-sexual in orientation, as it is most likely that, while engaged in such practices, the sexual fantasies driving the process are elsewhere.

Related to this is the fact that a wide variety of props and ancillary material may provide a stimulus to the sexual act. If straightforward intercourse between a man and a woman is taken as the sexual norm, then practices other than this may be said to deviate from the norm. As there are few reliable data on the range of activities that normal individuals engage in, it is strictly speaking not possible to pinpoint where normal deviation ends and formal sexual deviancy begins.

This chapter does not concern itself with gender orientation, sexual object preference, or the perversity or otherwise of sexual practices, as the taking of drugs or therapy with drugs reveals little about these issues. It is perhaps worth noting in passing, however, that Roland Kuhn's first English language article on imipramine (Kuhn 1958) and the recent *Listening to Prozac* (Kramer 1993) both describe cases of deviant sexual activity that were transformed by antidepressant treatment into more orthodox behaviour. The reason why this might happen is at present a matter for speculation, and if this does happen, it seems highly likely that just the opposite can also happen (Kafka 1995).

THE FEMALE SEXUAL RESPONSE

Like men, women have an erectile response, which involves clitoral engorgement and tumescence. This can spread to involve engorgement of the labia and vaginal walls. As with men, there may potentially be two components to this: a spontaneous rhythmic one and a psychogenic one that arises in response to the presentation of erotic material. Whether or not both are differentially affected is unknown. The extent to which diabetes, multiple sclerosis, trauma or other disorders affect these functions is also unknown, almost certainly because, to a greater extent than with men, a woman's sexual activity can still proceed even though aspects of functioning may have become deranged.

Women have a wider distribution of erectile tissue than men; for example, the nipples have erectile material and, in general, a large area of skin may become sensitised to touch in women in a way that does not happen as clearly in men.

As with men, there is also in women a twin-component ejaculatory response. The first component involves the release of fluid from the walls of the vagina, which derives from an increasing congestion of the blood vessels to the vagina: fluid literally transudes into the vagina. This fluid helps to lubricate and thereby facilitate sexual conjunction. Its absence is likely to produce dyspareunia – uncomfortable or indeed painful intercourse. A further amount of fluid is released on orgasm proper. An increase in vaginal lubrication is probably the single most reliable and observable component of the female response. It is not clear to what extent drug treatments may inhibit or enhance this.

In women, orgasm proper is not as clearly tied to an ejaculatory event as it is in men. It is tied to some extent to a set of sequentially arranged contractions of the pelvic floor and vaginal walls, which have their counterpart in the set of muscle contractions in men that lead to ejaculation. Because there is a less clear-cut ejaculatory event, in women there has traditionally been a broader focusing on the quality of sexual arousal than on the specifics of orgasm.

As with men, the quality of orgasmic episodes may vary considerably. It is perhaps important here to distinguish between the actual physical quality of an orgasmic event and its pleasurable significance. An event may involve an orgasm and be both pleasurable and among the most significant sexual encounters, but yet have a lesser orgasmic intensity. Conversely, a meaningless encounter may involve an intense orgasmic outcome. It is not clear what specific factors make for intensity of orgasmic outcome.

In women, as with men, there is also sexual libido. When in full flood, libido in either sex is easy to recognise in that it leads to a mental state dominated by thoughts and fantasies of sexual activity and heightened awareness of others as potential sexual partners or stimulants to sexual activity. However, while such mental states happen to all of us on occasion, in the normal course of events attempting to judge the state of our libido is more difficult. A person's libido is intact if they are noticing as sexual objects members of whichever sex they have been used to noticing as sexual objects in the past. Libido is intact if, when someone walks down the street, they find themselves aware of others as men and women rather than just as people. Libido is low if there is little or no spontaneous sexual fantasising.

All of these factors – libido, orgasm and female potency – come together in the case of sexual fantasies, orgasmic dreaming and masturbation, when the various elements of the sexual response can be disentangled from the 'faking' that may occur in conjugal situations. Orgasmic dreaming corresponds to the male wet dream or nocturnal emission. It consists of a semi-awakening to find oneself aroused and on the verge of or immediately post-orgasm. If it is happening more or less frequently than before, while on a particular drug, the question arises as to whether the drug may be playing some part in the change. Very much the same thing is true of sexual fantasising. Masturbation, to some extent, offers a chance for an individual to become aware of the various components of their sexual response and to determine, in the case of a change, which element is most affected.

21

Effects of drugs on aspects of sexual functioning

NORADRENERGIC EFFECTS

The central factor that determines potency is blood supply to the relevant tissues. In general, blood supply increases during sexual activity, leading to tumescence. Anything that interferes with this will compromise performance. Anything that improves this will enhance performance. One of the main controls on blood flow is the sympathetic system, and increases or decreases can be brought about by stimulating or blocking a variety of receptors on which noradrenaline acts, either in the penis and vagina or in the brain (Segraves 1989, Sullivan & Lukoff 1990).

Many tricyclic antidepressants, as well as the selective noradrenaline reuptake inhibitor reboxetine and a number of antipsychotics, produce erectile problems by this means. These are transient effects in most people but can be longer lasting in others – in both women and men. Some of the antipsychotics produce effects on potency by this means that are quite separate to the effects on libido they also produce. Chief among these has been the 'brewer's droop' associated with thioridazine. This appears to come about because of an action on α_1 receptors, which reduces blood supply to the sexual vasculature. The incidence of this problem with other antipsychotics remains uncertain, although a number of them can cause retrograde ejaculation.

Noradrenergic inputs to sexual functioning are mediated through the sympathetic system. This system handles 'psychogenic' responses – lubrication or tumescence in response to sexual stimuli. There is also a parasympathetic system input, mediated by acetylcholine, which handles the rhythmic inputs to sexuality – the rhythmic increase and decrease in tumescence that takes place, usually unobtrusively, throughout the day and night. Tricyclic antidepressants and antipsychotics, with their anticholinergic effects, may affect either of these.

A great many compounds used mainly for the control of blood pressure may lead to a reduction in noradrenaline output and hence to a reduced ability to vasodilate the sexual blood vessels. These include clonidine, guanethidine and methyldopa (Aldomet).

The effects of agents active on α-adrenergic receptors are generally antagonised by agents active on β-adrenergic receptors. In this case one might expect beta-blockers, such as propranolol, to interfere with sexual potency, and there are some reports that this is the case, although it is unlikely to be a common effect, as there are far more α receptors in the sexual tissues than there are β receptors.

SEROTONERGIC EFFECTS

While erectile responses depend critically on the action of noradrenaline on its receptors, the dopamine and serotonergic systems appear to affect the threshold for ejaculatory or orgasmic responses. While not actually responsible for erections, effects on these systems may, however, make erectile and ejaculatory/orgasmic responses more or less likely.

The development of the selective serotonin reuptake inhibitors (SSRIs) and growing awareness of the changes in sexual functioning associated with their use have triggered off renewed interest in this area and increased understanding of the various mechanisms involved. In brief, serotonin inhibits orgasmic functioning. In practice, S_1 agonists, such as buspirone, and S_2 antagonists, such as cyproheptadine and yohimbine, bring orgasm forward, whereas S_1 antagonists and S_2 agonists, such as LSD, delay it. There is a profound interplay between the sexual hormones and serotonin in this area, such that the sexual hormones mediate their effects by leading to increases or decreases in serotonin synthesis, while serotonin in turn does not act other than in the presence of a normal hormonal milieu (Kafka 1995).

DOPAMINERGIC AGENTS

It can be very difficult to tease apart libido, potency and orgasmic functioning. A change in one will tend to affect the others. But where serotonin seems to be responsible for orgasm, and noradrenaline and acetylcholine to be responsible for potency, dopamine appears more responsible for libido.

Thus cocaine, the psychostimulants generally, L-dopa, apomorphine, amantadine, pergolide and bromocriptine, all of which enhance dopaminergic functions, have been reported to bring about increases in libido. Conversely drugs that reduce the effects of dopamine in the brain tend to antagonise sexual functioning generally, as well as decrease libido. The most obvious such compounds are the antipsychotics. Well over 50% of individuals taking antipsychotics have impairment of sexual functioning of some sort. This appears to be dose related, so that the higher the dose of an antipsychotic, the more likely the sexual problem. One of these agents, benperidol, has been marketed for the management of hypersexuality, although there is little evidence to suggest that it has any more marked effects on libido and potency than any of the other antipsychotics.

The effects of dopamine antagonists are complex. There may be a direct action through the dopamine system, but dopamine blockade also leads to an increase in prolactin levels and this can produce amenorrhoea, gynaecomastia and a reduction in libido. The use of quetiapine, which has a much less marked effect on prolactin, may make it possible to tease apart these direct and indirect dopaminergic contributions.

SEX HORMONES

Another group of drugs that has effects on libido is the sex hormones, particularly testosterone. Testosterone may lead to increases in libido in both men and women, and, indeed, in women the androgens (male sex hormones) appear to be primarily responsible for libido. A number of takers of contraceptive pills report a decrease in libido, which may stem from an alteration in the ratio of androgen to oestrogen, so that there are proportionately fewer androgens. The ratio of androgen to oestrogen, in both men and women, is also what is likely to determine the incidence of side effects from hormonal preparations. These can include excessive sexual interest and drive or 'masculinisation' – an increase in male secondary sexual characteristics, such as facial hair.

OPIATES

Broadly speaking the opiates, heroin, morphine, pethidine, etc., have been associated with a decrease in sexual libido. However, the acute use of opiates such as papaverine is associated with enhanced sexual performance and there are opiate receptors in the sexual tissues. The apparent contradiction can probably be best explained in terms of the reduction in libido that occurs as a consequence of long-term opiate use, leading to a more general impairment of health and nutritional status. It may also be partly a secondary impairment of libido rather than a primary impairment, in that the consuming focus of appetitive interest has become the getting and taking of opiate drugs, and this displaces sexual libido from its usual place in the emotional economy.

TRADITIONAL APHRODISIACS

For millennia there has been a search for agents that would reliably enhance sexual functioning (Meyer 1986). In general, this has tended to mean agents that increase male potency, although some agents such as cocaine may increase sexual interest quite separately from any effect on potency (see below). Among the agents quoted most consistently as being aphrodisiac is ginseng, especially powdered ginseng root, which probably acts to increase noradrenaline release.

Another widely cited aphrodisiac is cantharides, also called Spanish Fly, which is composed of the dried and ground parts of the *Cantharis vesicatoris* beetle. This can be sprinkled on the penis and it leads to erections by virtue of being an irritant. It can also be taken orally and, when excreted through the kidneys, leads to irritation of the genitourinary passages, which in turn makes erections more likely or prolonged. As it is a frank irritant, the effects are unpleasant.

A wide range of other herbs and vegetables have been cited as aphrodisiac, including garlic, leeks, khat (quat; Abyssinian tea), licorice and sea-foods, especially oysters. In Japan, the puffer fish or fugu is used. Shark fin is sought after elsewhere in the Orient, while eels enjoyed the same reputation in the Occident. In the West Indies, the conch is the seafood most used as an aphrodisiac.

YOHIMBINE

While ginseng and cantharides are better known aphrodisiacs, the agent for which the best evidence was available, before the advent of the SSRIs and sildenafil (Viagra), was yohimbine. This compound, which is derived from the bark of the Yohimb tree, has a long-standing reputation as an aphrodisiac. Its use, however, was discouraged owing to doubts about its efficacy and a concern about possible side effects. However, recent studies appear to have laid these doubts and concerns to rest, showing that about two-thirds of men with erectile difficulties respond to it, without troublesome side effects (Reid et al 1987, Riley et al 1989). The theoretical side effects are an increase in blood pressure or in anxiety. These can happen but appear to be infrequent. The response seems better in cases where there appears to be a psychogenic component to the problem, but is not absent in straightforward cases of organic impairment.

In the case of yohimbine, it seems likely that benefits are brought about by a combination of actions on receptors for noradrenaline and serotonin. It is both an α_2-adrenergic antagonist and an S_2 antagonist. Both of these systems appear to affect the threshold for erectile and ejaculatory responses, so that, while not actually responsible for erections, effects on these systems may make erectile responses more or less likely.

TRAZODONE

A compound with a very similar profile, and which is more widely available at present, is trazodone (Molipaxin). This has been in use in recent years as an antidepressant. One of its notable side effects has been priapism (sustained erections). While this side effect has been widely publicised, what has been less touted is the fact that a great number of people, male and female, show an enhancement of sexual interest and potency while taking trazodone.

Priapism, which can be a complication of any of these treatments, involves erections that fail to reduce over several hours. At present, it is considered that any erections lasting longer than 8–12 h warrant medical attention. The problem is that if such erections are not reduced, there is a risk of damage to the penis owing to a compression of the blood supply to its component tissues, which can lead to cell death. The reduction of priapism involves aspirating blood from the penis by syringe, usually accompanied by the injection of drugs, which leads to vasoconstriction (closing down) of the blood vessels in the area.

NEFAZODONE AND CYPROHEPTADINE

Nefazodone (Dutonin) is another antidepressant that has potent S_2 blocking effects, and as such can be expected to facilitate orgasms and perhaps, as a consequence, increase libido. It is very similar in its profile of actions to both trazodone and cyproheptadine, which was first developed in the 1950s. This agent increases appetite and improves sleep, but failed to find a niche after development – other than as a tonic. It would now seem that, along with trazodone, yohimbine and nefazodone, it facilitates orgasm and enhances libido.

BETHANECHOL

The role of the cholinergic system in erectile and sexual functioning is at present less certain than that of the monoamine systems. A series of cases has been reported of sexual dysfunction precipitated by a range of different agents that has proved to be responsive to the addition of bethanechol (Myotonine). Bethanechol also appears to have a place in impotence or erectile failure stemming from back injuries. This may have something to do with the fact that the parasympathetic nerves to the sexual areas travel in nerves from the sacral area of the spine. Bethanechol has also been reported in some cases to reverse problems produced by antidepressants or neuroleptics. This raises the possibility that the anticholinergic drugs, which are widely used in clinical practice, might also produce sexual dysfunction more widely. One effect that anticholinergic drugs are likely to have is a drying of secretory responses, such as the lubricant fluids produced by both men and women during arousal, making sexual interaction less comfortable.

GLYCERYL TRINITRATE (GTN)

This compound has been used for years for the treatment of angina. Until recently, it was available as a pill that was put beneath the tongue when chest pain started or was likely. It was quickly absorbed from there and eased pain by dilating the coronary arteries. However, once absorbed into the system, GTN remains active for several hours and leads to the dilatation of a range of arteries throughout the body. This latter action brings about its most troublesome side effect: headaches.

In an attempt to overcome this problem, a number of companies have produced GTN paste and GTN patches, which can be applied to the chest wall. The drug is absorbed through the skin and leads to a preferential dilatation of the coronary arteries. Once the pain has gone, the patch can be peeled away and further absorption stopped. Application of such patches to the penis has been reported to bring about vigorous erections.

TRANSCUTANEOUS ABSORPTION

Perhaps related to the above are anecdotes reported from a variety of places that the sprinkling of various compounds on to the penis may lead to erectile responses. In this case, everything depends on the preparation of the compound. Capsules that can be opened up may be of use where tablets would not be. The antidepressants have been among the compounds used for this purpose. Dosulepin (dothiepin), in capsule form, appears to be useful. However, other compounds, even though in capsule form, appear relatively ineffective and, indeed, may cause side effects such as local irritation. At present it is not certain whether drugs that produce useful effects do so by virtue of an irritation they cause, or whether they are absorbed transcutaneously and act that way.

INTRAPENILE TREATMENTS

One way to get over the problem of absorption through the skin of the penis is to inject compounds into the body of the penis, which is termed the corpora cavernosa (= the cavernous bodies – one for each side). This is done by plunging a needle into the side of the penis about an inch back from the tip. Surprisingly, it is relatively painless. The method was first described in 1982.

The initial compounds administered in this way were papaverine, which is a smooth muscle dilator, and sometimes a combination of papaverine and phentolamine, which increases noradrenaline release from sympathetic nerve endings. More recently prostaglandin E1, which is found naturally in the sexual tissues and whose levels are increased during sexual activity, has been used. This appears to lead to a lower incidence of priapism. The preparation that has displaced most others is intracavernosal alprostadil (Caverject). Alprostadil is a prostaglandin E1 analogue which inhibits α_1-adrenergic receptors in the penis.

Apart from priapism, the side effects of intracavernosal injections include bruising, discomfort and, more seriously, the production of plaques or nodules. Essentially these latter indicate a proliferation of scar tissue at the site of injection. The exuberant growth of scar tissue is something that can occur after a wound or a burn. If it happens on the penis, it can lead to distortion of its shape. This, however, seems to be relatively rare (Kirby 1994).

Alprostadil has also been developed in a form that allows insertion of a slim stick containing the drug into the urethra (Muse). The side effects of this are penile irritation or burning, bleeding from the penis, or swelling of the groin or legs. Faintness or dizziness may also occur.

The use of prostaglandins to stimulate erectile function in this manner raises the possibility that many analgesics, such as aspirin or other drugs used to treat arthritic conditions, which act to inhibit prostaglandin synthesis, might in susceptible individuals lead to impairment of performance. Any screening of people with difficulties should therefore check for this possibility.

VIAGRA

Viagra has joined Valium and Prozac as a brand name, which defines an epoch. In this case the epoch is not so much one in which treatment of sexual dysfunction became more successful, as an era in which it became possible to talk about sexual functioning and its management.

Viagra is sildenafil. In the penis, nitric oxide increases the activity of cyclic guanosine monophosphate (cGMP), which dilates the smooth muscles of the penile blood vessels. Sildenafil inhibits phophodiesterase type 5 (PDE-5), which breaks down cGMP. This mechanism of action means that nitric oxide release must take place for sildenafil to work, i.e. sexual stimulation must take place and must take effect. This is different, for instance, to alprostadil, which works regardless of whether there is sexual stimulation.

Viagra is licensed for use for impotence in men. This does not mean that it has effects only in either impotence or men. It was originally discovered as part of a series of clinical trials aimed at seeing whether its vasodilating effects might be useful in angina, following the successful use of nitrates such as

GTN for this purpose. Its sexual effects were noticeable by normal people (i.e. people in trials of Viagra for heart conditions who had nothing wrong with their sexual functioning). It follows that Viagra may potentially have effects in most of us, including women. Trials in dyspareunia have apparently not demonstrated significant effects, but this may say more about the heterogeneous nature of dyspareunia than it does about the effects of Viagra.

The commonest side effects of Viagra are headaches and flushing. A proportion of people, probably up to 10% of takers, have a temporary alteration in colour vision, which leaves everything tinged with blue for some hours. Dyspepsia has also been reported.

DYSPAREUNIA AND ANORGASMIA

As outlined, there is a complex of functions involved in ejaculation and orgasm. While ejaculation itself is a peripheral act, in both men and women, it is linked intimately to a central event, orgasm, so that disruption of one set of functions tends to compromise the other. It is also difficult to disentangle this complex from general questions of libido. Drugs that reduce potency can also be expected to interfere with orgasm and ejaculatory responses (Segraves 1989, Sullivan & Lukoff 1990).

While there are areas of overlap, there are also clear differences between erectile and orgasmic functions that have become more apparent with the widespread use of the SSRIs. The commonest effect of the SSRIs on sexual functioning in both women and men is a delay of orgasm. There are varying estimates of the frequency with which this happens and the severity of any problem it may cause, but the data sheets for the agents involved suggest that up to 80% of individuals taking an SSRI or clomipramine may experience changes in sexual function.

For men this may be a benefit rather than a problem, as surveys suggest that up to one-third of men may have problems with premature ejaculation. Contrary to popular mythology, premature orgasm is something that may afflict women also, although the extent of the problem is unknown. Cases of premature ejaculation/orgasm may be treated with an SSRI, whether or not there is concomitant depression. In this case, a small dose of an SSRI, such as paroxetine 20 mg or clomipramine 10 or 25 mg taken 1–2 h before sexual relations may make an appreciable difference to the length of time for which erection can be sustained before orgasm.

When used in higher doses the SSRIs and clomipramine may lead to a failure of ejaculation in men or anorgasmia in women. In some men there may be complete erectile failure. Discontinuing these drugs may also lead to problems, with complaints of anorgasmia, for example, being replaced by problems with uncontrollable spontaneous orgasms.

Spontaneous orgasm also appears to be a side effect of SSRIs in a small proportion of takers. This seems to happen because we are all 'wired up' slightly differently. Thus a few people given a beta-blocker, which slows heart rate in over 90% of cases, will find an increase in their heart rate.

In cases of spontaneous or drug-induced anorgasmia or retarded ejaculation, a number of serotonergic antagonists, such as cyproheptadine, may help, but in theory buspirone should also help. Bethanechol has also been reported to be helpful. Whether buspirone or cyproheptadine taken in modest doses shortly before sexual activity will act as specifically as the SSRIs, or whether they have to be taken regularly, is at present uncertain.

ANTIAPHRODISIACS

As outlined, the oestrogens antagonise the effects of androgens on libido. Accordingly they are sometimes given to suppress sexual libido. Ordinarily this is likely to happen only if an individual's sex drive is such that it has been getting them into trouble. Clinically, however, one occasionally meets men who in the past have been given oestrogens for nothing more than worries about masturbation, with shocking consequences such as a relatively permanent development of breast tissue. There was also a not uncommon use of antipsychotics such as benperidol in the 1960s and 1970s to curb what was seen as sexual promiscuity in younger women.

Two other agents are sometimes given for more serious sexual problems: cyproterone and medroxyprogesterone. These are synthetic antiandrogens that block brain androgen receptors. They produce a decrease in libido, a reduction in sperm count, an impairment of erectile capacity and a decreased ability to achieve orgasm, but do not produce overt feminisation. Their use is largely restricted to men convicted of sexual crimes.

The steroid hormones are closely related to the sex hormones – more closely to the oestrogens than to the androgens. A not infrequent side effect of steroid therapy, therefore, may be a loss of libido along with breast development or milk production.

A number of diuretics (agents that assist in the excretion of body fluid, which are often used in cardiac failure or hypertension) are also closely related to the steroid hormones. The use of some of these, especially spironolactone and aldactone, may also lead to loss of libido. All diuretics may lead to sexual problems in about 5% of users. Given that other antihypertensive agents, such as propranolol and centrally acting agents such as clonidine or α-methyldopa may also cause sexual problems, impairments of sexual functioning, it would seem, are a potential complication of any treatment for hypertension (although the effects of angiotensin-converting enzyme (ACE) inhibitors in this regard are at present unknown).

Antihistamines have also been reported to have an inhibitory effect on sexual functioning. The antiulcer treatments, cimetidine (Tagamet) and ranitidine (Zantac), have been reported to reduce vaginal lubrication, to cause increased breast size in both men and women, and to reduce libido generally.

Appendix 21.1
Male sexual functioning questionnaire

Drugs being taken

1   2
3   4

Circle any options that apply to you.

1. **Have you had any change in sex drive lately?**
   An increase   A decrease   No change to normal

   If there has been a change lately, does this bother you?
   Not at all   A little   Definitely bothered   Extremely bothered

   If there has been a change, do you think it is related to the drugs you are on?
   No   Possibly   Probably   Definitely

2. **Lately, have you been fantasising about sexual matters?**
   More often than before
   Less often than before
   About the same as before

   If there has been a change lately, does this bother you?
   Not at all   A little   Definitely bothered   Extremely bothered

   If there has been a change, do you think it is related to the drugs you are on?
   No   Possibly   Probably   Definitely

3. **How likely has sexually explicit material been to cause you to become sexually excited lately?**
   More likely   Less likely   About as often as before

   If there has been a change lately, does this bother you?
   Not at all   A little   Definitely bothered   Extremely bothered

   If there has been a change, do you think it is related to the drugs you are on?
   No   Possibly   Probably   Definitely

4. **Erections may be more or less vigorous and sustained. How have your erections been lately?**
Better and longer lasting than before
Weaker and more short lived than before
About the same as before

If there has been a change lately, does this bother you?
Not at all   A little   Definitely bothered   Extremely bothered

If there has been a change, do you think it is related to the drugs you are on?
No   Possibly   Probably   Definitely

5. **Spontaneous erections happen regularly during the night. Has this been happening to you lately?**
More frequently
Less frequently
About as often as before
Don't know

If there has been a change lately, does this bother you?
Not at all   A little   Definitely bothered   Extremely bothered

If there has been a change, do you think it is related to the drugs you are on?
No   Possibly   Probably   Definitely

6. **The commonest difficulty with an orgasm is 'coming' too quickly. Has this been happening to you lately?**
More frequently
Less frequently
About the same as before

If there has been a change lately, does this bother you?
Not at all   A little   Definitely bothered   Extremely bothered

If there has been a change, do you think it is related to the drugs you are on?
No   Possibly   Probably   Definitely

7. **Another problem with orgasms can be difficulty in 'coming'. Have you noticed this happening to you lately?**
More frequently than before
Less frequently than before
About the same as before

If there has been a change lately, does this bother you?
Not at all   A little   Definitely bothered   Extremely bothered

If there has been a change, do you think it is related to the drugs you are on?
No   Possibly   Probably   Definitely

8. Sometimes you may have what feels like a normal orgasm but nothing comes out. You may notice that your urine is cloudier than usual. Has this happened to you lately?
   More frequently than before
   Less frequently than before
   As often as before
   Don't know

   If there has been a change lately, does this bother you?
   Not at all   A little   Definitely bothered   Extremely bothered

   If there has been a change, do you think it is related to the drugs you are on?
   No   Possibly   Probably   Definitely

9. **How often have you been masturbating lately?**
   Less often than before
   More often than before
   About the same as before

   If there has been a change lately, does this bother you?
   Not at all   A little   Definitely bothered   Extremely bothered

   If there has been a change, do you think it is related to the drugs you are on?
   No   Possibly   Probably   Definitely

10. **What amount of pleasure do you get from orgasms lately?**
   More pleasurable than before
   Less pleasurable than before
   Unchanged

   If there has been a change lately, does this bother you?
   Not at all   A little   Definitely bothered   Extremely bothered

   If there has been a change, do you think it is related to the drugs you are on?
   No   Possibly   Probably   Definitely

11. **Orgasms may happen spontaneously (for no obvious reason). Has this been happening to you lately?**
   No
   More often than before
   For the first time ever

   If there has been a change lately, does this bother you?
   Not at all   A little   Definitely bothered   Extremely bothered

   If there has been a change, do you think that it is related to the drugs you are on?
   No   Possibly   Probably   Definitely

12. **How would you describe your sex drive compared to that of other people?**
A stronger than average sex drive
A weaker than average sex drive
An average sex drive

13. **How would you describe your interest in sex compared to that of other people?**
Like sex more
Dislike it more
Like it about the same as others

14. **If there have been changes in your sex life caused by drug treatment, have you considered stopping the drugs?**
Yes   No

Appendix 21.2
Female sexual functioning questionnaire

Drugs being taken

1	2
3	4

Circle options that apply to you.

1. **Have you noticed any change in your sex drive lately?**
   An increase
   A decrease
   No change to normal

   If there has been a change lately, does this bother you?
   Not at all   A little   Definitely bothered   Extremely bothered

   If there has been a change, do you think it is related to the drugs you are on?
   No   Possibly   Probably   Definitely

2. **How often have you been fantasising about sexual matters lately?**
   More often than before
   Less often than before
   About the same as before

   If there has been a change lately, does this bother you?
   Not at all   A little   Definitely bothered   Extremely bothered

   If there has been a change, do you think it is related to the drugs you are on?
   No   Possibly   Probably   Definitely

3. **How likely has sexually explicit material been to cause you to become sexually excited lately?**
   More likely than usual
   Less likely than usual
   About the same as before

   If there has been a change lately, does this bother you?
   Not at all   A little   Definitely bothered   Extremely bothered

   If there has been a change, do you think it is related to the drugs you are on?
   No   Possibly   Probably   Definitely

4. **Moistening of the vagina (lubrication) is a common sign of sexual interest. How often has this been happening to you lately?**
More frequently than before
Less frequently than before
About the same as before

If there has been a change lately, does this bother you?
Not at all   A little   Definitely bothered   Extremely bothered

If there has been a change, do you think it is related to the drugs you are on?
No   Possibly   Probably   Definitely

5. **Sex can sometimes be painful. How painful has it been lately?**
More painful than before
Less painful than before
About normal for me

If there has been a change lately, does this bother you?
Not at all   A little   Definitely bothered   Extremely bothered

If there has been a change, do you think it is related to the drugs you are on?
No   Possibly   Probably   Definitely

6. **It can be difficult to have an orgasm. Have you had this problem lately?**
More frequently than before
Less frequently than before
About the same as before

If there has been a change lately, does this bother you?
Not at all   A little   Definitely bothered   Extremely bothered

If there has been a change, do you think it is related to the drugs you are on?
No   Possibly   Probably   Definitely

7. **Orgasms are normally pleasurable. The pleasure, however, is not always quite the same. How pleasurable have your orgasms been lately?**
More pleasurable than before
Less pleasurable than before
Unchanged

If there has been a change lately, does this bother you?
Not at all   A little   Definitely bothered   Extremely bothered

If there has been a change, do you think it is related to the drugs you are on?
No   Possibly   Probably   Definitely

8. **Orgasms may happen spontaneously (for no obvious reason). Has this happening to you lately?**
No   More often than before   For the first time ever

If there has been a change lately, does this bother you?
Not at all   A little   Definitely bothered   Extremely bothered

If there has been a change, do you think it is related to the drugs you are on?
No   Possibly   Probably   Definitely

9. **How often have you been masturbating lately?**
More often than before
Less often than before
About the same as before

If there has been a change lately, does this bother you?
Not at all   A little   Definitely bothered   Extremely bothered

If there has been a change, do you think it is related to the drugs you are on?
No   Possibly   Probably   Definitely

10. **Have you noticed any change in breast size or tenderness recently, other than the kind of changes you normally get with your periods?**
Increased size
Increased tenderness
Decreased size
Decreased tenderness
No change in size
No change in tenderness

If there has been a change lately, does this bother you?
Not at all   A little   Definitely bothered   Extremely bothered

If there has been a change, do you think it is related to the drugs you are on?
No   Possibly   Probably   Definitely

11. **How regular have your periods been lately compared to normal?**
Less regular
Less frequent
More frequent
No change to before

If there has been a change lately, does this bother you?
Not at all   A little   Definitely bothered   Extremely bothered

If there has been a change, do you think it is related to the drugs you are on?
No   Possibly   Probably   Definitely

12. **Compared with normal, how painful have your periods been lately?**
Increased   Decreased   Unchanged

If there has been a change lately, does this bother you?
Not at all   A little   Definitely bothered   Extremely bothered

If there has been a change, do you think it is related to the drugs you are on?
No   Possibly   Probably   Definitely

13. **How would you describe your sex drive compared to that of other people?**
A stronger than average sex drive
A weaker than average sex drive
An average sex drive

14. **How much do you like sex compared to other people?**
Like sex more
Dislike it more
Like it about the same as others

15. **If there has been a change in your sex life lately that you think has been caused by your drugs, have you considered halting your drugs?**
Yes   No

References

Kafka MS (1995) Sexual impulsivity. In: Hollander D, ed. Impulsiveness and aggression. Chichester, UK: John Wiley.

Kirby RS (1994) Impotence: diagnosis and management of male erectile dysfunction. British Medical Journal 308: 957–961.

Kramer P (1993) Listening to Prozac. New York: Viking.

Kuhn R (1958) The treatment of depressive states with G22355 (imipramine hydrochloride). American Journal of Psychiatry 115: 455–464.

Meyer C (1986) Herbal aphrodisiacs from world sources. Glenwood, IL: Meyerbooks.

Reid K, Surridge D, Morales A et al (1987) Double-blind trial of yohimbine in treatment of psychogenic impotence. Lancet i: 421–422.

Riley AJ, Goodman RE, Kellett JM, Orr R (1989) Double blind trial of yohimbine hydrochloride in the treatment of erection inadequacy. Sexual and Marital Therapy 4: 17–26.

Segraves RT (1989) Effects of psychotropic drugs on human erection and ejaculation. Archives of General Psychiatry 46: 275–284.

Sullivan G, Lukoff D (1990) Sexual side effects of antipsychotic medication: Evaluation and interventions. Hospital and Community Psychiatry 41: 1238–1241.

Management of dependence and withdrawal

Physical dependence type I

INTRODUCTION

The issues of dependence and withdrawal have come up repeatedly through these pages. They are a primary concern of any taker of psychoactive medication.

It has been traditional to distinguish between physical dependence and psychological dependence. Physical dependence is the state that produces withdrawal syndromes. The classical instances are alcohol-induced delirium tremens and opiate-induced cold turkey. These are intensely physical states with shakes, palpitations, sweating and sometimes even convulsions and death.

Psychological dependence, in contrast, has often been thought to be purely a psychological thing that does not involve anything physical in the brain. It gives rise to symptoms of craving that leads addicted individuals to start taking a substance again, often after they have gone through the horrors of a withdrawal, which one might have imagined would have scared any reasonable person off taking the particular drug again.

These old ideas, however, are giving way to a welter of new discoveries. Before considering the implications of recent research, we must exclude a type of physical dependence that occurs with a great number of drugs and that is ordinarily of little consequence.

REBOUND SYMPTOMS AND WITHDRAWAL REACTIONS

Many drugs cause rebound symptoms once they are discontinued. Receptors blocked by drug antagonists become hypersensitive. When the blocking drug is then removed, these receptors are flooded with the normal neurotransmitter and they respond vigorously. It may take 48–72 h for them to settle back down to normal.

Examples of this are the rebound phenomena that may occur with beta-blockers, such as propranolol. Propranolol rebound may lead to palpitations, sweating and flushing. Cholinergic rebound in response to anticholinergics may produce poor sleep and nausea or vomiting. These syndromes are not serious. They clear up quickly and without consequence.

This has traditionally been thought to be quite different to the physical dependence that produces full-blown withdrawal reactions in response to alcohol, the barbiturates, the benzodiazepines and the opiates. Of these compounds by far the most dangerous withdrawal syndrome is produced by alcohol. In its full-blown form, delirium tremens, this can still be fatal. Very few alcohol-dependent individuals now ever have delirium tremens, although many think that having experienced the 'shakes' that go with alcohol withdrawal, or perhaps even having the fits that may occur or having heard voices, they must have had the DTs.

The least serious is probably opiate withdrawal, which has a fearsome reputation but is never fatal – except historically where medical zeal has intervened (Bakalar & Grinspoon 1989). In between lie benzodiazepine and barbiturate withdrawal. These may lead to delirium and fits but rarely, if ever, death. The benzodiazepines seem to lead to marked withdrawal only in susceptible individuals when given in high doses for sustained periods.

BRAIN PHYSIOLOGY

Understanding withdrawal syndromes needs some appreciation of the physiology of the brain. In 1954 Marthe Vogt discovered noradrenaline in brain cells. This was the first demonstration that neurotransmitters existed in the brain, which had until then been thought to operate only electrically. In 1964, it was shown that neurones containing noradrenaline formed a system within the brain that has its roots in the most primitive parts of the brain, the pons and the medulla oblongata, which are responsible for vital functions such as breathing, cardiac activity and arousal. As cell bodies that contain noradrenaline stain blue, the 'nucleus' of noradrenaline-containing cells came to be known as the locus coeruleus (the blue spot).

This system extends up through other areas of the old brain into the cortex of the brain areas. It is paralleled as it goes by another system, termed the raphe system, which uses serotonin (5HT) as its neurotransmitter. In general, these two systems act in a complementary fashion. Where the noradrenergic system arouses, the 5HT system sedates. In addition to its role in sleep, breathing and cardiac functioning, the locus coeruleus has a role in vigilance, alerting us to things going on around us (or within us, such as a full bladder) that may be of interest or a potential threat. It is in this role that it plays a part in anxiety, which is a state of hypervigilance in which we get ready to fight or flee.

Interference with these systems produces the withdrawal reactions noted above for opiates and, to a greater or lesser extent, the dependence on alcohol, barbiturates and benzodiazepines. Before finding out exactly how, another phenomenon of drug use needs to be considered. This is tolerance.

TOLERANCE

For a number of psychoactive drugs, over time it may be necessary to take more of the substance to induce the same effects. For example, 100 mg morphine given to someone unaccustomed to taking it would be a large amount, sufficient even to kill as a result of respiratory depression. However, for a chronic opiate abuser doses of 4000 mg can be tolerated without undue suppression of breathing (Baker & Tiffany 1985, Jaffe 1989).

This phenomenon, not surprisingly, is called tolerance. This is what happens when the sedative effects of benzodiazepines wear off. It happens with alcohol. It happens with some of the side effects of antidepressants and antipsychotics, so that they produce less in the way of a dry mouth after a while. (We will pick up the issue of whether it happens with the central effects of the antidepressants and antipsychotics later in this section.)

Early attempts to explain tolerance focused on an aspect of the metabolism of barbiturates. Like morphine, barbiturates can be taken in ever-increasing doses, with the subject becoming progressively more tolerant as the dose rises. It was discovered that the level of an enzyme in the liver, which is responsible for the breakdown of barbiturates, increases with exposure to these drugs. Hence, it was argued, more and more of the drug has to be taken simply to achieve the level that was obtained initially. The development of tolerance of this type, it has been argued, is what leads to withdrawal reactions.

Comparable factors, it was thought, must be involved in opiate, alcohol and benzodiazepine tolerance and withdrawal reactions. However, it is now accepted that this is not what causes tolerance, and that the development of tolerance has no clear relation to withdrawal reactions. For example, a number of drugs, such as cocaine, caffeine, LSD and many others, may cause tolerance but yet do not lead to withdrawal reactions. It has also become clear that, far from being a purely physical matter, tolerance may involve a considerable amount of learning.

Living on a busy street or beside a train line produces a comparable phenomenon. When first exposed to the noise it may be deafening, but after a few days the sounds are hardly heard any more – unless a particularly large truck roars past the window or the train driver sounds the horn while going past. The person has become tolerant to the noise. No changes in enzyme levels or brain receptors need be postulated to explain what is going on. The brain has simply learned not to pay any heed to this particular event.

What seems to be involved here relates to survival. Organisms pay heed to novel events, until they have assessed the threat that such events pose. When they are judged to be harmless, less heed is paid to them. If the organism remains uncertain about what is going on, attention is maintained. This means that the event remains in awareness and is subjected to all the processing capacities that can be brought to bear on what is happening. Drugs are one such event. Like loud noise or unusual visual events, they bring about change in the internal milieu. While the change is novel and its significance uncertain, experimental animals and human beings react sensitively to it. If repeated administration proves harmless, reactions will be increasingly blunted.

The event being reacted to is rarely something as simple as a noise, but is rather the situation in which this noise occurs. In the wild, animals faced with novel sounds, sights or smells react not just to those stimuli but to an entire environment. The issue is not simply one of deciding whether the beast that makes that strange noise is dangerous or not, but rather whether the environment in which such beasts occur is a safe one. Or alternatively: 'I thought I knew what was going on around here, but it seems that I don't'.

This is particularly the case with drugs. Work on animals reveals that the animal assesses the environment in which drugs are being taken. For example, morphine has an analgesic effect on animals, but there are striking interactions between the environment in which analgesia is being tested and the amount of analgesia produced. If analgesia is tested for day after day in the same experimental situation, more and more morphine is required daily to bring about a constant level of analgesia.

However, if the environment is changed, much less morphine may be needed. Tolerance to higher doses can be rolled back by a change of environment – at least partly. The change of environment, it seems, makes the animal less certain that the drug-induced changes are something that can be safely ignored. This would seem inconsistent with purely biological explanations, such as altered receptor number or enzyme level.

Drinkers or drug takers are all aware of similar phenomena associated with the usage of alcohol and other drugs. Typically drinking in a particular environment at one point of the day, such as one's local in the evening, can lead to the development of an ability to handle quite large amounts of alcohol without becoming inordinately discoordinated or slurred of speech. However, having a drink over a business lunch or in the morning may go to one's head much quicker.

WITHDRAWAL SYNDROME

This account of the development of tolerance does not explain why some drugs should lead to withdrawal effects. Not hearing a train go past my window is not something that is likely to plunge me into a delirious state, but it does play a part, in that the drugs that cause physical symptoms of withdrawal all produce tolerance also. This leads to subjects taking them chronically, often ending up on very large amounts.

In the case of alcohol and the opiates, these drugs compromise locus coeruleus–raphe function. This, however, cannot be substantially compromised without death ensuing. These systems, as outlined above, are crucially concerned with the regulation of vital functions such as breathing, temperature and blood pressure – functions that cannot be turned off. Accordingly, the effects of drugs that would tend to turn such functions off must be counteracted. This is achieved by the locus coeruleus adapting to the threat by increasing its activity.

If the depressing stimulus of morphine or alcohol is then removed, the locus coeruleus is left hyperactive and it is this overactivity that constitutes the core of the withdrawal syndrome, with the subject overbreathing, becoming hyperthermic and having raised blood pressure. In the face of these internal events, happenings in the external environment are not as likely to be processed accurately if at all. This is what constitutes delirium.

Whether a drug interferes with the activity of the locus coeruleus or not is, however, a matter of accident rather than a question of the perversity of personal dispositions or any intrinsic evil in the compound. For example, the hallucinogens, cocaine and the amphetamines do not cause withdrawal syndromes of this type.

 User Issues

DETOXIFICATION FROM ALCOHOL

The current management of alcohol withdrawal traditionally involves the use of diazepam, chlordiazepoxide or chlormethiazole to suppress the manifestations of withdrawal. Locus coeruleus function will usually return to normal some 1–2 weeks after withdrawal from alcohol. There have been reports indicating that clonidine and calcium channel blockers may also be useful for withdrawal but, as management with minor tranquillisers is safe and established, it seems unlikely that these other agents will find much place.

There have now been two large studies in which alcohol-dependent subjects were detoxified and put on a regimen of either naltrexone or placebo. Both of these studies have indicated that those on naltrexone are less likely to relapse. The reason for this is at present uncertain, and it is not clear whether this effect holds for all types of alcohol dependencies or for a particular subset. Another agent, acamprosate, has also been shown to reduce relapse rates (see Ch. 23).

User Issues

DETOXIFICATION FROM OPIATES

The opiates suppress locus coeruleus function more directly than does alcohol or the benzodiazepines. Based on this, it was predicted that clonidine, which reduces locus coeruleus activity, would suppress the effects of opiate withdrawal. This has proved to be the case. The use of clonidine has been replaced in recent years by lofexidine, a related agent. These drugs offer significant benefit but do not completely abolish withdrawal symptoms from opiates.

Treatment with either lofexidine or clonidine starts at 200 µg twice a day, increasing up to 1.2 mg daily for clonidine in divided doses and 2.4 mg per day for lofexidine. It is maintained for 7–10 days and then reduced over 2–4 days.

More recently, there has been a trend to combine clonidine with the opiate antagonists naloxone or naltrexone (Preston & Bigelow 1985), which push opiate users into withdrawal more rapidly than would otherwise be the case. Using them, it is possible to shorten the length of time detoxification takes. An even more recent approach has been to give naloxone under general anaesthesia to produce rapid withdrawal with minimal distress. The whole procedure only takes a matter of hours (Loimer et al 1989), although residual symptoms may persist for some days.

User Issues

BARBITURATES AND BENZODIAZEPINE DETOXIFICATION

In the case of barbiturate withdrawal, individuals are switched to benzo-diazepines and withdrawn according to the schedule outlined in Chapter 12. Where the benzodiazepines are concerned, the schedule in Chapter 12 is standard practice at present, despite the development of the benzodiazepine antagonist flumazenil, which can precipitate a more rapid withdrawal.

Physical dependence type 2

INTRODUCTION

In 1954, Olds and Milner discovered that there appeared to be pleasure spots in the brain (see Olds 1959). Implanting electrodes in certain areas of the brain, and enabling a rat to stimulate that area by pressing on a lever that activated an electric current, produced in most brain areas nothing of note. In some areas, however, the rats seemed keen on the effects of self-stimulation; in some cases, if left to their own devices, they would self-stimulate to the exclusion of all else – this was most likely to happen in a degraded environment almost completely devoid of stimulation.

As mentioned, noradrenaline was discovered in the brain in 1954. In 1959, a second catecholamine, dopamine, was identified. This was shown to be deficient in patients with Parkinson's disease. Replacement therapy, using the dopamine precursor L-dopa, brings about substantial benefits to sufferers of this disease.

The later mapping of dopamine-containing neurones showed that they, like noradrenergic neurones, tend to originate in a discrete area – the ventral tegmentum. Some of these neurones run to strictly motor areas of the brain and constitute the nigrostriatal system. It is the loss of nerve cells in this pathway that leads to Parkinson's disease.

Other dopamine-containing neurones run to higher areas of the midbrain and to cortical areas. It appears that these are centrally involved in what is termed incentive learning – the kind of learning that occurs when an animal encounters a biologically important stimulus such as food or a potential sexual partner.

The ventral tegmental system seems to be closely associated with the pleasure systems discovered by Olds and Milner. However, the picture has become far more complicated. It now seems that, far from there being pleasure hot spots in the brain, there are areas of the brain that respond to familiar signals pleasurably and unfamiliar signals with displeasure. Pleasure seems to be at least in part a function of the familiarity of the message being relayed through the system.

CRAVING

Why do so many alcohol or opiate users return to their addiction after detoxification? If the terror of withdrawal were such a significant factor in producing chronic abuse, it might be expected that anyone with the least bit of wit would keep well clear of further involvement. What perversity or self-destructive impulse is it that leads to further abuse?

The traditional response to this problem was to distinguish between physical dependence and psychological dependence. It is usually argued that the latter is a state of mind, one that may stem from deep-seated psychological difficulties. It is this state of mind that some people see as the real problem with the addictions. While it is relatively easy with modern technologies to take in drug addicts and 'dry them out', it is a much more difficult problem to ensure they remain drug free.

When asked why they return to their habits, the usual response from sufferers is in terms of cravings. The notion of cravings seems to suggest a depravity or perversity in keeping with the social opprobrium accorded to addicts. It suggests some weakness on their part that fits in with the idea they have psychological difficulties. Current research suggests that this picture is quite wrong (Pickens & Johanson 1992).

It seems, increasingly, that cravings are a very tangible physical reality and that the form of dependence that is characterised by cravings is in fact a physical dependence of another sort. In favour of this argument is the fact that not all drugs of abuse cause cravings. Cocaine, the amphetamines, nicotine, alcohol and the opiates notably do, but LSD, phencyclidine, the psychedelic drugs generally and the benzodiazepines do not.

BEHAVIOURAL SENSITISATION

Experimental work on drug effects on the brain has revealed that continued administration of certain drugs, far from leading to tolerance appears to produce just the opposite effect, even when the environment is held constant. Indeed, in a mirror image of the production of tolerance, the holding of the environment constant, in these experiments, appears to facilitate the production of increasingly enhanced effects in response to certain drugs.

This phenomenon is called behavioural sensitisation (Hand & Franklin 1986, Jaffe 1989). Certain drugs induce it, others do not. Morphine is capable of inducing both sensitisation and tolerance within the one animal: the animal develops tolerance to some of the effects of morphine, such as analgesia, and sensitisation to others – one of which is the fact that continued intake becomes increasingly pleasurable.

Initial experiments suggested that morphine produced behavioural inactivity and was somewhat unpleasant. Animals who were linked up to electrodes connected to the so-called pleasure spots in the brain were less likely to self-stimulate themselves when given morphine. This ran contrary to the popular belief that opiates are pleasurable, even though, it should be noted, the experience of many people trying them for the first time is that they are not very pleasant.

Subsequent experiments demonstrated that morphine becomes increasingly pleasant to take. Chronic exposure to morphine in experimental animals gradually brings about increases in activity and self-stimulation. There is an odd aspect to this, which is that such increases are at their height some 3 h after morphine administration, in contrast to analgesia which is at a maximum 1 h after administration. Maximal brain levels of the drug also occur 1 h, and not 3 h, after administration. Furthermore, analgesia and the respiratory depression brought about by morphine can be antagonised by morphine antagonists, such as naloxone, but the pleasurable effects of the drug are not antagonised by these agents.

APPETITES

What is happening? It appears that morphine, alcohol, cocaine and the amphetamines feed into the brain systems responsible for the generation of and satisfaction of appetites, of which the ventral tegmental system outlined above is a component part. A moment's reflection should indicate that the last thing an appetitive system could do with is tolerance to the sight of food, drink or sex, for example – rather, just the opposite. In contrast to the effect of environmental cues in helping to bring about tolerance because they signal the non-threatening, or insignificant, nature of what is happening, environmental cues might be expected to lead to increased effects where appetites are concerned. That is, we will become increasingly sensitive to aspects of an environment that indicate the possibility of food or sex or drink. Such cues should lead to increased rather than decreased interest. Typically, however, we do not notice the accumulation of environmental prompts pushing us toward the consummation of an appetite, unless we have been removed from the environment artificially for a while. Try dieting, seriously, and you will become aware of all the prompts to eat in the environment – advertisements in magazines, smells of food, cooking, etc.

The effect of public houses and the cultures surrounding both drink and drugs provide a host of small prompts, each of which prime an appetite that has already been created. This can even extend to having one's appetite aroused by the sight of needles.

Once stimulated, appetites, while not imperative, have a way of grabbing attention. It is natural to bend our minds to the satisfaction of our appetites, when they require satisfying. As the weight of cues to indulgence builds up, we typically come closer and closer to behaving on automatic pilot. We less and less regard alternative cues in the environment. Thus the hacking cough is not registered as we light up another cigarette, or the number of meals and amount of food we take are not realised as we sit down for a little soothing snack, while we worry at the same time about our figure, and the children's Christmas presents get forgotten until the drink runs out.

The establishment of such appetites can be blocked. For example, giving morphine accompanied by dopamine-blocking drugs (antipsychotics) or naloxone does block the development of behavioural sensitisation. However, once appetites have been established, they cannot easily be extirpated. Neither opiate antagonists nor antipsychotics abolish cravings for opiates once they have become established.

It does not make sense that appetites could be abolished – controlled, perhaps, but not abolished. It is possible to manage one's appetite. For example, the amount of food habitually taken bears some relation to the amount of food felt to be needed. Thus eating a lot creates a big appetite. Decreasing one's intake can lead to reduced cravings. Similarly sexual appetites are to some extent set by the frequency of indulgence. The notion that some of us are born with greater sex drives than others has little solid evidence in its favour. But, even in the case of total abstinence, we would not expect our sexual appetite to vanish entirely.

However, while appetites, once established, may not readily be abolished, the notion of craving should not be taken to imply that something has been created that is insatiable and beyond human resources to combat. For example, opiate-induced craving, while a real phenomenon, does not appear to be uncontrollable. Rather, as the experience of American GIs returning home from Vietnam suggests, the vast majority of regularly indulging individuals can put aside the habit when they are removed from social situations conducive to it. Once removed from the environmental cues that prompt cravings, only a minority of individuals have overwhelming difficulties.

Current therapeutic strategies are increasingly leaning toward the management of cravings on the model of managing appetites for food, when these are disordered as in bulimia or anorexia nervosa. The issue is often one of helping the individual set a reasonable management strategy rather than having them insist on complete self-control. For example, subjects with bulimia will often plan to eat only one meal a day. This leaves them liable to be overcome by hunger pangs on some other occasion, leading to guilty and rushed snacks, which is unsatisfying and leads in turn to eating more and more food and feeling even more guilty afterwards. Management aims at recognising when an appetite has been stimulated and how to handle it at that point, in a manner that allows the individual to bring into play the usual controls we all have where appetites are concerned but regarding which we do not normally need to be aware.

PHARMACOLOGICAL MANAGEMENT OF APPETITES

The first treatment for alcohol problems was disulfiram (Antabuse). This operates on a behavioural principle and aims to abolish an appetite or help with its control. Alcohol in the body breaks down to an aldehyde compound and then to an acid. Disulfiram blocks the conversion of the aldehyde to the acid. This leads to an unpleasant increase in the amount of the aldehyde in the bloodstream, so that after a drink or two subjects taking disulfiram may feel extremely nauseated and/or have a severe headache. This experience is supposed to deter them from taking any more alcohol. In practice, if individuals want to drink, they simply do not take their disulfiram that morning.

A similar approach has been taken with opiate users. It is common in a number of centres for opiate users who have been detoxified to be put on maintenance naltrexone. This is supposed to block the pleasure that they would get from their drugs. There is some debate about how well it does this. Naltrexone can cause dysphoria, which, in the case of an opiate user, might make them liable to seek out relief. In all cases the use of naltrexone should be delayed until the user has been opiate free for at least 5 days because of the risk of precipitating withdrawal effects. The initial dose of naltrexone is 10 mg per day, increasing to 150 mg over 2 weeks. The effects of naltrexone last up to 3 days, and therefore dosing need be only every 3 days.

However, another use for naltrexone has emerged recently, which stems from the probable role of brain opioid systems in the genesis of appetites. A number of trials have now indicated that the use of naltrexone after alcohol detoxification reduces the risk of relapse, probably by reducing craving (Volpicelli et al 1992). This has led to it being licensed for this purpose.

Another drug licensed for the management of relapse in alcoholism is acamprosate. This acts on the γ-aminobutyric acid (GABA) system on which the benzodiazepines act. Whether it produces a direct anticraving effect or reduces cravings by being in some way anxiolytic is less clear. Naltrexone and acamprosate seem to work best for different patient groups. There is, however, very little clinical work aimed at mapping out which groups of patients will respond to which agent. This is not the kind of work that drug companies are likely to be inclined to do, as it would mean settling for a restricted segment of the market.

Finally, bupropion, a dopamine and noradrenaline reuptake inhibitor, marketed as an antidepressant in the United States (Wellbutrin), has recently been licensed under the trade name Zyban for smoking cessation. Again, this seems to work, in part at least, by minimising cravings for nicotine and cigarettes.

There is every reason for believing that each of these agents may in fact work for particular individuals, rather than for different conditions such as alcohol, opiate or nicotine dependency. Judicious clinical trials of each, even in the conditions for which they are not licensed, are appropriate. The rationality with which these drugs are used would be further enhanced by studies that pay heed to how takers who find the drugs effective say they are working.

PSYCHOLOGICAL FACTORS IN SUBSTANCE ABUSE

The induction of appetites and cravings used to be seen as psychological dependence. If it is, in fact, just as much a physical process as the dependence and tolerance that underpin withdrawal, is there any other psychology involved?

There almost certainly is (Bakalar & Grinspoon 1989). For example, LSD, phencyclidine and many of the new designer drugs do not cause either physical dependence or craving, yet they are abused – and increasingly so. Despite evidence that phencyclidine, for example, led to a considerable number of deaths and despite the fact that it did not lead to any obvious euphoria, during the 1980s it became – for a period – the second most common drug of abuse in the USA. Why?

Common to many of these drugs is the fact that they alter consciousness. As a result, they are interesting to take. They also permit an escape from reality. This suggests that two factors in their use will be a certain amount of playful activity and a need to escape reality.

As regards playfulness, there are two aspects to this. First, there is the notion that people will try something new simply because it is there, just as they will climb unclimbable mountains or run across continents. In addition, allied to these things 'simply being there', there is the matter of our innate curiosity. The other aspect to playfulness is that it is a means to handle boredom. For want of something better to do, humans will turn to virtually anything, no matter how dangerous it may be. Even Russian roulette, as Grahame Greene confessed, may be tried as a way of livening things up or structuring them. Indeed, it can often seem that everything that happens is just a game to counteract boredom, from intrepid mountain climbing to scientific endeavours, the writing of books or the taking of the most recently designed drugs.

When we are bored, we do things: we eat or shop. New clothes, books or records often seem to restore a sense of purpose to things. One of the central problems of treating alcohol and opiate dependence, aside from physical dependence of both types, is the question of what will the individual now do to structure their time. Frequently it turns out that keeping an alcohol-dependent individual away from pubs also means effectively abolishing their entire social life at a stroke. What are they to do with the yawning hole that opens up where their social life used to be?

From this perspective, the question of drug abuse becomes, to a large extent, a matter of accident, which stems from the fact that, at various points in life, some of the activities available to be sampled cause physical dependence and others produce cravings – just as it is an accident that some of the pursuits available to be taken up, such as motorcycling, have a high fatality rate.

Just as with motorbikes, it seems that if one can get through a playful–experimental stage between the ages of 15 and 25 years without having been too involved in high-risk pursuits or in taking of drugs with a high dependence potential, then one is not likely to be killed accidentally or to become substance dependent accidentally. It is not that playfulness diminishes after this age, so much as that the burden of commitments and responsibilities restricts for most of us the opportunities to participate.

DISINHIBITION

Along with the fear that drugs may cause dependence, there is a fear that they may change personalities by either abolishing the normal personality of an individual or by liberating demons from the unconscious. The adage *in vino veritas* is often taken to mean something like this. Both alcohol and benzodiazepines are supposed to disinhibit people. What is happening?

One thing that may happen, but which is relatively rare, is that these compounds, like almost any other drug that gets into the brain, may cause dissociative reactions. These are outlined in Chapters 2, 5 & 11.

The more usual disinhibition on alcohol is socially disinhibited behaviour, which may involve an inappropriate pinching of bottoms or, more seriously, violence towards one's partner. In such cases, it is typically argued that alcohol is a general depressant that depresses brain inhibitory pathways first. Accordingly, with an inhibition of inhibitions, there is supposedly a brief period of disinhibition before increasing levels of alcohol blot out all behaviour in a general stupor. The supposed inhibitory tracts that are especially sensitive to the effects of alcohol, benzodiazepines or barbiturates are rarely specified. If pushed, advocates of this position tend to suggest that activity of the frontal lobes of the brain is the first to be affected by alcohol, this being a brain region that has general executive or inhibitory control over all other brain regions. However, there is little evidence to support this scheme of things – other than the popular presumption that something like this must be the case. But must it?

There is no question that alcohol discoordinates and slurs speech. This can be demonstrated reliably in experimental situations and can be correlated precisely with the actions of alcohol on coordination centres, such as the cerebellum. Alcohol and benzodiazepines also reverse the inhibition that fear may cause, enabling someone to go on stage and give a lecture, for instance. But in the case of someone behaving outrageously in a public situation, who then gets some troubling news such as their house is on fire, they are liable to 'sober up' instantly – although they may still remain less than perfectly coordinated as they set about getting home. Or the social disinhibition that I show one evening may be quite different to the disinhibition I show the following evening, in contrast to the discoordination, which will be approximately the same.

An alternative account of what is happening is that, misled by the very real effects of alcohol on gait, coherence and anxiety, we also put other changes in behaviours down to the drug that are more properly seen as a function of the social situation in which it is taken. In general, there is a gap between our knowledge of what drugs reliably do and our difficulties in explaining the complexities of social interactions that can be exploited by both substance abusers and those who would put down societal ills to such abuses.

There are a number of factors that almost compel such an identification. There is, first, our tendency to seek an explanation for what is happening to us. This shows up well in placebo-controlled studies of drugs generally. It is the common experience of many investigators that a not inconsiderable number of subjects have to be withdrawn from such studies because of intolerable side effects of the placebo.

A probable explanation for this is that, of 100 subjects who enter a study, a number of them are bound to get obscure aches or physical complaints of some sort, on at least one occasion anyway. Such discomforts are borne none too happily in the normal course of events. We put up with them because it is not clear what the cause is and accordingly we have little option. But if they occur during a week when we are taking some new pill, it may be very difficult to believe that the pill is not responsible.

Applied to alcohol, such arguments yield the following picture. That alcohol itself does not disinhibit. That alcohol is commonly consumed in situations where the usual rules of restraint are altered. That alcohol, by altering the physical state, provides a cue that a certain state has been entered in which the subject has learnt that the usual rules of accountability do not apply. Thus, if after drinking I go home and beat my wife, I know that my friends, who know me for a basically decent sort, will not attribute what has happened to me but rather to the drink they saw me having – and the fact that I may have had a bit too much. This, it should be noted, is not an *in vino veritas* argument.

These issues also play a considerable part in the abuse of other drugs. In the case of cannabis, it is quite clear that takers have to 'learn' to get stoned. Initial taking of the drug produces the effects on perception that are typical of cannabis but not 'stoned' behaviour. It is subsequent smoking in the company of others who are 'stoned' that brings about stoned behaviour.

When it comes to the abuse of street drugs, generally, the analysis of urine samples indicates that users are often taking mixtures that contain a wide variety of white powders – and perhaps none of the particular white powder they think they are getting. Some of these extras may be other stimulants, such as strychnine, but the behaviour the users display will be behaviour appropriate to the culture surrounding the drug they think they are on.

Physical dependence type 3

HISTORICAL PERSPECTIVE

Until the 1940s, the main theories about addiction focused on the personality of the addict. Addiction was a matter of addictive and sociopathic personalities – low-lifes. This began to change only with a proposal by Abe Wikler that alcohol dependence was maintained by fear of the withdrawal state and the subsequent application of the same idea to opiate and barbiturate dependence. Wikler's idea that withdrawal was important revolutionised treatment of the addictions (Healy 2001).

The next breakthrough came in the 1960s following the work of Olds and Milner (see Olds 1959). This gave rise to the concept that certain drugs had an addictive potential. Animals might crave them. The concept of drug dependence emerged to explain why people became addicted to cocaine, amphetamine and other drugs that had few withdrawal effects associated with them.

ANTIPSYCHOTIC DEPENDENCE

But while all this was happening, in 1957 Leo Hollister conducted a placebo-controlled randomised controlled trial of chlorpromazine in tuberculosis. On discontinuing treatment 6 months' later, it became clear that up to one-third of those on chlorpromazine had a significant physical dependence and great difficulty in stopping the drug (Hollister 1998, Hollister et al 1960). By the mid-1960s, a large number of research groups had reported marked and severe physical dependence on antipsychotics. At an international meeting in 1966 the concept of therapeutic drug dependence was recognised (Battegay 2000).

The kind of problem that was recognised was as follows. People, commonly women, who take 1 mg trifluoperazine (Stelazine) per day for several months might be unable to get off this, ever again, in their lives (Tranter & Healy 1998). Another form this dependence took was tardive dyskinesia, which was first recognised on discontinuing antipsychotics. This set of disfiguring facial and sometimes truncal movements could last for years after the discontinuation of treatment (see Chs 1 & 2).

Despite this, the concept of therapeutic drug dependence vanished almost immediately after it was born. It was 30 years before another article on dependence on antipsychotics appeared. What had happened?

In the late 1960s the Western world was in upheaval, and student revolutions from the United States through Europe across to Japan were closely associated with antipsychiatry. Departments of psychiatry were occupied and research was brought to a halt. The new psychotropic drugs were a central part of what was happening. From the same laboratories that had produced the antipsychotics came LSD, the benzodiazepines and the oral contraceptives, all of which were transforming society. Previously drug treatment was a matter of treating diseases in order to restore a person to their place in the social order. These new drugs threatened the social order. They gave women freedom from men and they threatened to liberate the young from the social hierarchies imposed by their parents.

The establishment responded with a war on drugs. LSD, cocaine, amphetamine and a range of other drugs were scheduled. The supposed characteristic of the bad drugs was that they caused dependence, even though LSD, for instance, appears to produce neither physical dependence nor craving. If dependence was a characteristic of bad drugs, good drugs therefore could not cause it. The idea of therapeutic dependence vanished (Healy 2001).

The problem returned to haunt the establishment in the 1980s when benzodiazepine dependence was recognised. The initial response from psychiatric associations and other medical bodies was that there was no such problem. The subsequent response was to distinguish between dependence and addiction. This distinction was, strictly speaking, correct: the benzodiazepines do not lead to addiction in the sense that individuals will mortgage their houses and souls to get a supply of these drugs. However, this subtle distinction was lost on the public at large. Where before drug users had been seen as social outcasts, the new benzodiazepine 'addicts' were seen as victims of a medico-pharmaceutical complex (see Ch. 11).

The consequences of this are with us still. Buspirone, the first of the drugs active on the serotonergic system, was initially marketed as a non-dependence-producing anxiolytic (see Ch. 12). It never took off because, besieged by legal actions about the benzodiazepines, physicians were sceptical of the idea that there could be a non-dependence-producing benzodiazepine, while consumers had grown wary of the entire idea of treating the stresses of life chemically.

This meant that when the selective serotonin reuptake inhibitors (SSRIs) came on stream they were marketed as antidepressants rather than anxiolytics. Patients who, in the 1970s and 1980s, had so obviously been seen as cases of anxiety to be treated with an anxiolytic were, under the marketing weight of the pharmaceutical companies, transformed in the 1990s into clear-cut and obvious cases of depression to be treated with antidepressants.

In Japan the problem with benzodiazepine dependence never happened and, as a consequence, no SSRI is yet available on the Japanese market as an antidepressant. In Japan through the 1990s the antidepressant market remained a small one compared with the market in the West. In contrast, anxiolytics remained widely prescribed. In other words, the age of depression that we have had in recent years in the West, with depression being touted as one of the greatest causes of disability in the world today, stems from the conflicts about dependence on therapeutic drugs.

STRESS SYNDROMES

The concept of therapeutic drug dependence runs smack up against current concepts of addiction and dependency. Tardive dyskinesia is a clear example of a syndrome arising from dependence on antipsychotics or SSRI antidepressants. However, this syndrome is not obvious only when treatment is halted: it emerges during the course of treatment. In other words, it is a consequence of a drug acting as a stressor on the brain. For some individuals who are vulnerable to this particular kind of stress, the consequences are that some brain systems get 'pushed out of shape' and simply do not revert to normal on discontinuation of treatment (Healy & Tranter 1999).

When dependence on antipsychotics was first described during the 1960s, it was clear that neurological problems such as tardive dyskinesia could be precipitated, but these accounted for only about one-third of the presentations. In other cases patients had dysthymic syndromes, heat and pain dysregulation syndromes, stress insensitivity, disturbances of the autonomic system and other disturbances.

Given that negative syndromes are thought of as being part of schizophrenia, the emergence of stress syndromes of these kinds should make it clear that one of the consequences of these syndromes is that it becomes almost impossible after the first few months of treatment with an antipsychotic to know where the treatment begins and ends and where the disease begins and ends. This is not an argument against treatment. It is simply to state that the act of therapy changes people for ever, and that both the therapist and the patient need to be aware of this and to work together to manage the situation for the best.

A similar situation applies to antidepressants. In recent years dependence on SSRIs has come into focus. This appears to happen in up to one-quarter of individuals who take SSRIs. The problems on discontinuation can be marked, and may last for several weeks or months. As with antipsychotic and benzodiazepine dependence, the response of physicians to difficulties in discontinuing treatment is that this is simply a manifestation of the illness for which treatment was being given and that treatment should simply be restarted.

Just as with the antipsychotics, it seems that in the course of treatment with SSRIs the effects of treatment can wear off and may be replaced by a variety of other syndromes. These have been generically referred to under the heading of 'poop out', a term that refers to SSRIs seemingly losing their potency in the course of treatment. In fact, it may well be that treatment with SSRIs sets people up for a perpetual cycle of neurological difficulties. It is too early to say just yet.

However, importantly, discontinuation syndromes can be distinguished from new illness episodes. In the case of either the antipsychotics or SSRIs, for instance, problems that arise within a few days or weeks of discontinuing treatment should lead to suspicion that this is a discontinuation syndrome rather than a new illness episode. If the person has discontinued treatment while seemingly well, it should be several months before a new psychotic or affective episode appears.

Second, if, on the emergence of problems, re-instituting treatment leads to the problems clearing up quickly, this indicates a discontinuation syndrome until proven otherwise. In the case of new illness episodes emerging some months after treatment has been discontinued, the common clinical experience is that these respond slowly and often poorly to the treatment that helped the person to get well previously. Much higher doses of treatment may be needed.

Finally, if the pattern of symptoms shown by the person is somewhat different to the initial pattern of symptoms that they had, this again is good evidence for a discontinuation problem.

The consequences of therapeutic drug dependence (stress syndromes) are far reaching. Essentially, the recognition that severe dependence can happen on antipsychotics and antidepressants punctures a hole in all current theories of addiction and dependence:

- Tolerance is not required for therapeutic drug dependence to happen.
- The drugs do not have to be pleasurable or craved.
- The personality of the taker appears to play little part in what has happened.

Current biological theories of addiction stress the enduring brain changes that happen following intake of illicit drugs, but these enduring brain changes are no greater and certainly no longer lasting than the enduring brain changes brought about by antipsychotics or antidepressants. A disease model of addiction based on the idea that this is a disease because there are enduring brain changes after illicit drug use does not hold up unless it is conceded that treatment with antipsychotics or antidepressants also causes brain disease in a significant number of patients.

Addiction is a social concept. It is social in two senses. It is social in the sense that drugs of addiction are ones that society has deemed to be addictive – their addiction potential does not arise from some biological factor. Drugs of addiction are social in a second sense in that the previous chapters have shown the exquisite interplay between environmental and biological factors. Addictions of the kind that society is so concerned about, while having clear biological components, arise in degraded environments. Tackling these problems is unlikely ever to be simply a matter of treatment with a further drug.

References

Bakalar JB, Grinspoon L (1989) Drug control in a free society. Cambridge: Cambridge University Press.

Baker TB, Tiffany ST (1985) Morphine tolerance as habituation. Psychological Review 92: 78–108.

Battegay R (2000) Forty-four years in psychiatry and psychopharmaocology. In: Healy D, ed. The psychopharmacologists, vol 3, pp 371–393. London: Arnold.

Hand TH, Franklin KB (1986) Associative factors in the effects of morphine on self-stimulation. Psychopharmacology 88: 472–479.

Healy D (2001) The creation of psychopharmacology. Cambridge, MA: Harvard University Press.

Healy D, Tranter R (1999) Pharmacopsychiatric stress syndromes. With commentaries by Ashton H, Baldessarini R, Haddad P and by Anderson I, Hollister L, Tyrer P. Journal of Psychopharmacology 13: 287–290.

Hollister LE (1998) From hypertension to psychopharmacology: a serendipitous career. In: Healy D, ed. The psychopharmacologists, vol 2, pp 215–235. London: Arnold.

Hollister LE, Eikenberry DT, Raffel S (1960) Chlorpromazine in nonpsychotic patients with pulmonary tuberculosis. American Review of Respiratory Diseases 81: 562–566.

Jaffe JH (1989) Addictions: what does biology have to tell? International Review of Psychiatry 1: 51–62.

Loimer N, Schmid RW, Presslich D, Lenz K (1989) Continuous naloxone administration suppresses opiate withdrawal symptoms in human opiate addicts during detoxification treatment. Journal of Psychiatric Research 23: 81–86.

Olds J (1959) Studies of neuropharmacologicals by electrical and chemical manipulation of the brain in animals with chronically implanted electrodes. In: Bradley P, Deniker P, Radouco-Thomas C, eds. Neuropsychopharmacology, pp 20–32. Amsterdam: Elsevier.

Pickens RW, Johanson C-E (1992) Craving: consensus of status and agenda for future research. Drug and Alcohol Dependence 30: 127–131.

Preston KL, Bigelow GE (1985) Pharmacological advances in addiction treatment. International Journal of the Addictions 20: 845–867.

Tranter R, Healy D (1998) Neuroleptic discontinuation syndromes. Journal of Psychopharmacology 12: 306–311.

Volpicelli JR, Alterman AJ, Hayashida M et al (1992) Naltrexone in the treatment of alcohol dependence. Archives of General Psychiatry 49: 876–880.

Consent, abuse and liability

SECTION CONTENTS

Consent

INTRODUCTION

Over the past two decades there has been a shift within healthcare from an expectation that patients with medical problems should entrust themselves passively to the care of physicians to an expectation that they should cooperate in their own care, and even have some responsibility for the outcome of medical procedures they undergo. These changes are reflected in the terms we use: for instance, the word patient, which means someone who endures, is often replaced by terms such as client or consumer, which suggest a more active and discriminating participant in the medical process.

Informed consent was not an issue in medical practice 20 years ago. Today, it forms a central issue in a number of ethical codes applied to medicine, from the Nuremberg Code to the Helsinki Code, and others. It may seem immediately clear what informed consent is, but a moment's reflection will dispel this illusion.

In a key study carried out some years ago, volunteers were asked to participate in a study in which they were told that a drug was being investigated and they would be paid for participation in the study (Epstein & Lasagna 1969). They were given varying amounts of information about the drug's properties and expected side effects. The more information the volunteers were given, the less likely they were to take the drug, despite being offered money. When they found out that the drug being investigated was aspirin, most subjects said that what they now knew would not influence how likely they were to take aspirin when they went home for a headache or fever.

Despite its name, therefore, there seems to be a sense in which informed consent cannot be about being fully informed. Too much information can prejudice valid consent just as readily as too little. Rather than meaning fully informed consent, it would seem that informed consent must mean something more like valid or voluntary consent (Levine 1986). There are two key issues. One is whether the consent is voluntary. Another is the issue of adequate or appropriate information, which, in practice, cannot be separated from the question of comprehension on the part of the person being informed. Finally, there is an issue of legal competence.

VOLUNTARY CONSENT

When an individual attends for a consultation, there is an implicit assumption that they are seeking help and will take the advice offered by the doctor, psychologist or community nurse. In this regard, a prescription often seems to function in two ways: on the one hand as a treatment for a particular condition, but on the other as a symbol of the advice being offered. Taking a little piece of paper away with them from the surgery leaves the person feeling that they are not alone in trying to sort the problem out.

Arguably, however, the question of informed consent has come to prominence in recent years precisely because we no longer accept this as a proper and fitting way of going about things. We do not voluntarily consent to current practice. There is a problem in that a surgery or outpatient setting is not one that is conducive to any of us being able to articulate our concerns. We may be worried by the condition that has led us to seek help. We may be anxious when faced with the doctor, nurse, psychologist, or whoever. We may be aware of the queue of others after us, who need to be seen. Once the allotted appointment time of 10–15 min is up, it is often very clear that the doctor is wondering whether they are likely to get to lunch or to get home if all consultations during this session are going to take as long.

For these and other reasons, we often take the script. However, available evidence suggests that most people being treated with antidepressants, for instance, do not take them for longer than 4 weeks, despite recommendations that they be taken for 3–4 months. One reason for this may be that the pill prescribed does not suit them, but another reason that seems likely is that many people being treated do not voluntarily consent to the treatment and, once away from the pressures generated in clinical settings, they withdraw consent.

The lack of consent involved here probably does not reflect an opposition to drug treatment so much as an opposition to a style of treatment delivery, in which an authoritarian doctor decides what is best for a patient and issues instructions. Implicit in this authoritarian approach is the idea that medical science has developed to such an extent that there is something approaching certainty regarding the proper management of most conditions, and the doctor is an authority – or at least knows better than the patient – what they should be doing.

In contrast, a cogent case has been argued by a number of commentators in recent years that medical care should involve a greater acknowledgement of ignorance or uncertainty on the part of the practitioner and an invitation to collaboration (Bursztajn et al 1990, Kleinman 1988, Seedhouse 1991). According to this approach, treatment would be a matter of negotiation rather than one of instruction: a negotiation that would recognise that an illness is one event within the drama of someone's life and that, for a variety of reasons, rigid adherence to a treatment regimen, with all the side effects that may be entailed, may not be that person's top priority.

From this perspective, the issue of voluntary consent becomes a matter of good clinical practice. This is not something that can be properly defined at law. Even signed consent forms, in certain circumstances, may not be interpreted by a court as indicating valid consent, while on the other hand the lack of a signed consent will not necessarily be taken to indicate a lack of consent should someone apply for legal redress for a claimed injury.

The law is only a blunt instrument. Ideally a profession should give some indications about what it thinks on certain key issues. In this case, what would seem to be required are a set of statements about what psychotropic drugs do and what their role is in the management of nervous disorders. The problem in mental health work lies in getting the different professionals comprising a mental health team to come to some agreed form of words regarding the treatments they deliver. On a national scale it would be even more difficult to get all psychiatrists, for example, to agree amongst themselves on a common form of words for what the antipsychotics do. In the absence of such agreements, patients exposed to different mental health professionals are all too likely to be given quite different, even contradictory, views on the nature or purpose of their treatment. The possession of a book such as this can perhaps in some way redress this problem, by offering a clear set of statements with which their therapist may agree or disagree, and in the process reveal something of their approach to therapy.

A clinical style that is more likely to result in valid consent to taking the risks involved in any act of healthcare hinges, in my opinion, on an ability of healthcare professionals to live with explicit ignorance about the likely outcome of their interventions in the circumstances of their patient's life. The acknowledgement of ignorance and the sharing of knowledge and power that such an approach advocates is not one that all healthcare professionals agree is appropriate or one that all can live with easily, even in limited circumstances. This book, however, has been written in the belief that such an approach is necessary.

INFORMATION AND COMPREHENSION

As regards the act of informing someone about the risks and benefits of treatments, how much information needs to be on offer? Most commentators come down in favour of informing the taker of a drug of the significant risks associated with treatment rather than making them aware of every possible risk. There are a number of issues here.

One is the question of being able to make an informed judgement of whether to consent to treatment or not. A bald list of side effects or complications is unlikely to help any of us to make up our minds. In contrast, meeting someone who is taking the drug or who has undergone the treatment in question is more likely to offer a tangible example of the issues involved.

The issue of a real-life flesh and blood example rather than abstract lists also brings home the fact that, in making decisions, there is often a question of isolation involved. It is not an easy matter for anyone to be faced with 'facts' in clinical settings, which often bring with them implicit requests to make our minds up soon, without the benefit of prior knowledge of the issues involved. Where psychotropic drug taking is concerned, this isolation and the disempowerment that it brings about could be managed by encouraging prospective drug takers to visit local user groups or MIND branches, or by having advocates on wards.

Groups such as MIND have been seen as hostile to medical practice in the past. Where indeed they are hostile, caution is indicated, but even there a pattern of more frequent referral might encourage a more collaborative approach. This could only be good for the community in general. The role of the community at large in accepting medical practices is often overlooked. A century ago there was much more commonality of understanding and interest between medical practitioners and those they sought to treat. With the relentless progress of technical developments in the latter half of the twentieth century, this community of understanding has all but disintegrated. In the case of the benzodiazepines, the controversies were fuelled in part by the larger non-drug-taking community deciding against these drugs.

A further important point is whether the information that is given comes with implicit or explicit permission to return with further concerns and queries at a later date, or even the permission to consult a third party. In this case, the privileges of the wealthy, who think nothing of seeking further advice elsewhere if they are not happy with what they have paid for, contain a pointer to the state of affairs that would be desirable for all.

Finally, on the question of information, there is the issue of comprehension. Clinical settings are often very stressful and there is a good deal of research to suggest that only half of the information imparted in a consultation is retained afterwards. One way to overcome this would be to copy letters sent to the patient's general practitioner, detailing what has happened at the consultation, to the patient also. This would give patients an opportunity to remind themselves of the recommendations that were made and give them a chance to review these recommendations in a less stressful setting (Fitzgerald et al 1996, Healy 1995).

The language in which recommendations are made may pose its own problems. The practice of medicine, as with the practice of anything else, involves the comprehension of a jargon. This jargon becomes so commonplace to practitioners that they often forget that the terms they use may be effectively meaningless to the person they are seeing. A term such as schizophrenia, for example, is likely to suggest something akin to a split or multiple personality disorder to most lay people – a condition that would not, on the face of it, appear to be appropriately treated with drug therapy.

In clinical trials, for example, I have regularly found that, despite what may have seemed to me to be clear instructions, a patient may simply not grasp that, of the two pills they are taking, only one is active. Another issue is the question of antidotes. For instance, many patients do not appreciate that the anticholinergic drugs they are taking (see Ch. 3) are actually reversing changes brought about by the antipsychotic drug they are also taking.

 User Issues

LEGAL COMPETENCE

Where mental health matters are concerned, the question of legal competence revolves around the issue of whether the person has been detained compulsorily in a hospital and for treatment against their wishes. Detention assumes that the patient is not, at the time of detention, capable of validly consenting to what appears to be the best available treatment for their condition. All too often, the interpretation put on the status of a detained patient is that he or she can be forced to take treatment. This is not the case. The forcible administration of medication, whether the individual is a voluntary or detained patient, may provide the basis for a legitimate claim of assault. Conversely, in circumstances where it is clear that there is an emergency – someone has been violent or is clearly threatening injury to themselves or others – this assault may be justifiable, whether or not the individual has been detained under the Mental Health Act.

The grey area is where mental health staff suspect that problems may be brewing and that a patient may soon become violent. A concern about potential trouble is more likely to lead to an earlier intervention with medication in circumstances in which there are staff shortages or where staff training is such that there is little confidence in non-pharmacological methods of managing difficult behaviour. The forcible administration of medication in these latter circumstances may well amount to an assault.

Far from permitting such assaults, the spirit of detention under the Mental Health Act is that patients thereby detained should be treated as though their relatives were constantly present. The treatment should be such that a relative would be likely to approve were they present to witness what was happening. The Act was, after all, enacted to protect patients. It is not there to legalise assault in certain circumstances.

Having said this, it should be recognised that what actually happens often depends on the persuasive skills of staff members. Many individuals have considerable skill at persuading others to go along with a sensible course of action. There are probably a number of components to such skills, ranging from sheer physical presence and/or force of personality to a number of other tricks

continued

of the trade. Such skills appear to me to be in danger of being lost, and the current over-reliance on pharmacological methods of treatment tends to militate against the development of such skills. The heavily prescriptive nature of recent Codes of Practice enacted under the Mental Health Act may also be having an effect on the confidence of staff to act in the best interests of patients.

COMPLIANCE

There is a very considerable overlap between the areas of consent and compliance. Those who do not consent to treatment are unlikely to comply with it afterwards. Many people, when they consent, do so only provisionally. For instance, a consent to antidepressant treatment will often involve an agreement to take the medication only until some improvement appears; it will not in the first instance have meant to the patient an agreement to go on taking medication for months or years.

In response to indications of poor compliance with antidepressants, the pharmaceutical industry has gone some way down the road to provide the simplest possible regimens – one pill a day in the case of some of the SSRIs. This, however, should not be thought of as the answer to problems with compliance. The issues involved in non-compliance hinge primarily on relationships and education, not on whether the pills come in a once-a-day formulation. Current research suggests that the greatest single determinant of compliance is the quality of the relationship between the patient and their keyworker or prescriber. This is caught best by William Osler's famous quip that the distinguishing feature of human beings is their propensity to industrially self-medicate: in other words, patients often have much more faith in their pills than in their therapists. It may speak volumes for their relationship with their therapist if, against this background, they choose to give up treatment.

Another important element in the equation is an individual's personal situation. Becoming a patient may be just one more episode in a personal drama – a drama that may involve getting or holding down a job, sexual relations, driving safely, and so much more (Kleinman 1988). Nursing staff and other mental health keyworkers may be much more aware of this than their medical colleagues, and could probably do a great deal to minimise confrontations by emphasising difficulties with side effects.

One of the weapons a patient or their keyworker can use in the face of medical power is the weapon of data. Filling up rating scales such as the LUNSERS (Liverpool University Side Effect Rating Scale) (Day et al 1995) is a way to face a physician with data; if the physician is being as scientific as they claim, this tests how they will respond to data. A more specific version of the same would use specially designed rating scales for each problem being faced by the patient (see Fig. 25.1). Using scales such as this, the individual (perhaps helped by a keyworker) would rate how much difficulty they were having from voices, for instance, and how much from a side effect such as weight

Self-assessment questionnaire

Usual experiences/problems (enter your own problem)

[1] Today, how much have you had paranoid feelings/low mood, etc?

Not at all ☐☐☐☐☐☐☐☐☐ A great deal

[2] Today, how much have you heard voices?

Not at all ☐☐☐☐☐☐☐☐☐ A great deal

Distress caused by unusual experiences/problems

[1] Today, how much have you been distressed by your paranoid feelings?

Not at all ☐☐☐☐☐☐☐☐☐ A great deal

[2] Today, how much have you been distressed by voices?

Not at all ☐☐☐☐☐☐☐☐☐ A great deal

Side effects (enter your own side effect)

[1] Today, how much have you had agitation caused by your drugs?

Not at all ☐☐☐☐☐☐☐☐☐ A great deal

[2] Today, how much have you had dry mouth/sexual dysfunction, etc?

Not at all ☐☐☐☐☐☐☐☐☐ A great deal

Attitudes to medication

[1] Today, I have felt that my medication:

Has not helped at all ☐☐☐☐☐☐☐☐☐ Has helped a great deal

[2] Today, I have been distressed by my side effects:

Not at all ☐☐☐☐☐☐☐☐☐ A great deal

Figure 25.1 Rating scales used to determine a person's experience while taking psychotropic medication.

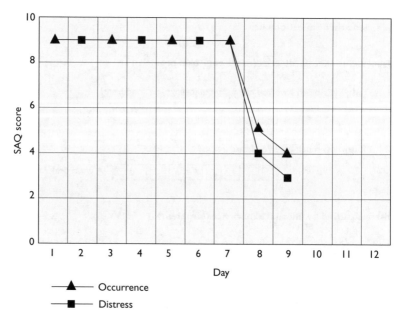

Figure 25.2 Occurrence and distress caused by paranoid feelings, as rated by self-assessment questionnaire (SAQ).

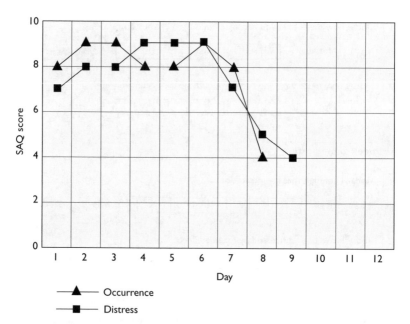

Figure 25.3 Occurrence and distress caused by voices, as rated by self-assessment questionnaire (SAQ).

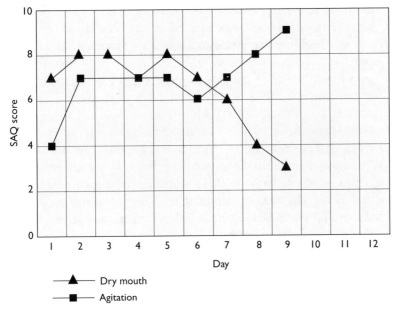

Figure 25.4 Dry mouth and agitation as rated by self-assessment questionnaire (SAQ).

gain, stiffness or sexual dysfunction. The progress of problems stemming from both the illness and the treatment could be charted over the course of several weeks in this fashion and presented to the prescriber (Figs 25.2–25.4). If the prescriber refuses to respond to these data, or if their behaviour is not manipulable by feedback of this sort, it may be time to change prescriber.

PRESCRIBING

The role of prescribing in issues of compliance and consent also needs to be considered. A prescription, initially, was an order to a pharmacist to dispense a particular medication, but until quite recently it was not the only way a patient could obtain medication. Most drugs, including thalidomide for example, were sold over the counter (OTC). Alternatively, based on an earlier prescription, a patient could go back to the pharmacist for virtually endless repeats.

The situation effectively changed following the thalidomide disaster and the amendments to the Food and Drugs Act in the USA in 1962 (Healy 1997). Before 1962, there had been resistance to the idea that the US Food and Drug Administration (FDA) should have the power to make new drugs available on prescription only. The prescription-only category had been introduced in 1914 to control the availability of drugs such as cocaine and the opiates. In 1951, it was extended to restrict the availability of the first really effective agents, the new antibiotics. This seemed odd to many. Why should a system designed for addicts be applied to free citizens? Since this system was copper-fastened in place in 1962, all of us have effectively been forced to hand over control of our healthcare to professionals in a way that we did not have to do before.

In recent years, some of the new 'wonder' drugs have become available OTC – the histamine H_2 blockers such as cimetidine and ranitidine, for instance. Is there any reason why the SSRIs or antipsychotics could not also be available OTC? With respect to safety and possible interactions with other drugs, the SSRIs are at least as safe as the H_2 blockers. If chlorpromazine had been available OTC, it seems a safe bet that it would never have been self-prescribed by users in the megadoses that were administered by clinicians during the 1960s, 1970s and 1980s. The hazards stemming from high-dose use are something that users would be unlikely to have inflicted upon themselves. It is more likely that the regimens users would have opted for would probably have been pretty close to what medical opinion 40 years later seems to be coming around to recommending as optimal.

Sold OTC, the antidepressants would probably have been marketed as tonics rather than antidepressants: they improve sleep, appetite, energy, etc. Seen in this light, they might be far more acceptable to many people. Part of the appeal behind alternative medicine and the use of health foods is that this kind of management leaves control of health in one's own hands and there are not the same disease implications. If you are stressed or burnt out – something we all are from time to time – you can take St John's Wort. To get Prozac, you have to be given depression first of all.

The prescription question is bound up with the question of disease. In 1962, the FDA attempted to minimise the risks of treatment by restricting the use of drugs to those who were genuinely ill, so that any risks brought about by a drug could be weighed in the balance of clear benefits also produced. In the case of depression, it would seem that many people simply do not accept a disease model of depression: they do not consent to treatment on these premises and, as a consequence, they very often do not comply.

Pharmacological abuse

When chlorpromazine was first introduced, doctors prescribed and patients took what they were given. The prescription of a medicine now, however, is much more likely to be based on the assumption that a patient should understand the condition for which the prescription is given, the nature of any treatment, its duration, its chances of success and the risks of side effects. Patients should be free to ask for any information they want from the prescriber, who will respond genuinely.

Clearly, respect for the autonomy of the patient has to be balanced against a respect for the autonomy of others. Uniquely in psychiatric practice it is necessary on occasion to give treatment without consent, but society has put mechanisms in place to compensate for a patient's loss of autonomy in such situations (Brabbins et al 1996, Ormrod 1987). The argument below does not apply to emergency situations or to the small number of situations facing all practitioners that amount *de facto* to a community treatment order, where clinicians may be operating with partial or grudging consent from patients. The argument is aimed at situations, particularly with antipsychotics, where a paternalistic approach to patients may involve an insidious loss of autonomy, which may be counter-therapeutic and ethically dubious.

THE PROBLEM

Consider the following. Many patients, when first admitted to hospital, will be started on medication regimens that they will not know exceed *British National Formulary* limits and greatly exceed the regimens that have been shown by research to be optimally effective. They are unlikely to know that there is rarely a pharmacological justification for the co-prescription of two different oral antipsychotics or for a combination of both an oral and depot antipsychotic. They may not clearly know that the anticholinergic agent they are taking has been given as an antidote to the side effects of the primary medication. If they do know this, they are unlikely to know that, quite commonly, it would be possible to avoid the need for an anticholinergic agent or about the difficulties that these agents may cause in their own right, if the doses of the primary medication were lowered sufficiently. If they are on a combination of antidepressants and antipsychotics, they almost certainly will not know that their 'depression' may be a consequence of treatment with antipsychotics and, as such, will not be responsive to antidepressant medication.

Doubts have been expressed as to how often, in practice, patients validly consent to many prescribed regimens, and growing concerns have prompted a working party of the Royal College of Psychiatrists to issue guidelines covering some aspects of prescribing (Thompson 1994). Against this background, it seems possible that in clinical practice betrayals of trust occur, and indeed that situations may arise that are 'abusive'. It may be instructive, therefore, to consider to what extent dynamics that are familiar from other areas of abuse might apply.

As in other forms of abuse, a 'victim' of 'abusive prescribing' may be dependent on the 'abuser' (Healy et al 1998). This dependence may be brought about by virtue of an unavailability of psychiatric services in the victim's area other than through the prescriber, and by virtue of the unavailability of psychotropic compounds other than by prescription. The victim, therefore, may have to maintain an interaction with the perpetrator and may in the process have to cope with the fact that the perpetrator at some level may be or may be deemed to be showing concern for them. A common response to this point is that there is a difference between the intent to take advantage of children found in child abuse and the worst that clinicians can be accused of, which is adherence to out-of-date treatment practices: doctors do not casually or deliberately 'violate' their patients. In my opinion, this probably overestimates the degree of conscious intent to harm in many cases of child abuse and almost all cases of sexual harassment and underestimates the harm that can be done by clinicians 'who know best'.

As with other forms of abuse, there will necessarily be a low incidence of disclosure to others, for a number of reasons. First, it is necessary to disclose the illness in order to disclose the abuse, and victims will ordinarily be reluctant to do this. Second, there may be a legitimate fear of reprisals should complaints be made, which many patients suspect might take the form of an increase in the dose of the treatment being complained about. Third, a status as a victim of abusive prescribing will not be sought out as it risks further stigmatisation of the victim as a 'loser'. Fourth, there are difficulties in ventilating feelings or perceptions in this area as demonstrating nervousness and problems, and the interpretation of these as a consequence of a prescribed regimen, leaves the subject open to the perception that all that has been demonstrated is the problem that led to the initial prescription.

Indeed, a further problem is that many individuals may not explicitly make the connection between their treatment regimens, their capacity to change that regimen and the way they are feeling (Healy & Farquhar 1998, Sharp et al 1998). It may only be when they are evaluated by another prescriber that they become consciously aware of a connection between their treatment and symptoms such as anxiety, depression, demotivation, fatigue, a variety of psychosomatic symptoms, nervousness, impulsiveness, irritability, weight gain, sexual disturbances, suicidality, emotional blunting and other problems.

Finally, if a patient complains, there will often be a lack of support from significant others. This, as in other forms of abuse, may be important in its own right. Indeed, there may be considerable external pressure on the individual – from relatives and friends as well as from mental health professionals – to accommodate to the situation and to internalise blame. This will lead to a sense of defectiveness on the patient's part or denial of the difficulties that are being experienced. Thus the patient may request that their prescription for an anticholinergic not be discontinued in the apparent belief that this is a tranquilliser in its own right and indeed the more effective of the 'two tranquillisers' they are on. In this case, the idea that my doctor would do me no harm inhibits recognition of the fact that the anticholinergic is in fact treating difficulties produced by the antipsychotic.

As with other forms of abuse, unpredictability may make things worse, as may the duration of the abuse, the extent to which the abuse pervades all aspects of the subject's life, and the extent to which prescribing is seen as reactive to conflicts rather than aimed at rational and agreed therapeutic ends. Particular difficulties are raised in the case of violent incidents in clinical settings. In such circumstances mental health staff risk assuming the role of both judge and jury.

Ongoing abuse has also traditionally found justification from evidence that the discontinuation of treatment leads to serious problems. This is invariably interpreted as a re-emergence of the illness, a situation that, ethically, all but demands the resumption of treatment. However, there is a considerable body of evidence to indicate that what is typically taken as a new illness episode following a reduction or discontinuation of medication may in a large number of cases be evidence of a dependence syndrome (see Chs 1 & 24) (Tranter & Healy 1998). It is known that clinicians routinely fail to warn patients about the risk of tardive dyskinesia owing to their own emotional discomfort at raising this possibility. Probably for similar reasons, they appear to have managed to ignore evidence indicating the existence of tardive dysthymias and other drug-induced stress syndromes. Clearly, clinicians seem in practice all but unable to inform their patients of these significant risks.

PRESCRIPTION 'RIGHTS'

Some of this potential for abuse may arise from the prescription-only status of psychotropic medicines. A significant reason for the extension of prescription-only arrangements to all medicines in the 1950s lay in an assessment that the amount of information regarding the proper use of the new medications was too extensive to fit on the label and that making the drugs available only on prescription would ensure that any information a patient needed would be given to them by their prescriber.

One consequence of prescription-only status is that it is not only when a patient has been formally detained that a prescriber is given more than the usual amount of power in determining the outcome of a clinical condition. Every writing of a prescription involves a potential deferral to a medical opinion in a manner that does not happen when people manage their own conditions by non-pharmacotherapeutic means or by means of over-the-counter medications or health food supplements. The potential for abuse in prescription-only arrangements was recognised by Senator Estes Kefauver, who chaired the hearings that led to the 1962 Amendments to the US Food and Drugs Act, when he noted that 'he who orders does not buy and he who buys does not order' (cited in Healy 1997, Ch. 1).

Potentially abusive prescribing of the type outlined probably applies in the case of all medications, given recent indicators that drug-induced conditions are now the fourth leading cause of death and may lead to up to one-third of admissions to hospital (Lazarou et al 1999). The issue, however, probably applies with extra force in the case of the psychotropic agents, in that the problematic effects of medication are most likely to be pernicious in this domain. The recent development of mental health advocacy recognises the potential for abuse in current mental health services. But where the women's movement has been able to lobby effectively for a consideration of sexual abuse and harassment both on a legal level and in terms of raising conscious-ness in society, mental health patients have fewer levers available to them and would seem to be even more vulnerable.

The doctrine that medical practices are all but immune to prosecution if a significant minority of the profession can be shown to practise similarly means that, in the case of abusive prescribing, a legal recourse is unlikely to be helpful in all but the most extraordinary cases. This will be the case even though the documentary proof of abuse in the form of a prescription record is likely to be available in a way that evidence in the case of child abuse or sexual harassment rarely is. Few people will want to take legal action, anyway, partly because they may fear it will affect their relations with all prescribers and not just with one.

AWARENESS OF THE PROBLEM

As with sexual harassment and other forms of abuse, there has been a tendency to put up with the situation as an inevitable fact of life. Many will think that the extent of and consequences of abusive prescribing hinted at here are overstated, even though the Royal College of Psychiatrists considered it neces-sary to issue a position statement on high-dose prescribing of antipsychotics

(Thompson 1994). Many will feel that, if things were this bad, more would have been made of the problem before this. The failure to recognise the problem may stem from the extent to which we ourselves have been abused. Most medical and nursing staff, while training, will have been instructed by their superiors at various times to administer doses of medication that they considered were unwarranted. Most colleagues I trained with will have seen haloperidol narcosis being administered to young female patients who were not unduly disruptive. This involved giving haloperidol 10 mg intravenously every hour for several days at a stretch. In the hospital where I worked until the mid-1990s, the standard regimen on which all admitted psychotic patients were commenced – even frail women in their sixties – was haloperidol 10 mg four times daily. Regimens of up to 1000 mg per day of flupentixol (equivalent to 20 000 mg chlorpromazine) were not uncommon in the management of young women until recently (Bogeso & Pedersen 1998).

Indeed, it is a moot point as to whether some (although clearly not all) of the benefits of monotherapy with clozapine may not stem from the fact that, in such circumstances, some of the patients most at risk of prescription abuses are much less likely to be poisoned than they once were (see Ch. 1). The experiences of researchers working with healthy volunteers here are of relevance. Some researchers have, for example, made videos of the effects of small doses of antipsychotics on these subjects, who are transformed so much that they appear to be indistinguishable from patients who are thought to have schizophrenia with predominantly negative features. Similar outcomes have been recorded using rating scales such as the Positive and Negative Symptoms Scales: volunteers develop 'negative' symptoms. In the main, these findings have not reached the public domain owing to concerns among researchers that their impact would damage healthy volunteer research.

Our group, however, has published findings in this area. We found that a single 5-mg dose of droperidol given blind to healthy volunteers invariably produced severe agitation and dysphoria, as well as suicidality in some (Healy & Farquhar 1998, Jones-Edwards 1998). The effects in a number of individuals lasted for up to a week. Alcohol and taking to bed, in an effort to minimise external stimulation, proved the best management strategies. These behaviours when undertaken by patients, of course, are regularly taken as indicators of illness. The views of patients that a considerable part of the problem may be drug induced are regularly discounted.

A vignette may bring some of the issues home. MC is a 65-year-old well-educated articulate woman who became depressed for the first time in her life. She had concomitant osteoporosis that restricted the choice of antidepressant medication that might have suited her. She was accordingly put on sertraline. After several weeks on this she developed chest pain, probably anginal, and breathlessness. After attendance at a clinic, I wrote to her general practitioner recommending a change from this antidepressant. He did nothing. A follow-up letter copied to the patient, suggesting that this was SSRI-induced angina and an SSRI-induced respiratory dyskinesia, again advising a change of medication from SSRIs, also had no effect. The doctor's interpretation was that the angina was unrelated to her treatment. He interpreted her breathlessness as panic attacks, and therefore as evidence that she should continue with treatment and preferably with an SSRI. The woman herself continued with treatment, afraid that if she stopped, given her evident problems, and had to call her general practitioner out in an emergency and he were to find that she had gone against his instructions he would refuse to treat her when she really needed it. The general practitioner was finally persuaded to change to a non-SSRI, and after several weeks MC's chest pains and breathlessness cleared up.

This vignette illustrates how dependent people can become in therapeutic situations. In recent years, there has been an increase in antidepressant prescribing to children, with estimates that there are several million prescriptions per year in the USA alone (Fisher & Fisher 1996). This increase has taken place even though most of the randomised trials of antidepressants that have been undertaken in adolescent and childhood populations have shown no benefit of antidepressants over placebo. There is an ethical issue as to whether this kind of treatment should take place at all in the face of so much negative evidence but, more to the point, children are almost certainly even less capable of maintaining their perceptions of drug-induced abnormality in the face of contradictory interpretations from adult clinicians. The potential for abuse, therefore, would seem to be even greater in such situations.

THE MANAGEMENT OF ABUSE

As with other situations of abuse, the adverse effects of abusive prescribing will remain invisible so long as the existence of abusive prescribing remains unacknowledged. If recognised, it may be possible to put a cost on the consequences of such prescribing. This cost may be substantial, if increased hospitalisation, compromised compliance and decreased employment in either the job market or the voluntary sector are taken into account.

Recognition may make it possible to remedy the situation. The potential for abuse is inherent in all therapies and, in practice, may occur to a greater extent in psychotherapeutic exchanges than in routine pharmacotherapy. The question of abuse in therapy formed the heart of the Osheroff case, in which an individual who was depressed was treated for 9 months with psychotherapeutic approaches that had not been shown to work. Subsequent treatment with antidepressants brought about a prompt improvement in his condition, but this was too late to save his marriage or his job. The issues were debated at length in the pages of the *American Journal of Psychiatry* (Klerman 1990, Stone 1990). In brief, there was no agreement that therapy should necessarily follow evidence of efficacy, but there was agreement that persistence with one therapeutic line, in the face of a lack of progress without a genuine review of other options, was indefensible. This would apply even where the therapy being delivered has been shown to have some evidence of efficacy.

Some lessons may be drawn from the Osheroff case. It can be suggested that it would now be prudent for all therapists, including pharmacotherapists, to specify what outcomes they are aiming at, the period of time for which they are likely to persist in a particular course of action in the face of non-response or partial response, and what other treatment options they would consider should the current course of treatment fail to deliver the expected benefits. Exactly these recommendations were written into a recent British Association for Psychopharmacology consensus statement on prescribing for childhood and learning disability indications (Healy & Nutt 1997).

However, it is possible to go further. Just as the Mental Health Act is supposed to sanction the treatment that would be given to the detained patient as if their relatives were present to witness what was being done, so also, if the prescription-only status of psychotropic agents is not revoked, therapists ideally should do pharmacotherapy with the genuineness they would bring to bear if a medical relative or advocate were present with the patient to monitor what was happening.

Liability

DRUG-INDUCED INJURY

Liability for drug-induced injuries did not become an issue of general concern until quite recently. However, a number of drug-induced problems – from thalidomide in the 1960s to Opren and diethylstilboestrol in the 1970s – have caused widespread public disquiet and led to increasing awareness of issues to do with liability. In psychiatry, the first big concern in the UK focused on the question of benzodiazepine prescribing, while in the USA the paramount issue was tardive dyskinesia in individuals taking antipsychotics. The question has become an emotive one, with some commentators who survey the problem referring to the appalling frequency of drug-induced injury, while others comment on its astonishing rarity. Whatever the absolute frequencies of problems, contrary probably to public belief, the evidence suggests that the larger the pharmaceutical company, the better its practice regarding drug safety is likely to be (Braithwaite 1984).

Drug-induced problems may stem from the toxic effects of a drug, from toxic effects caused by an impure additive, or from allergic reactions to the drug or its additives. Problems may also stem from overprescribing. For instance, in the case of someone who dies from a resistant bacterial infection, a relative could claim that the subject's death arose in part from the excessive prescription of antibiotics that contributes to the production of resistant infections. In the case of the antipsychotics, problems may be brought about by the overuse of these drugs, although this overuse, far from being promoted solely by drug companies, stems in part from the current politics of mental health: deaths have resulted from rapid tranquillisation often by harassed staff in psychiatric units.

The question of liability is something of a rolling log on which companies, prescribers and drug takers try to maintain a footing. In addition to attempting to produce increasingly safe compounds, companies try to restrict liability by hedging their data sheets with warnings and lists of side effects, so that if something goes wrong either the prescriber or the consumer will be to blame, on the basis that they were warned beforehand if they chose to notice. Against this, in the pursuit of markets, rather than make novel compounds drug companies often manufacture drugs that are closely related to other compounds on the market in an attempt to gain a share of what is obviously selling well. This minor manipulation of a molecule may confer no additional therapeutic benefit but may produce unsuspected side effects.

When it comes to determining whether a particular drug has been responsible for a particular injury, it can be extremely difficult to decide with confidence what has actually happened. Questions that arise are, for example, whether it is known that the individual actually did take the drug that supposedly caused the problem? Did they take anything else? Did the individual have any pre-existing disorder that made an unfortunate reaction to a compound more likely?

The majority of drug-induced disorders resemble disorders that happen naturally anyway. For example, benzodiazepine withdrawal produces anxiety. Anxiety is common. One can question whether all that is happening in the case of withdrawal is a re-emergence of the anxiety that led to the individual being put on treatment in the first instance. In the case of tardive dyskinesia, dyskinesias that are indistinguishable from those caused by the drugs occur in individuals who have never had antipsychotics. Even the limb deformities produced by thalidomide occur naturally. Drug-induced injury often involves a change in the frequency of something rather than an entirely novel development. For reasons such as these, the occurrence of adverse events to a drug is rarely taken automatically as indicating that the drug has caused the problem.

Even if it is agreed that the drug has caused the problem, questions arise as to whether the prescriber should have prescribed for the problem in the first instance. If not, then they share a part of the blame. Did the taker implicitly or explicitly agree to run the risk that is involved in all drug taking? Did they contribute to their own injury in any way – by altering the amount of salt in their diet, perhaps, while taking lithium?

In the case of a possible suicide consequent on antidepressant (see Ch. 5) or antipsychotic-induced akathisia, for example, it is not clear exactly where blame might lie in individual cases. It may not be possible, given our current state of knowledge, to produce antidepressants or antipsychotics that will never produce akathisia or dysphoria, and hence the drug induction of suicidal behaviour is at present an inherent risk of drug taking. This puts an onus on prescribers to warn patients of this possible side effect and what to do should it develop. The particular interest in the cases of SSRI-induced akathisia is explicit company denials that their drug could lead to akathisia or suicide. What do these company denials do to liability?

There are three principles that can be applied to all drug taking, as outlined in Box 26.1 (Dukes 1996, Dukes & Swartz 1988).

Box 26.1 Principles of drug taking

First Principle

No drug or drug treatment can be guaranteed in advance to be entirely safe. Risks are inevitable and justifiable provided they are not disproportionate to the purpose that the treatment is supposed to serve.

At present, society as a whole deems that risks such as tardive dyskinesia may be justifiable against the backdrop of an otherwise irremediable illness such as schizophrenia. But what of tardive dyskinesia consequent on the prescription of a neuroleptic for anxiety or a sedative neuroleptic as a hypnotic?

Second Principle

No party can reasonably be blamed for doing their best, even if injury is one of the consequences.

The issue here, of course, may depend on being able to show that one has done one's best; herein lies the importance of documenting advice given, etc.

Third Principle

Responsibility is carried by anyone on whom one is entitled to rely.

This includes the nurses who hand out medication who have a responsibility to get the drug and dose right, the pharmacist to dispense the right medication, and potentially anyone who acts as an authoritative source of advice regarding the benefits or hazards of medication, including your mother.

RISKS AND BENEFITS

The idea that one of the cardinal principles of medical practice is that a healer should 'first of all do no harm' is appealing, but it is a very poor description of medical practice. In the case of drug treatment, no treatment is possible unless risks are taken. No drug is safe. Treatment is a matter of weighing risks and benefits. The discovery of anaesthesia crystallised this dilemma. When first introduced (and still today), it was known that some people would die from the anaesthetic. There were many who had problems with the idea that some lives would intentionally be put at risk in order to benefit others, but the same is true of practically all treatments today. There is therefore a need to ensure that the person being treated is going to derive a clear benefit from treatment such that it is justifiable to take certain risks. For example, in the case of someone with cancer, it may be justifiable to take the very considerable risks associated with chemotherapy, but it would not be reasonable to give chemotherapeutic agents to someone with a cold or depression.

The antihypertensives provide a good case. There are very few people who absolutely need antihypertensives to lower malignant increases in blood pressure caused by hypertensive disease. However, there are legions of people who have some increase in blood pressure, and increased blood pressure is associated with an increased risk of heart attacks or strokes as a consequence. Some individuals may have raised blood pressure only as a result of the anxiety of attending their doctor. Increases in blood pressure are, furthermore, only an indication that a disease process may be operative. One option in such cases is repeated monitoring with a recourse to treatment only if the situation worsens. For those with minimal increases in blood pressure, the risk of likely problems is so small that one can legitimately ask whether the cost in side effects (impaired sexual functioning) is worth it.

Until 1960 calculations of risk and benefit were made by the consumer. Since all drugs were made available on prescription only, in the case of the antihypertensives for instance, these calculations have typically been made for patients by clinicians – who are often on automatic pilot. A great deal of prescribing is almost automatic; it is difficult for it not to be when, for instance, the latest research indicates that hypertension is a risk factor for heart disease and there happens to be available a means of mitigating the risk. It takes considerable discrimination to appreciate that the risk may be quite minimal, and indeed less than the risks posed by the drug. An even greater skill is needed to impart this state of affairs to the patient. In such circumstances it behoves all the members of a health team to have a good grasp of what drugs can and cannot do, as some may be better able to influence particular patients than others.

CLINICAL TRIALS AND LEGAL JEOPARDY

The prozac story

In clinical studies before its launch in 1988, Prozac was associated with akathisia and agitation, occurring with sufficient frequency and intensity to lead to recommendations that benzodiazepines be co-prescribed with it in clinical trials (Healy 1999a). Leading textbooks on the clinical profile of psychotropic agents mention Prozac's well-known propensity to cause akathisia. Akathisia has been implicated as a mechanism whereby Prozac may, in certain circumstances, lead to violence and suicide (see Ch. 5). The physiological mechanisms by which this happens are relatively well understood, yet Lilly's presentation of the side effects of Prozac from their clinical trials database contains no mention of akathisia.

Emotional flatness or blunting is a not infrequent side effect of treatment reported by patients on Prozac. Arguably, this effect is all but intrinsic to the mode of action of the drug, which generally reduces emotional reactivity. It has been reported in observational studies, where it has been linked to other potentially harmful behaviours (Hoehn-Saric et al 1990), yet nothing resembling emotional blunting appears in the clinical trials side-effect database for Prozac.

There is a good deal of published and unpublished evidence that SSRI use is associated with a higher rate of suicidal ideation early in the course of treatment than other antidepressants, strongly suggesting that treatment may induce suicidality in some. Whether or not the reader believes that an antidepressant could induce suicidal ideation, it is a fact that treatment-emergent suicidal ideation is not recognised by any code in current clinical trial systems. It is not recorded as a side effect of Prozac in Lilly's database.

These examples point to a number of problems with the side-effect data from clinical trials. One is the failure of systems to cope with 'new' problems. Another is the current dependence on self-reporting methods for the collection of data on side effects. In the case of the SSRIs it would seem that these methods detect only one in six of the side effects detected by systematic checklist methods (Rosenbaum et al 1998).

If the side-effect profile of a drug drawn from clinical trials were used just for marketing purposes, there might be little problem with this state of affairs. We could all take them with a grain of salt. After all, clinical trials indicated that sexual dysfunction on SSRIs occurred at a 5% rate when in fact the true rate was probably closer to 50%. These profiles have, however, also been used in academic debate and for legal purposes to deny that claimed adverse effects are happening (Healy 1999b).

Against this background, it would seem that any patients entering into any clinical trials of any kind of medication where side-effect data are collected by spontaneous reporting methods are putting individuals who may subsequently suffer a drug-induced adverse event into a state of potential legal jeopardy. The consequences for prescriber liability are also uncertain.

Health service professionals have been in the business of encouraging patients to participate in clinical trials, arguing that it is almost a civic duty to do so – although they are much less likely to participate themselves in trials or to encourage their own family members to do so. But, in fact, participation of any of their patients at present is probably doing themselves or their families an injury: pharmaceutical companies seem prepared to argue that, because data on a particular side effect were not collected in their clinical trials, this proves the side effect does not happen. It may be time to stop participating in trials that may yield thousands of pounds per patient for the clinician running the study but only increased legal jeopardy for the rest of us.

A refusal to participate might have many positive benefits. At present companies are reluctant not to have a UK arm to their studies. If it becomes difficult to perform trials in Britain, the companies are likely to amend their consent forms to include a statement that side effects collected by current methods could be used for marketing but for no other purposes. Alternatively they could introduce better side-effect collection methods, which would both enhance the scientific information provided by clinical trials and minimise the risks of jeopardy.

References

Bogeso K, Pedersen V (1998) Drug hunting. In: Healy D, ed. The psychopharmacologists, vol 2, pp 561–580. London: Arnold.

Brabbins CA, Butler J, Bentall R (1996) Consent to antipsychotic medication for schizophrenia: clinical, ethical and legal issues. British Journal of Psychiatry 168: 540–544.

Braithwaite J (1984) Corporate crime in the pharmaceutical industry. London: Routledge & Kegan Paul.

Bursztajn HJ, Feinbloom RI, Hamm RM, Brodsky A (1990) Medical choices: medical chances. London: Routledge.

Consumers Association (1995) Risk benefit analysis of drugs in practice. Drugs and Therapeutics Bulletin 33: 5.

Day J, Wood G, Dewey M, Bentall R (1995) A self rating scale for measuring neuroleptic side effects. British Journal of Psychiatry 143: 129–150.

Dukes MNG (1996) Social, economic and pharmacological aspects. In: Healy D, Doogan DP, eds. Psychotropic drug development, pp 94–102. London: Chapman & Hall.

Dukes MNG, Swartz B (1988) Responsibility for drug-induced injury. Amsterdam: Elsevier.

Epstein LC, Lasagna L (1969) Obtaining informed consent: form or substance. Archives of Internal Medicine 123: 682–688.

Fisher R, Fisher S (1996) Antidepressants for children. Is scientific support necessary? Journal of Nervous and Mental Disease 184: 99–102; commentaries 103–108.

Fitzgerald F, Healy D, Williams B (1996) Shared care. Some effects of patient access to medical communications. Journal of Mental Health 6: 37–46.

Healy D (1995) Involving users in mental health services in the era of the word-processor and the database. In: Crosby D, Barry M, eds. Community care: evaluation of the provision of mental health services, pp 209–231. Aldershot, UK: Avebury Press.

Healy D (1997) The antidepressant era. Cambridge, MA: Harvard University Press.

Healy D (1999a) Guest editorial: A failure to warn. International Journal of Risk and Safety in Medicine 12: 151–156.

Healy D (1999b) Clinical trials and legal jeopardy. Bulletin of Medical Ethics 153: 13–18.

Healy D, Farquhar GN (1998) Immediate effects of droperidol. Human Psychopharmacology 13: 113–120.

Healy D, Nutt D (1997) British Association for Psychopharmacology consensus statement on childhood and learning disabilities psychopharmacology. Journal of Psychopharmacology 11: 291–294.

Healy D, Savage M, Thomas P (1998) Abusive prescribing. OpenMind September: 18.

Hoehn-Saric R, Lipsey JR, McLeod DR (1990) Apathy and indifference in patients on fluvoxamine and fluoxetine. Journal of Clinical Psychopharmacology 10: 343–345.

Jones-Edwards G (1998) An eye-opener. OpenMind. September: 13–14, 19.

Kleinman A (1988) The illness narratives. New York: Basic Books.

Klerman GL (1990) The psychiatric patient's right to effective treatment: implications of Osheroff vs Chestnut Lodge. American Journal of Psychiatry 147: 409–418.

Lazarou J, Pomeranz BH, Corey PN (1999) Incidence of adverse drug reactions in hospitalized patients. Journal of the American Medical Association 279: 1200–1205.

Levine RJ (1986) Ethics and regulation of clinical research. New Haven, CT: Yale University Press.

Ormrod R (1987) Therapy, battery and informed consent. Psychiatric Bulletin 11: 185–186.

Rosenbaum JF, Fava M, Hoog SL, Ashcroft RC, Krebs W (1998) Selective serotonin reuptake inhibitor discontinuation syndrome: a randomised clinical study. Biological Psychiatry 44: 77–87.

Seedhouse D (1991) Liberating medicine. Chichester, UK: John Wiley.

Sharp HM, Healy D, Fear CF (1998) Symptoms or side effects? Methodological hazards and therapeutic principles. Human Psychopharmacology 13: 467–475.

Stone AA (1990) Law, science and psychiatric malpractice: a response to Klerman's indictment of psychoanalytic psychiatry. American Journal of Psychiatry 147: 419–427.

Thompson C (1994) The use of high-dose antipsychotic medication. British Journal of Psychiatry 164: 448–458.

Tranter R, Healy D (1998) Antipsychotic discontinuation syndromes. Journal of Psychopharmacology 12: 306–311.

The marketing of tranquillity

SECTION CONTENTS

The ethical industry

INTRODUCTION

Before the second half of the nineteenth century, the dominant medical and popular notions of disease rested on a humoral theory of disease, first put forward by Hippocrates in Greece and later by Galen in Rome. According to this theory, there were four humours – phlegm, choler, bile and sanguine – and diseases resulted from an imbalance of these humours or between the humoral state of the individual and conditions in the environment (Vogel & Rosenberg 1979). The idea that masturbation or menstruation might lead to disease or madness stemmed from this theory, in that both involve a loss of secretions and therefore entail a disruption of the internal balance of the humours. As this was being done in an uncontrolled or injudicious way, the outcome was liable to be dysharmony.

A version of this theory survives to this day in the Chinese notions of yin and yang, which are popular in complementary medicine settings, and in the three dhosas of Ayurvedic medicine. In both yin and yang and the four humours systems, what is aimed at is a state of harmony. Treatment consists of efforts to restore balance or internal equilibrium. Until the nineteenth century this was done by regulating diet, by bleeding, purging, inducing vomiting, raising blisters (in which noxious vapours could collect), or by giving a variety of tonics – agents that were stimulant or strengthening in some way. Diet and tonics of various sorts remain the most popular methods today.

Among the drugs used for nervous problems were black hellebore (a drastic purgative) and white veratrum, which produced vomiting. Shaving of the head was also employed in order to let the vapours out. Oleum cephalicum (oils for the head), which would blister the shaven scalp, were used. Iron was also in use, literally to strengthen the constitution. Camphor was a popular stimulant and bromides were used as sedatives (Sneader 1990).

These treatments may sound odd now, but essentially what physicians aimed at was to mimic the body's own reactions: sweating, bleeding, purging, vomiting, the passage of water, etc. Producing what we would now call side effects like these seemed to be the obvious thing to do and, far from suing the way patients might do nowadays, these side effects were taken as a welcome sign that the treatment was working.

Against this background, a large industry flourished and aimed at satisfying consumer needs (or profiting from their misery), through the provision of tonics, elixirs, and so on. The market was almost entirely consumer led as numerous plays, novels and operas, such as Donizetti's *L'Elixir d'Amour* attest. It was a regular feature of village life that the peddlar of medicines would come around with a range of potions for sale. Individuals regularly treated themselves with such compounds. Even when quite seriously ill, it was common until the twentieth century for afflicted individuals to have a go at treating themselves first.

In the nineteenth century, patent medicines emerged – medicines containing 'secret' remedies. These were marketed vigorously in the popular press, and a great number of the techniques underpinning modern advertising developed in an effort to sell these compounds. Their success became an increasing problem in orthodox medical circles and amongst regulators (Liebenau 1987). The patent medicine industry still survives today in over-the-counter (OTC) medicines, and most clearly in the health food industry, whose food supplements are 'drugs' by another name. Some modern examples of this are the burgeoning phenomenon of smart drugs outlined in Chapter 19 and the growth in nutraceuticals such as lipid-lowering spreads.

The modern pharmaceutical industry took shape in the early twentieth century as a reaction to these patent medicines. The newer drug companies that emerged, and which survive today, termed themselves 'ethical' companies in contrast to the patent medicine industry. The term ethical needs some clarification. These companies saw themselves as being ethical, in that they were prepared to purify the compounds that went into their preparations and were willing to specify exactly what a medicine contained.

THE MAGIC BULLET

The development of specific theories of disease was the most significant factor affecting the outcome of competition between the ethical and patent pharmaceutical industries. The discovery by Pasteur of bacteria and their role in infection led to a growing belief in specific causes for specific diseases. The key breakthrough came with the development of diphtheria antitoxin, in 1896, which led to the eradication of diphtheria.

Allied to this, there was during the nineteenth century an increasing awareness that the many natural herbs and compounds that appeared to be helpful in the treatment of disease all contained specific compounds and that it was these compounds rather than the whole herb that were the curative factors. For example, it turned out to be the morphine in the poppy rather than the entire poppy that was helpful, the digitalis in foxglove, and the salicylic acid in the bark of the willow tree (*Salix alba*). Other developments, such as the increasing use of anaesthesia for ever more specific surgical procedures, fostered the idea of specific illnesses and correspondingly the idea of specific cures. The growing trend found a notable expression in Paul Ehrlich's concept of the magic bullet. Magic bullets would enter the body and act on a disease process specifically, leaving all other metabolic processes undisturbed (Pellegrino 1979).

The antibiotics have come closest to this ideal in practice. The idea, however, has taken hold that all modern drugs are magic bullets of some sort, and this leads many, if not all, of us who are prescribing or taking drugs to believe that we are taking something that will work specifically on just one faulty piece of the human machinery.

The reality, however, is quite different. It is not just that most drugs, particularly psychotropic drugs, may cause side effects but rather that they all act on a great number of body systems. For instance, the calcium channel blockers have therapeutic actions on almost every system in the body. The antipsychotics may be used as anxiolytics, antipsychotics, antidepressants, antipruritic agents or antiemetics. The marketing by modern drug companies militates against a recognition of this state of affairs.

Initially the ethical companies aimed at purifying natural compounds, such as digitalis, salicylic acid or morphine from the poppy. The great advantage of purification was that the amount of a drug given could be controlled. In the case of foxglove, for example, crushing and administering the plant may help cardiac failure – if the dose is right – but it may be poisonous if the dose is too high. In principle, if there is an active ingredient in a natural compound it should always be possible to establish what it is and to purify it.

The next step was involvement in the manufacture of entirely synthetic organic compounds. The development of the barbiturates was a significant step forward in this regard. The production of chlorpromazine, in the twentieth century, was a laboratory-based exercise of this nature that was spectacularly successful. There are a number of potential drawbacks to this enterprise, however. The increasing recognition of an ever-growing number of distinct receptors, and the ability to synthesise compounds that will bind to each of these relatively specifically, seem to be leading to a situation in which the cart is getting put before the horse. An ever-increasing number of compounds is being developed in laboratories – the only problem is that it is not clear what illness they are supposed to be treating. We have a range of magic bullets and seem programmed to believe that there must be appropriate illnesses for each of them. From this comes the need for companies to market their compounds in what is becoming an ever more crowded marketplace.

A further aspect of the current situation is that, despite the rhetoric of magic bullets, the last thing the pharmaceutical industry actually wants – arguably – is a series of drugs that clear up the problem. The best selling compounds are the antihypertensives, lipid-lowering drugs and, until recently, gastric acid-reducing agents, together with the antidepressants, most of which lower the risk of stroke or suicide from occurring rather than curing the disease. Indeed, it would seem that, in the case of the use of antibiotics for ulcers or improving diet for heart disorders, the weight of evidence the industry brings to the table sometimes works against the recognition of solutions to the problem.

THE INTERFACE BETWEEN ETHICS AND MARKETS

In 1906, in an attempt to curb the production of the more dangerous patent medicines, what was later to be the Food and Drug Administration (FDA) was set up in the USA. The operation of the FDA led to the removal of many patent medicines from the market and to the demise of a large number of small companies producing such compounds. This removal of competition arguably fostered the growth of the ethical industry (Liebenau 1987).

With the agreement of the ethical companies, the FDA began to put in place a set of regulations aimed at forcing the manufacturers of pharmaceuticals to disclose the ingredients of their medicines and to provide demonstrations of efficacy and safety. Based on these high standards, drug companies can be sued.

This, of course, is appropriate, but it should be borne in mind that no other branch of the health service has to meet such stringent criteria or is open to such liabilities. For example, the producers of a new psychotherapeutic approach or its practitioners cannot easily be held legally responsible for the fact that the therapy does not cure or that great distress may be occasioned by over-zealous administration. To this day, there is no evidence that psychoanalysis, for instance, brings about specific responses in any condition of the order of magnitude that drugs are obliged to provide before they can be marketed.

This does not apply only to psychotherapy. New surgical procedures are not regulated before use in the way that drugs are. Surgeons are free to work out new operative interventions and to go ahead and try them out on patients without prior evidence of efficacy or safety, although this rarely happens without some previous experimentation on animals and a good theoretical rationale beforehand. Similarly, at present, large-scale changes are being effected in the health services of Great Britain and other Western countries without any evidence that they will improve health. Who will be sued by the relatives of those who die as a result?

Given the notable disasters that have occurred with some drugs, especially thalidomide, the pharmaceutical industry, in contrast to all other aspects of the health services, is landed with the task of proving what amounts almost to extreme safety. Until recently there was evidence that some companies faced with these regulations might massage the data, but the fact remains that current procedures do much to ensure that compounds coming to market are as safe as can reasonably be expected. Herein lies a rub.

When new compounds are produced there is a prima facie case for conducting a series of open studies in clinical populations to establish their actual effects in humans as opposed to the effects proposed by current theories or by extrapolation from animal experiments. This, however, is not the way the modern pharmaceutical industry works.

Given the costs of demonstrating efficacy and safety, and the liabilities involved in selling drugs, the modern production of a drug requires a prior determination of market returns balanced against liabilities: on what basis might we be sued and how much is this likely to cost? The initial requirement of demonstrating profitability acts as a mould into which subsequent developments must fit. This leads to a number of strategies and a number of consequences.

DRUG DEVELOPMENT

One strategy is that drug companies attempt to determine, early in the process of a drug's development, what kind of drug it is: is it an antidepressant, antihypertensive, antipsychotic, or what? The reason is that the company must make calculations regarding potential market size and liabilities should things go wrong. This can be done only if it is known what the drug is likely to do. Accordingly, while new drugs could be developed in a manner that produces safe compounds, with the aim of leaving it to clinicians or consumers to establish what these compounds do by prescribing and taking them, this is not how development happens.

There is a further aspect to this. Advance information about the compounds that a company has may have a substantial impact on the company's share price. Stockbrokers employ analysts to pore over the proceedings of pharmacology conferences for indications of what may be forthcoming. Based on this there may be considerable shifts in market capital. Several years ago, it was rumoured that Glaxo had a new antischizophrenic compound, a serotonin S_3 antagonist, ondansetron. This produced substantial advances in its share price. Even though ondansetron never made it, this issue of defining a market early in the development process, because of potential effects on share price, is of increasing importance (Marsh 1989).

As a consequence, companies have a predilection for the 'rational' development of drugs. Rational development in this context means that the drugs are produced as the consequence of some theory that predicts the nature of reality and how to intervene in it to obtain desired effects. It includes the development of drugs through a set of procedures that involve screening compounds for desired effects on animals. It also involves aiming at drugs that conform to theories that were developed on the basis of a previous generation of drugs.

A great deal of work is therefore done before drugs are marketed – a great deal of 'science'. Increasingly, the impression has developed that all the 'science' has been done before a drug comes to the marketplace, and all that remains is for a clinical trial to confirm the predicted benefits. This belief that drug development is a rational process and that all the significant science has been done before a launch is, however, at odds with the evidence.

Against this background, observations such as those made on the anti-dyskinesia effects of the calcium channel blockers (see Ch. 3) are unsettling. Such observations are likely to pose serious problems for companies, in that they upset the balance sheet of profits and potential liabilities. They indicate that very fundamental observations may have been overlooked. Far from being grateful when new observations are pointed out and new uses indicated, drug companies are liable to be less than enthusiastic.

Given what is at stake, as outlined above, a company must try to take all the steps it can to define its market and then to realise that market. In such a process, the interesting observations of consumers or their keyworkers are a problem, even where, as in the case of the calcium channel blockers, they appear to offer the prospect of increased sales. They do so, but at an uncertain cost. If these drugs are entering the brain, what else might they be doing that might be a potential liability?

There is an important consequence of the need to be profitable. There is considerable public disquiet about drug companies. They are held to treat victims of drug-induced disorders poorly. They are believed to spend inordinate sums of money selling their products to doctors, attempting, it may seem, to brainwash doctors or to bribe them with free conferences in exotic locations or with under-the-counter gifts. Reading about current practices in a book such as *Cured to Death* is liable to put one off taking drugs entirely (Melville & Johnson 1982).

There is substance to all of these complaints. In part, however, the issues come down to the term 'ethics'. In order to comply with the ethical norms that they themselves have played a part in setting, drug companies must expend a considerable amount of money before a drug comes to market, establishing its safety and efficacy. From the time of first seeking a licence for the product, they are entitled to a patent lasting for around 20 years. During this time they have a monopoly on the production of the compound. Depending on how long it takes to get from applying for a licence to the time of launching on to a market, a company may at the most have 10 years free from competition in which to recoup its investment. The return on any one drug may also have to cover the costs of development of other drugs, whose development is aborted for one reason or another. Furthermore, when it finally comes to a launch, it is likely that compounds that have got this far will have to penetrate an already crowded marketplace.

As drug companies are businesses, this leads to a need for intense marketing following a launch. This marketing has all the characteristics of any other marketing enterprise, from automobiles to washing powders. There is market surveillance beforehand, to determine what sales pitch will work. There are a variety of post-launch strategies that have been worked out for other industries and applied equally to medical practitioners. This is an inevitable hazard of the modern way to develop drugs, but it seems to run against our wishes that medicine in general not be a business and that all concerned with it be motivated by a wish to relieve suffering rather than any desire for money.

Another consequence of strategies to ensure profitability is that a fundamental observation has been overlooked, one that is of central concern to this book. The fact is that the development of most psychotropic drugs so far has come about serendipitously and by clinical observation rather than by a process of 'rational' development, and this is likely to remain the case for some time.

There is another way to put this. Clinicians assume that the compounds they are given and have been told are anxiolytics and antidepressants are just that. They, accordingly, ask their patients the question: 'Did it improve your depression?' Psychopharmacologists assume that what is important about a compound is what receptor it acts upon and therefore they ask: how did it get that individual better? The question that is not being asked, and indeed is being obscured by current clinical practice, is: what did it do to you? What did you notice while you were taking that drug? Questions such as this, if asked more routinely, would be liable to lead to important discoveries. Questions such as these would be obviously scientific questions to ask, but the current thrust of drug development strategies make them unwelcome to both drug companies and academics.

In 1956, just after chlorpromazine was developed, there was a conference involving clinicians, basic scientists, industry personnel and all those interested in further drug development to look at how to move forward. Most parties agreed on a need for clinical trials, rating scales and a range of screening tests for new drugs. But Ed Evarts from the National Institutes of Mental Health in the USA pointed out that chlorpromazine would have done as much to control the behaviour of patients with dementia paralytica (tertiary syphilis) as it did for those with dementia praecox (schizophrenia). If the drug companies had gone down the same route to develop new drugs for that as they were now proposing to do for schizophrenia, a therapy and research establishment would have grown up around producing variations on chlorpromazine, and the benefits of penicillin for this condition would never have been discovered.

29

Evidence-biased psychiatry

RANDOMISED CONTROLLED TRIALS

The randomised clinical trial (RCT) came into psychiatry in the 1950s (Healy 1991a, Rawlins 1990). The evidence from placebo-controlled trials was meant to act as a brake on over-enthusiastic claims of what a drug could do. It was meant to stop therapeutic bandwagons. Used in this way, RCTs have recently brought a halt to debriefing after trauma by showing that the benefits claimed for debriefing just cannot be demonstrated when compared with non-intervention. Clinical trials show what treatments do not work; they cannot show what works. A positive result for a trial means that it is simply not possible to say that this treatment has no effect (Healy 2001b).

However, instead of providing a brake on therapeutic enthusiasm, a belief has developed that RCTs show that treatments work. The results are increasingly used to persuade clinicians that they have a duty not just to detect conditions but to persuade patients to go on treatment. All new antidepressants and antipsychotics now undergo a series of clinical trials of this sort, but, far from pushing forward science, clinical trials have become a marketing tool. Results are pored over in detail, with the details of side effects being of most interest, as marketing strategists decide on which aspects of the compound to emphasise, given the profiles of their competitors.

If a fraction of the amount of money and effort that is put into clinical trials were to be put into attempts to specify the range of effects that a compound may have (other than the target clinical indication), the causes of science and therapeutics might be much better served. Instead, the costs of such trials significantly increase the overall costs of new drugs and lead to the need for companies to engage in aggressive marketing practices of the sort that get the pharmaceutical industry a reputation for being unethical.

All of this is well known, but there are in fact much bigger problems with the evidence from RCTs than is usually realised. RCTs originated within epidemiology. They are a legitimate shortcut that enables companies to recruit hundreds rather than thousands of subjects to trials – but at a cost. The cost is that there is no guarantee that the trial sample is representative of the rest of the population. Many epidemiologists have considerable misgivings about the capacity of randomisation to overcome the problems of external validity that result from the sampling methods adopted by this approach. The problems inherent in RCTs are compounded in company-sponsored RCTs, which explicitly recruit samples of convenience: they want young and fit subjects who are not particularly ill. This approach means that trials such as this may show that the treatment has an effect, but these trials offer no guarantee that this effect will translate into clinical practice.

Why would companies settle for trials like this? The answer lies in the fact that such trials will suffice to get a drug through the regulators: the Food and Drug Administration (FDA) in the USA and the Medicines Control Agency in the UK. The public and health professionals tend to see the regulators as a watchdog guaranteeing the efficacy and safety of medicines. This is not their role. The role of the regulator is to accept or otherwise that this product labelled as butter or an antidepressant actually is butter or an antidepressant as claimed. In order to do this in the case of an antidepressant, the regulators simply have to see some result from some trial that would make it impossible to say that this drug has no effect in depression. But licensing a drug on this basis says nothing about how good an antidepressant it is or how safe it is in the longer run. The decision to use the treatment clinically at present can be based only on clinical judgement; it does not follow from the fact that regulators have permitted a drug on to the market. Companies, however, portray approval by the FDA to mean that the drug can all but be put in the drinking water.

There is a further problem in psychiatry, where trials of treatments never look at whether patients get back to work or are less likely to commit suicide, etc. The trials all look at changes on rating scale scores. There are four potential domains of measurement: (1) observer-based disease-specific rating scales, such as the Hamilton Rating Scale for Depression (HAM-D) – scales where the clinician rates symptoms of particular interest; (2) patient-based disease-specific rating scales, such as the Beck Depression Inventory; (3) observer-based non-disease-specific scales of global functioning; and (4) patient-based non-disease-specific scales of global functioning (Quality of Life/QoL), where patients rate areas of functioning they are interested in.

It might be possible to feel more confident that a treatment was likely to work generally if a clear treatment effect could be demonstrated on rating scales from all four domains of measurement. As a matter of fact, however, there is not a single antipsychotic or antidepressant that has been demonstrated to have treatment effects across all these domains. In the case of the antidepressants, demonstrations of treatment effects have been largely on the basis of scales such as the HAM-D, where the clinician rates the patient on symptoms of particular interest. In the case of trials with SSRI antidepressants, QoL scales have been used in possibly up to 100 trials, with data from fewer than 10 reported.

From the patient's point of view, therefore, there is little evidence the treatment is working. If convincing scores on rating scales across the range of domains of measurement were available, there would still remain the problem of factoring in the evidence of discontinuation syndromes before anyone could begin to say whether it was a good idea to take a treatment or not.

As with other epidemiological studies, RCTs essentially provide evidence of associations. But, as in studies of smoking and lung cancer, or of diet and cardiac disorders, this kind of evidence points to a link between events rather than an explanation of how or why these events may be linked. In the case of RCTs, arguably, evidence that links drugs to a therapeutic outcome often obscures the mechanisms whereby these events are linked by deflecting our attention away from what the drug actually does to bring about the association. For antidepressants, for instance, it is inconceivable that noradrenaline reuptake inhibitors and serotonin reuptake inhibitors do the same thing, but calling them both antidepressants because RCTs have shown them both to be 'antidepressants' obscures the differences between them.

Prescribing without knowing what potentially beneficial effects an agent produces is not likely to lead to either rational or good practice. If we do not know what these diverse agents do to get depressed patients better, how can we know which of them to select to give to the patient in front of us? Results from studies with healthy volunteers suggest that 50% of people prescribed an antidepressant in fact get the wrong drug for them.

Depression is a relatively simple case. The apparently clear-cut effects on HAM-D scores in short-term trials of antidepressants have contributed to the impression that it is possible to assess the efficacy of our treatments in complex conditions such as manic-depressive disease or schizophrenia – but consider the problems in bipolar disorders. No one rating scale can be used in a condition that cycles from one pole to its polar opposite. Using frequency of episodes as an endpoint, thousands of patients would have to be recruited across multiple centres and sustained within an experimental protocol for years in order to produce a convincing demonstration of prophylaxis. This simply cannot be done. Even the resources of the largest pharmaceutical companies have not enabled trials like this to happen. As a result, current anticonvulsant 'mood stabilisers' are underpinned by evidence of a treatment effect in depression or in mania, but not by evidence of effects in patients with manic–depressive disease. In the same way, there is no evidence on the extent (if any) to which antipsychotics – new or old – work for schizophrenia over and above their treatment effect in acute psychotic states.

There is little question that the drugs we have do useful things. But, compared with the period before chlorpromazine was first introduced, we now detain three times more people, we admit 15 times more people, and people with most conditions spend more time in a service bed now than before the introduction of chlorpromazine (Healy et al 2001). Part of the reason for this is simply that we channel more people and more problems in the direction of the health services than we ever did before. But when treatments really work, they get rid of disorders as penicillin did with dementia paralytica: they do not lead to ever greater rates of admission. The evidence of trials indicates that our treatments can do beneficial things but, for one reason or another, they often don't.

MARKETING THE EVIDENCE

In the real world, the problems with the evidence are even graver than hinted at above. First, clinical trials that do not favour a company's interest are frequently not reported. This leads to a situation where the greatest single determinant of outcome of a published study appears to be its sponsorship (Freemantle et al 2000, Gilbody & Song 2000). Second, as mentioned above, there is no obligation on companies to report all the data from within trials that are published. In the case of the SSRIs, for example, there has been almost universal non-reporting of QoL data. Finally, there is an over-reporting of favourable studies. At international meetings and in peer-reviewed journals, senior experts in the field who have had no participation in a study present data from company trials in a manner that leaves others attempting to meta-analyse the results, confused as to how many trials there actually have been. A recent estimate has been that this process leads to a 25% overestimate of the efficacy of new antipsychotics, for instance (Huston & Locher 1996, Rennie 1999).

Aside from the under-reporting, selective reporting and over-reporting, an increasing proportion of the treatment literature is ghost written. This applies particularly to material appearing in journal supplements as the proceedings of satellite symposia or consensus conferences. These articles commonly have the names of senior figures in the field on them, but it is by no means clear that these experts will have even seen the article to which their name is attached. Based on a survey of review articles on the use of antidepressants in depressions complicated by physical disorders, my estimate is that up to 50% of the review articles, appearing in respectable journals, on new drugs or aspects of their use either appear in supplement form, are ghost written or are written by company personnel.

Surely mental health professionals are now trained to review papers and assess the literature critically. Indeed, their duty under prescription-only arrangements is to determine the true hazards of new agents and to distinguish hype from genuine advances. Unfortunately, prescription-only arrangements also mean that the full weight of the pharmaceutical industry can be borne to bear on a very small number of purchasers as opposed to having to be deployed across an entire marketplace. It would be a mistake to believe that this weight will be without influence. How else can we explain the wholesale switch from tranquillisers in the 1980s to antidepressants in the 1990s with the same patients being diagnosed as having anxiety disorders in one decade and depressive disorders in another – and in all likelihood rediagnosed as anxiety disorders, to be treated with anxiolytics (rather than tranquillisers) in the near future as the SSRIs come off patent? In the case of the antipsychotics, an earlier generation of weakly neuroleptic antipsychotics was replaced with a generation of neuroleptics. The past 5 years, however, has seen a wholesale switch from neuroleptics back to a group of compounds that, in terms of receptor profile and efficacy, are indistinguishable from the generation of earlier antipsychotics. Neither of these switches can be justified on the basis of clinical trial evidence.

TREATMENT EFFECTS

RCTs demonstrate main effects and side effects. By convention, the main effect of antidepressants is taken to be on mood, and their effects, for example, on sexual functioning are designated as side effects. In fact, sexual functioning may be more reliably affected by an SSRI than mood. Where up to 200 patients may be needed to demonstrate a treatment effect for an SSRI in depression, as few as 12 patients may be needed to demonstrate efficacy for premature ejaculation. Evidence of the potentially beneficial effects of SSRIs on aspects of sexual functioning was kept almost entirely out of the public domain by companies for two decades. This should make it clear that the designation of a main effect of the compound is essentially an arbitrary decision, related to company economics and far from value-free (Healy & Nutt 1998).

The licensing system was put in place to constrain the claims that companies can make, not to regulate clinical practice. Increasingly, however, there has been confusion on this point and many clinicians feel that they can prescribe compounds only for their licensed indication. This confusion has come about since the 1962 amendments to the US Food and Drug Act, where the requirements for drug licensing moved from demonstrations of treatment effects to demonstrations of effects for particular disease conditions. With the restriction of drug treatments to disease states, companies have marketed medical disease models more aggressively as a means of selling compounds. This helps to further the link between the claims that a company can make regarding its compound and perceptions that clinicians may have of the appropriate use of those compounds, and it leads to an indiscriminate usage of many drugs for 'depression' on the basis that they have been demonstrated to be antidepressants. In fact, a licence is an acknowledgement that a treatment effect can be demonstrated – not that the treatment works. It can be issued even if the majority of patients to whom the drug is given in clinical trials fail to show this effect, as was the case with a number of the SSRI antidepressants.

THE MEDICALISATION OF NERVOUS PROBLEMS

The perception now is that new evaluative methods have pushed out bad medicines from the arsenal. In fact, there is every reason to suspect that RCTs are pushing good therapies out of healthcare. Psychiatric units that once had active occupational therapy units and social programmes are now reduced to boring sterile places where only things that have been 'shown to work' happen. Patients are not exercised, nor taken out on social activities, nor involved in art, music or other therapies. If they leave hospital for psychosocial reasons, it is likely to be because of boredom. One reason for this is that RCTs (as currently interpreted, allied to the patenting system) provide evidence that can be used for lobbying purposes. In contrast, other non-specific approaches will remain like placebo, undeniably but unprovably effective and as a result unsponsored.

Much of the above could be countenanced if RCTs had done something to control the *furor therapeuticus*. There is little evidence for this. In recent years there has been a mass medicalisation of a range of nervous conditions in primary care. Only time will tell how appropriate such medicalisation is. But what is clearly inappropriate is the current lack of monitoring of the therapeutic impact of intervening in these conditions. In practice, based on weak evidence of treatment effects, we have done a great deal to detect such conditions and to advocate that subjects are given treatment, but little to monitor whether treatment has in fact delivered the desired result. Because these agents have been shown by RCTs to 'work', we have promoted a situation, virtually free of warnings, where primary care prescribers and others, besieged by the mass of community nervous problems and all but impotent to do much for these, have been trapped by the weight of supposed scientific evidence into indiscriminately handing out psychotropic agents on a massive scale.

There have been moves in recent years by the Cochrane Centre and leading medical journals to encourage companies to publish all their data. The implication appears to be that if all the data are published, the field will become scientific. In fact, publication of all the data will only produce acceptable business practice in contrast to the currently unacceptable business practice: the systematic concealment of data about a new car, for example, would constitute bad business practice rather than bad science. It will take considerably more than more transparent publication practices to produce good science.

30

The marketing of psychiatric disorders

OBSESSIVE–COMPULSIVE DISORDER

The clinical trial has had another consequence. It enables the marketing of psychiatric disorders in a way that other drug development methods would not. In Chapter 10, the role of clomipramine in obsessive–compulsive disorders (OCDs) was noted. This agent was produced in the hope that by clorinating imipramine a more effective compound would be produced. Clomipramine is effective and many psychiatrists think it is among the more effective tricyclics, but it is probably also more toxic than the others are. It has more side effects, especially effects on sexual functioning. It is associated with a greater number of unexplained deaths. This faced Geigy, its manufacturer, with a marketing problem.

Studies had suggested to Geigy that clomipramine was anxiolytic. It seemed good for both phobic and obsessional disorders. However, the market for the treatment of anxious or phobic depressions was at that time being targeted by the producers of the monoamine oxidase inhibitor (MAOI) antidepressants. Clomipramine was therefore steered toward OCD. A great deal of research supports its beneficial effects in OCD (Beaumont 1996). Indeed, for a long time there was no research supporting any other treatment for obsessional states, but the fact that there was no research supporting a usefulness of other drugs for obsessional disorders does not mean that other compounds may not be useful. It is in the lack of research on other compounds that the rub lies.

There are two problems. One is that there is good reason to believe that other drugs, and in particular the antipsychotics, in sensitive doses, can be beneficial in obsessional disorders. Until clomipramine, however, no company had any incentive to develop the OCD market: there just did not seem to be enough people with the condition to warrant the development costs. All this has now changed. Until the mid-1980s, estimates of the prevalence of OCD in the general population stood at something like 0.05%; now it is thought that up to 3% of the population may have it. The recognition of the condition has gone up partly because of company encouragement based on their perception that the change in market size now warrants their interest and efforts. So what is happening here?

Following the success of clomipramine, the SSRI companies had an incentive to sell OCD in the belief that, if they increased its recognition, the sales of their compounds would follow. This, it should be noted, is not necessarily a bad thing, as it can be argued that until very recently OCD was seriously under-recognised.

The example of clomipramine and the SSRIs used in the treatment of OCD shows drug companies listening to some rather minor research, the outcomes of which suited their interest. In this and other cases they then cultivate the germinating seedling. At present, an increasing proportion of clinical research is closely tied to the marketing of compounds. As non-commercial research becomes increasingly difficult to get funded, particularly for relatively uncommon conditions such as obsessional disorders, the funding that might come from drug companies becomes ever more attractive. Where OCD was concerned, effectively from the early 1970s to the mid-1980s the only research being funded was by Ciba-Geigy – the company, in practice, was marketing OCD rather than just clomipramine.

The question of who is listening to the outcomes of research, what resources they have, and what interests they might have in promulgating the results of that research, is becoming an increasingly important one in science generally but perhaps in psychiatry in particular. For example, exposure therapy for obsessional disorders has had in comparison far fewer resources pushed its way, even though it is probably more beneficial than the SSRIs for obsessional disorders. The field must inevitably become distorted if information about SSRIs is facilitated but that about exposure therapy is not.

The development of science is popularly thought to be the result of heroic scientists working against the odds to push back the frontiers of knowledge. This is the view found in the histories written of scientific developments, which tend systematically to ignore the economic or commercial basis to scientific developments and enterprises. Nowhere is this truer than in medicine, where the idea that medicine might have associations with business is viewed with abhorrence. Those involved in health are supposed to be motivated by the loftiest of motives – how else could one face suffering humanity and live with one's conscience? Without wishing to question anyone's motives or integrity, it has to be pointed out that the evidence suggests that the reality is quite different. Not different just occasionally, but radically different – in principle.

THE MARKETING OF SOCIAL PHOBIA

Up to the mid-1960s, the MAOIs had been the most popular antidepressants. Then the 'cheese effect' was discovered. There was a dramatic slump in the sales of the MAOI antidepressants, from which they have never recovered. However, many of the clinicians who used MAOIs regularly were not prepared to accept that these drugs were not antidepressants. If they were not as effective for conventional depression, the argument was that they must be suitable for other forms of depression. Conveniently, there was a body of evidence to hand that could be used. From the start of the 1960s, there were suggestions that these antidepressants were specifically beneficial for a variety of atypical depressions, usually those with prominent anxiety features.

The concept of atypical depressions flourished during the 1970s and 1980s, even though no form of atypical depression with a specific response to MAOIs was ever substantiated. The concept should have vanished down the plughole of interesting but irrelevant concepts, but it didn't, in great part because it provided a marketing niche, seized on and used for the advertising of MAOIs.

What advertising? An increasingly large proportion of the scientific literature supplied to prescribers and other mental health professionals is supplied to them by drug companies. In many instances, this is an uncomplicated provision of information, in the form of free literature searches and other facilities. But this trend has its downside. Companies will rarely spontaneously provide information that might not be supportive of their product. In contrast, the appropriate supportive studies are rapidly forthcoming. This lends a bias to the clinical enterprise. It also leads to concepts such as atypical depression surviving when they might otherwise have vanished into oblivion (Healy 1997).

More recently there were reports that individuals with social phobia (see Ch. 10) showed a response to MAOIs. This led to efforts to develop a social phobia market to benefit moclobemide. As recently as 1990, social phobia was all but unrecognised in the UK or the USA; now there are estimates that 3% of the population may have it, with up to 10% of the population exhibiting a milder form. Social phobia is not being manufactured, but what is being supported are campaigns to make general practitioners and others aware of the latest information on this condition and to make the public aware that they may have a condition that could benefit from treatment.

Moclobemide failed to obtain a licence for social phobia, but paroxetine has done so and other companies producing SSRIs are likely to obtain licences also. Some good will be done by the increased recognition of cases of social phobia that will result from company efforts to educate clinicians. Some harm will be done by the unmonitored treatment of patients with agents that may make some of them suicidal. This will be a particular issue in the case of people who are shy rather than socially phobic and who are treated with SSRIs by mistake. The power of companies can be seen in one more small detail.

Social phobia has become social anxiety disorder, in part it seems to suit the marketing needs of SmithKline Beecham.

ALPRAZOLAM AND PANIC DISORDER

In 1964, Donald Klein suggested that within the subset of phobic/anxiety disorders there was a condition he termed panic disorder (see Klein 1996). This was a state of almost pure physical panic, without many apparently psychological features such as avoidance behaviour. He proposed that it might be an anxiety state particularly liable to respond to drug treatment. In 1980, DSM-III formally recognised the existence of panic disorder, which at this point was not a widely known entity. Today it is practically the best known neurotic disorder. People on the street will often describe any anxiety problem they have in terms of panic attacks – when most anxiety is quite different to panic attacks, which should not last longer than a minute. How did panic disorder come to be so widely known?

In the mid-1970s, Upjohn brought out a new short-acting benzodiazepine, alprazolam. This was just as the storm clouds were beginning to gather on the benzodiazepine horizon. Panic disorder was a way of appearing to avoid marketing a benzodiazepine for anxiety (Sheehan 2000). It appeared to be using a drug for the most severe form of anxiety. Upjohn funded a major research enterprise to demonstrate the efficacy of alprazolam for panic. The funding was spectacular. The research was good and participants, as should be the case in an ideal world, were given support for the presentation of their findings at a variety of meetings worldwide. The results suggested that alprazolam was better than placebo and this led to a licence for alprazolam for the treatment of panic attacks. How much better it was than placebo or other available treatments such as imipramine is another thing. Upjohn's sales boomed, in great part simply because all their efforts led to a dramatic increase in the recognition of the condition. Even the language on the streets with which we describe our nervous problems changed as a consequence of Upjohn's influence (Healy 1996).

THE MARKETING OF DEPRESSION

From these examples, it may seem that companies have been seizing upon some dubious disorders of lesser importance, but the very same process was involved with the first antidepressants. There was considerable company reluctance initially to market any antidepressants in the late 1950s as no one could see a sizeable enough market. The only people who were thought to be depressed were in mental hospitals, where electroconvulsive therapy (ECT) was the optimal treatment for them. The company that took the plunge and made the market was Merck, with amitriptyline. Merck committed itself to selling both amitriptyline and the concept of what an 'antidepressant' might treat by buying up 50 000 copies of a book by Frank Ayd (1961) on the recognition and treatment of depression in general medical settings. They made videos of how to interview depressed patients, and distributed these. In other words they sold depression. Nevertheless the recognition of depression and the use of antidepressants remained unexciting from a marketing point of view until the 1980s and the emergence of the SSRIs (Healy 1997).

This is rather startling now, when depression has become the common cold of psychiatry. But how did it become the common cold of psychiatry? In the late 1980s and early 1990s, both the Royal College of Psychiatrists in the UK and the American Psychiatric Association mounted campaigns to make professionals and the public aware that the condition is common and the diagnosis frequently missed. These campaigns depended in part on financial support from the pharmaceutical industry. There is nothing intrinsically wrong with this, but it so happened that company support was not disinterested. A new generation of drugs, the SSRIs, was about to emerge (Healy 1991b).

An interesting story lies behind the failure of buspirone to make inroads into the anxiolytic marketplace, outlined in Chapter 12. This made it clear that it would be very difficult to market a tranquilliser in the post-benzodiazepine era, largely because of concerns about the dependence potential of anxiolytics. The SSRIs could have followed down the buspirone route, but they didn't. They became antidepressants instead, even though at the time of registration as antidepressants there were no clinical trials that showed they worked in hospital patients with depression.

This developmental sequence did not happen in Japan where, as of the year 2000, there were no SSRI antidepressants on the market. Fluvoxamine was launched at the end of 1999 – as a treatment for OCD. In Japan, the antidepressant market remains the same size as the antidepressant market had been in the West up to the mid-1980s. In Japan, in contrast, the anxiolytic market remains robust. The critical difference lies in the fact that benzodiazepine dependence never became a problem in Japan.

As the SSRIs are safer in overdose than the earlier tricyclic and MAOI antidepressants, it became a feasible proposition to take the findings from social psychiatry and advise general practitioners that there are several times as many untreated depressives as was formerly thought; to educate them to recognise that patients with conditions presenting as anxiety, who had been given benzodiazepines up till then, often stemmed from an underlying depression; to reassure them that current evidence suggests that antidepressants (in contrast to anxiolytics) need to be taken chronically, in order to reduce the risk of relapse, and that this is a reasonable thing to do as the SSRIs are not dependence producing. From the beachhead of depression, then, raids could be launched on the hinterlands of anxiety. Whether or not the SSRIs are antidepressant rather than just anxiolytic is almost unimportant.

Two things may lead to a state of affairs where depression sinks back to the levels seen in the 1980s. A new generation of psychotropic agents coming through, which act on substance P, neuropeptide Y or sigma receptors, will be marketed by companies as anxiolytics rather than antidepressants – if they can. Few members of the public make any identification between the terms anxiolytic and tranquilliser. The second possibility is that SSRIs and some other psychotropics, which have gone off patent, will be sold over the counter. Should that happen, companies will market them in the way that St John's Wort is marketed: as agents for stress and burnout rather than for depression. A disease concept is only needed for marketing through prescription-only arrangements.

31

Marketing and the ethics of resource allocation

INTRODUCTION

The cost of drug treatment is ever escalating. Very often new compounds, such as the SSRIs, are no more efficacious than older agents are, even though they may cost substantially more. Increases in cost can be justified on the basis of the need to cover research, development and marketing overheads. They may also be justified in terms of the newer compounds offering better safety or quality-of-life profiles. Consequent benefits in terms of increased compliance and reductions in associated costs, such as intensive care facilities for drug overdoses, when included in the equations of a cost–benefit analysis may also reduce somewhat the discrepancy in costs. Based on a range of factors such as these, pharmacoeconomic models can make it seem as though drugs costing several hundred or several thousand pounds a year are actually cheaper than drugs costing less than £100 a year. This is largely voodoo science.

Some increase in cost provides little in the way of ethical difficulty. However, more recently a range of drugs has been developed whose costs are of an entirely different order to previous agents. So great are the increases that health workers are faced with a novel ethical problem. Use of these agents, especially in a climate of indicative budgets, may entail cutbacks in other services. It may lead to a requirement to choose between treatments or a trend to allocate treatments to some rather than to all of those who may benefit. Consider the following drugs and procedures.

CORONARY ARTERY BYPASS SURGERY

In 1964, the first coronary artery bypass operation was performed in the United States. By 1985, it was the most common elective surgery there (Halperin & Levine 1985). The procedure was introduced to relieve the pain of angina pectoris, which it certainly did in a number of instances. The increase in the number of patients undergoing surgery, however, was based on what appears to have been an implicit understanding that this operation would cure angina – a claim that has never been proven.

Despite this lack of proof, by 1985 the costs of the operation and the supportive services surrounding it were estimated at something of the order of $5 billion – a not insignificant proportion of the US healthcare budget. It seems probable that this state of affairs resulted in part from hospitals gearing up to do such operations and then finding it more cost-effective to do more of them. The acceptance of this position may in turn have depended partly on there being an ever-increasing number of surgeons whose livelihoods depended on the operation, who were as a consequence vigorous advocates of its desirability.

In short, this development probably depended to a great extent on decisions that were made intuitively, without the basis for the decisions being made explicit. In situations of limited options for healthcare, an option for the extensive provision of expensive procedures, such as coronary artery bypass surgery, must inevitably mean that other service possibilities will not be funded. It behoves us, therefore, to make explicit the basis for our treatment options.

ERYTHROPOIETIN AND INTERLEUKIN 2

A number of recently developed high-cost drugs have also reached public attention. One of these in the UK was interleukin 2, the withholding of which on the basis of cost from a patient with cancer in Christie's Hospital, Manchester, at the end of 1990, led to one of the first public outcries about failures of health services to provide a new treatment. Interleukin 2 appears, on the basis of current evidence, to improve quality of life and length of survival in patients with particular carcinomas. However, it is not life saving, and in the early 1990s it was costing in the region of £2500 per patient per year.

There have been similar debates within hospital settings regarding other compounds such as β-interferon for multiple sclerosis. Another of these is erythropoietin (Recormon), an analogue of naturally occurring erythropoietin, which when given to patients with chronic renal failure appears to be quite clearly life enhancing. Its use poses problems. We appear to feel obliged to commit large amounts of money to keep patients with kidney failure alive with renal dialysis and transplantation programmes, even though the quality of life available is often poor. Recormon can significantly enhance that quality of life but yet it is likely to be withheld in many instances on the basis of its cost, which is in the region of £4–6000 per year.

TISSUE PLASMINOGEN ACTIVATOR

In contrast to Recormon, tissue plasminogen activator (tPA) is a genetically engineered compound, which has been prescribed extensively in the USA for fibrinolysis following an acute heart attack, in preference to an alternative, streptokinase, despite the fact that it costs 10 times more. It became widely used before its efficacy was looked at in some of the largest clinical trials in medical history, which compared the effects of tPA, streptokinase and anistreplase for fibrinolysis following myocardial infarction (O'Donnell 1991). The results indicate that all three agents are equivalent in fibrinolytic activity but that streptokinase is superior to tPA by virtue of being less likely to cause subsequent spontaneous cerebral haemorrhages.

Following the publication of these results in the USA, current affairs programmes, investigating why tPA should have been prescribed so widely in the United States at an increased burden to the health services of $100 million per year, suggested that its sales may have involved a triumph of marketing over research. It was suggested that the makers of tPA, Genentech, may have used questionable tactics 'to keep a competitor's drug from gaining popularity' (O'Donnell 1991, p 1260).

The significance of these compounds is that the adoption of any of them, or more problematically a number of them, would seriously compromise funding in other areas of healthcare. The differences in benefit obtained from use of each of these compounds point to the fact that not all new and costly developments are necessarily equivalently good (Brody 1995). In the case of the above drugs, none is a breakthrough on the scale that penicillin or chlorpromazine was. Erythropoietin is life enhancing and possibly should be funded, but the case of tPA is of dubious benefit.

CLOZAPINE

Psychiatry is not immune to such issues. Indeed, perhaps the most interesting resource allocation issues surround clozapine (Healy 1993a). This drug was launched in the UK in January 1990. It costs over £2000 per annum in the UK and up to $9000 per annum in the USA. An unspecified proportion of this cost stems from blood tests that must be taken weekly for 18 weeks after the institution of treatment and fortnightly thereafter because of a risk of reduced white cell counts (agranulocytosis). A large part of the cost, however, has arisen from the company attempting to profit from the compound.

Clozapine was introduced with claims that it was a breakthrough in the treatment of schizophrenia – the first significant advance in the pharmacological management of schizophrenia for more than 20 years. Claims such as these inevitably led to pressure on healthworkers from families with schizophrenic members, concerned to get the best possible treatment for their relative and who did not see why they should be denied the benefits of any significant medical breakthrough on the basis of cost.

However, the overall picture in the case of clozapine is ambiguous. Clozapine is not a new drug. It was first manufactured in 1958. Promising clinical trials during the 1970s were aborted, when a number of deaths occurred as a consequence of agranulocytosis in Finland and malignant hyperthermia in Japan. Interest in re-introducing it grew, however, not because it was better than other agents – in standard clinical trials it was equivalent to other agents – but because it did not cause tardive dyskinesia, which had become a huge legal problem in the USA (Healy 2001a).

Clozapine was repackaged as a treatment for resistant schizophrenia. This led to a trial in which patients were recruited who were initially refractory to treatment and who were subsequently resistant to a 6-week course of haloperidol 60 mg daily. Subjects were then randomised to treatment with either clozapine or chlorpromazine in doses of up to 1800 mg per day. Of those on clozapine, 30% responded, whereas only 4% of those taking chlorpromazine subsequently responded.

As pointed out in Chapter 1, current evidence suggests that antipsychotic regimens higher than the equivalent of chlorpromazine 400–600 mg a day or haloperidol 30–40 mg per day are associated with significantly worse outcomes. One implication of these findings, therefore, is that higher doses of conventional antipsychotics had produced treatment resistance in susceptible individuals. There is also evidence that there are a number of individuals who are susceptible to developing akathisia, nervousness, dysphoria and tension, even on low doses of antipsychotics. These individuals appear to have a poorer outcome than those not experiencing such symptoms (Healy 1993a).

It is quite possible that the clozapine trial design helped to select a group of subjects who would show a poor response to conventional dopamine D_2 blockade. If this is the case, it is hardly surprisingly that such subjects should show a better response to clozapine, by virtue of its inability to bind to D_2 receptors to the same extent. One of the morals of the story, perhaps, is that there are treatment-resistant patients who could profitably be tried out on a drug-free regimen, or on minimal doses, or perhaps on psychostimulants. This rarely, if ever, happens, however.

In the face of the costs of clozapine, a number of hospitals in the USA and the UK have attempted to draw up guidelines to limit the number of people who can be prescribed clozapine at any one time and to delineate the period of time that should be considered a reasonable trial period, after which a failure to respond would lead to a discontinuation of treatment. For the first time, there was a perceived need to allocate resources between treatment options and within patient populations. Mental health professionals were being called upon to act as gatekeepers for society's resources – asked to balance their duty to individual patients against a duty to society.

It may be a historical accident that clozapine came to be seen as effective as it is. Had haloperidol been banned at one point and later reintroduced, it would have been particularly effective in populations unresponsive to clozapine and hailed as a breakthrough. But whether a historical accident or not, clozapine has achieved the reputation of being more effective than other second-generation agents that have followed in its wake. Despite this, its price has influenced the cost of these new agents. It set the going rate. Olanzapine, in particular, comes in at £3000 per annum for the 20 mg that is regularly prescribed. This is despite the fact that it can cause tardive dyskinesia, causes dramatic weight gain and possibly diabetes. There is little reason to believe that it marks any improvement over chlorpromazine or other agents of this generation of compounds.

Compared with clozapine, the SSRIs priced at £300 per annum seem relatively inexpensive. The problem here lies with the potential size of the market. A few years ago the annual bill for all psychotropic drugs (excluding clozapine) for a 50-bed district general hospital unit was of the order of £20 000 (Johnstone et al 1995). This has now greatly escalated, but the profits for companies and the cost to the health service still come from treatment in the community. If 5–10% of the population could be diagnosed as having depression and all were to take SSRIs, the bill would be astronomical. Quite apart from the monies involved, there is a further issue here: it is by no means clear that the mass treatment of general practice depression with antidepressants of any sort, old or new, expensive or not, would do much for the health of the population.

OUTFLANKING PSYCHIATRISTS

The 1960s saw the development of antipsychiatry. Psychiatrists who advocated physical treatments were faced with patient groups, such as MIND, and other mental health professionals who resisted them and their treatments. Currently, however, any psychiatrist not advocating the latest physical treatment is likely to be pilloried by patient groups. The pharmaceutical industry has recognised that patient groups can be among the most effective lobbyists for a new treatment, and it has penetrated established patient groups and set up or helped to fund new patient groups where these did not exist previously. These include the group Childhood Hyperactivity and Attention Deficit Disorder (CHADD) for attention-deficit hyperactivity disorder (ADHD), as well as groups for obsessive–compulsive disorder, social phobia and depression groups.

Industry personnel are sent to meetings on how to establish patient groups, how to work with such groups, how to place information on the internet, and how to use public relations agencies effectively. Public relations agencies work on placing articles in newspapers. Patient groups lobby members of parliament. In all cases, the mantra of why should we be denied the latest most effective treatments on the basis of cost is hugely effective.

Mental health teams are also courted. Where once it was only consultant staff who were taken out to meals or to conferences in exotic locations, it is now common practice for meals to be put on for mental health teams in the belief that community psychiatric nurses will have influence with general practitioners and consultants. The best drugs do not win the day. The ones that win are the ones produced by companies that can put sales representatives on the ground to meet doctors and others. The bottom line is marketing, and the best marketing is done through 'friendship'.

32

Nemesis or nirvana?

PERCEPTIONS OF PROGRESS IN PSYCHIATRY

The ethical pharmaceutical industry developed in the early years of the twentieth century. These and subsequent decades were a time of remarkable improvement in the health of people in the industrial democracies. The infant mortality rate fell, life expectancy increased and a number of scourges, such as tuberculosis and diphtheria, were largely eradicated. To a large extent technological developments in medicine – and perhaps pharmaceutical developments in particular – have been credited in the popular mind with bringing about these improvements.

The reality, as Thomas McKeown (1979) has demonstrated, was more complex. The drop in mortality rate from a variety of infectious diseases antedated the development of antibiotics, vaccines or any specific drug therapies. It resulted in the main from improved nutrition, the alleviation of overcrowding and public works programmes such as the provision of better sanitation. The increasing development of 'high tech' medicine, which has grown more spectacular with every decade since the Second World War, has done little to extend the basic improvements in healthcare brought about at the turn of the twentieth century.

Public perceptions of progress in psychiatry are the same as perceptions for other medical developments. The introduction of antipsychotics and antidepressants is credited with bringing about our current programme of emptying and closing large mental hospitals, by enabling the treatment of psychological disorders in the community. The reality is more complex. The closure of the large hospitals owes a great deal to administrative changes. Until the early 1950s many of the large asylums followed a policy of lumping patients together in wards regardless of diagnosis (Browne & Healy 1992, Valenstein 1986). A great deal was done by separating the mentally ill from the mentally handicapped, older subjects from younger individuals, chronic patients from those with acute disturbances, and the milder problems from the more severe ones. This led to the development of a wider range of treatment strategies for specific problems and a change in morale within the psychiatric services, to which the advent of chlorpromazine contributed (Healy 2001a).

What else of a non-specific or 'low tech' nature can be done or needs to be done now? There is a range of issues. Among the most important are the questions of child abuse – both sexual and physical abuse, but also mental torture and psychological cruelty – as well as domestic violence (Healy 1993b, McGhee & Wolfe 1991). It increasingly appears that programmes aimed at prevention of such abuses would lead to a reduction in morbidity in later life.

The process of randomised placebo-controlled trials that has been used to show that specific high-tech approaches work for certain conditions also reveals that non-specific treatments work. In trials of antidepressants, where 50% respond to the antidepressant, up to 40% respond to a placebo. What this means in practice is that, unlike the treatment of infection with an antibiotic, when it comes to the treatment of nervous conditions neither the antipsychotics or antidepressants are so specific that they will knock out the 'psychic infection' that an individual has regardless of the circumstances in which treatment is given. The rapport that patients have with those looking after them plays a big part in the likelihood of response to treatment and in the quality of that response.

Bamboozled by the evidence that antidepressants can be shown to add something over and above the benefits that can be got from a good-quality therapeutic relationship, we are at risk of forgetting that without the bedrock of a good-quality relationship they may not work at all. The psychotropic drugs should have made psychopharmacotherapy possible; the risk is that they will result in the staffing of the mental health service with psychopharmacological technicians. Physicians will become prescribers, who are increasingly insensitive to the dynamics of the relationships in which prescribing takes place.

Other non-specific developments that might be as therapeutic, if not more so, than the specific benefits of drug treatment include the provision of detailed information regarding drug therapies to those who take psychotropic medicines. As this book illustrates, the harmful effects of such drugs on a person's life may entirely outweigh any benefits they may confer. The trend toward providing such information, as well as moves to allow individuals access to their case notes, appear to be part of the Zeitgeist. Intuitively it would seem that enabling individuals to take control of their own lives in this way and to make their own decisions would be a good thing. There is considerable philosophical justification for such a position (Bursztajn et al 1980). However, this trend runs counter to the prevailing mechanical models in medicine – models that often underpin current drug company research and business programmes. It remains to be seen what the outcome of this potential clash will be.

IN THE BALANCE

The eating disorders appeared within psychiatry in the 1870s. Since then they have increased markedly in frequency, first in the 1920s and subsequently in the 1960s, when new variants such as bulimia nervosa emerged. These increases have given rise to a great number of theories aimed at accounting both for the nature of the eating disorder syndromes and for the reasons for their increase. These theories have for the most part involved almost exclusively biological, psychological or sociocultural views.

A biological perspective emerged early in the century with work on endocrine input to syndromes involving anorexia. There was a return of biological thinking in the late 1980s, when all of psychiatry went biological, with a number of groups demonstrating that dieting can produce neuro-biological changes, raising the possibility that the process could become self-sustaining.

This biological turn provided a serious challenge to the views that had become dominant during the 1950s and 1960s, which were psychodynamic. From this viewpoint, anorexia nervosa was seen as evidence of a rejection of a pregnancy wish, or as involving oral sadistic wishes and a reaction formation against incorporation wishes, or as stemming from conflicts within the family between daughter and mother. These psychodynamic views got the standard 1990s update when a possible contribution from child sexual abuse was noted.

The emergence of bulimia nervosa and the explosion in the frequency of the eating disorders during the 1960s and 1970s focused attention away from intrapsychic theories and oriented them toward a larger social and cultural picture. The argument went that sociocultural factors shaped the syndrome. Such formulations focused attention on the role of women in Western societies, as for the better part of the twentieth century the eating disorders appeared to be confined largely to Western societies. This perception gave rise to arguments that the eating disorders reveal a form of contemporary control over the female body. These perceptions had fed directly into the powerful feminist movement of the latter part of the century.

This brief overview of theories on the eating disorders suggests that a number of influences play a part in the generation of these syndromes. Fashion, pressures on women, whether overt or internalised, or what used to be termed neurotic difficulties, as well as biological factors triggered by an initial fasting, may all play a part in establishing and shaping the syndrome. The above theories, however, have generally been mutually exclusive. In addition, it is not clear that any one theory can explain the epidemiology of the disorder, its appearance in certain cultures at certain points in time and its later transformation into syndromal variants. Nor is it clear that any one theory provides a unique factor that can stabilise syndromal presentations.

All theories to date, however, have neglected a development that occurred in parallel with the eating disorders. The first weighing scales began to appear in the 1870s. Their use in medical and other settings led to data that persuaded the insurance industry for the first time that obesity, which had formerly been seen as a sign of health, was actually a risk factor for future ill-health. This led to increasing campaigns by insurers along with physicians to extol the virtues of thinness. It led to the establishment of norms for body weight and shape – one more set of norms to sit alongside the many different sets of norms that were emerging in the West at this time. The weighing scales also made it possible to know exactly whether a regimen aimed at increasing or reducing weight was having the desired effect.

The 1920s saw the emergence of the first weighing scales that could be bought and placed in the home. These became a regular feature in chemist shops or other retailers. In the 1960s small portable weighing scales appeared, which could be placed discretely in the bathroom. It became possible for most houses to have such a scale. The growth in the weighing scale industry, in fact, parallels the growth in the frequency of anorexia nervosa. The weighing scale factor also neatly accounts for the apparent cultural distribution of the syndrome such that it appears first in Western settings and subsequently migrates to non-Western settings, being found first of all amongst the wealthier classes. It also helps to explain why immigrants to Western cultures should develop the syndrome so rapidly. However, the really important aspect to the story is that, notwithstanding the fact that eating disorders may occur even in the blind, it is all but impossible to see how such disorders could mushroom to affect up to 30% of the healthy population in the absence of weighing scales.

The eating disorder story points to the role of norms and our responses to them, as a new factor in human behaviour. It provides a dramatic metaphor for the problems of maintaining equilibrium once we establish a set of norms and step on the balance. It illustrates how feedback from one area of our lives, which offers seductive possibilities of control, can become also imperious and how subjects may lose the ability to contextualise these inputs into the rest of their lives. Figures from one area of our life can trump impressions from other areas of life and make it very difficult to maintain a wise balance among our competing priorities.

Something similar seems to be happening at present with the data from clinical trials. Rather than simply indicating that this treatment has an effect, these data seem to trump all else so that we sign up to new pharmacotherapies on the basis of these figures, despite the visible degradation in the social environment of our treatment facilities that is occurring apace. The only psychosocial reason that is likely to lead to a patient leaving hospital now is boredom. We need a means to rediscover wisdom (Healy 2001a).

Something like this may underpin that increasing use of SSRIs and stimulants for children. Companies do not market to children. But, as checklists of various sorts are increasingly used in all areas of our lives, parents become aware of how their children may differ from the norm on some item of a checklist and worry about the risk this poses for their child's future development. They and their clinicians mistakenly believe that the results from trials on SSRIs or stimulants will generalise readily outside the trial situation, and they seek help to minimise the risks they perceive. Inadequate and poorly understood sets of figures seem to offer a route to salvation and very few people seem to meet health professionals these days who can persuade them otherwise.

LIFESTYLES OR DISEASES?

The emergence of Viagra since the last edition of this book is significant for many reasons. The obvious one is that it marks a point where it became possible to discuss sexual issues and treatments more openly. But of longer-term significance, perhaps, was that this was a point where company executives began to talk openly about lifestyle agents rather than treatments for a disease.

It was not the focus on sex that led to talk about lifestyles. What was different about Viagra that enabled executives to begin to talk about lifestyles was the reliability of the responses it produced. Nine or 9.9 times out of 10, it produced the desired effect. This was in contrast to the antidepressants, for instance, which produce the desired response only about 5 times out of 10 at best.

Unlike the antidepressants, Viagra produced quality outcomes. For anyone working in healthcare, quality until recently meant a situation in which the relationship between professional and patient was warm, understanding and intuitive. But this is not what the word means industrially. From the point of view of pharmaceutical companies, quality refers to reliability. Big Mac hamburgers are quality hamburgers in this sense: they are the same every time. What companies want are drugs that will equally reliable. And once drugs become this reliable, it becomes possible to jettison talk about diseases and replace it with talk about lifestyles.

Are we about to produce a whole new generation of antidepressants or anxiolytics that are so much more reliable soon? No. There will be no great change in the drugs we have, but what will happen is that the use of neuroimaging to see whether drugs are working or not and pharmacogenetic testing to check for adverse effects before treatment will make the next generation of drugs much more reliable. At this point, it will become possible for psychopharmacology to follow the path plastic surgery took as it evolved into cosmetic surgery. Plastic surgery began as a set of very unreliable procedures to repair the injuries inflicted by war. As it became more reliable, however, it burst out of the constraints of medicine to become cosmetic surgery (Haikan 1998). A somewhat similar fate may await psychopharmacology and all of us.[a] As techniques become more reliable there will be increasing pressure to develop a less medically and more lifestyle oriented psychopharmacology – a cosmetic psychopharmacology.

---

[a] The argument outlined here was put forward in the leading American bioethical journal (Healy 2000), published by the Hastings Center. It turned out that Lilly was a major funder of the Hastings Center and, following this issue of the journal, withdrew its funding.

References

Ayd FJ (1961) Recognition and treatment of the depressed patient. New York: Grune & Stratton.

Beaumont G (1996) The place of clomipramine in psychopharmacology. In: Healy D, ed. The psychopharmacologists, vol 1, pp 309–328. London: Arnold.

Brody BA (1995) Ethical issues in drug testing, approval, and pricing. New York: Oxford University Press.

Browne I, Healy D (1992) In conversation with Ivor Browne. Psychiatric Bulletin 16: 1–9.

Bursztajn HJ, Feinbloom RI, Hamm RM, Brodsky A (1980) Medical choices, medical chances; how patients, families and physicians can cope with uncertainty. London: Routledge.

Freemantle N, Mason J, Phillips T, Anderson IM (2000) Predictive value of pharmacological activity for the relative efficacy of antidepressants drugs. Meta-regression analysis. British Journal of Psychiatry 177: 292–302.

Gilbody SM, Song F (2000) Publication bias and the integrity of psychiatry research. Psychological Medicine 30: 253–258.

Haikan E (1998) Venus envy. A history of cosmetic surgery. Baltimore, MD: Johns Hopkins University Press.

Halperin J, Levine R (1985) Bypass. New York: Times Books.

Healy D (1991a) The ethics of psychopharmacology. Changes 9: 234–247.

Healy D (1991b) The marketing of 5HT: depression or anxiety. British Journal of Psychiatry 158: 737–742.

Healy D (1993a) Psychopharmacology and the ethics of resource allocation. British Journal of Psychiatry 162: 23–29.

Healy D (1993b) Images of trauma. London: Faber & Faber.

Healy D (1996) Psychopharmacology in the new medical state. In: Healy D, Doogan DP, eds. Psychotropic drug development, pp 13–40. London: Chapman & Hall.

Healy D (1997) The antidepressant era. Cambridge, MA: Harvard University Press.

Healy D (2000) Good science or good business? Hastings Center Report 30: 19–23.

Healy D (2001a) The creation of psychopharmacology. Cambridge, MA: Harvard University Press.

Healy D (2001b) The dilemmas posed by new and fashionable treatments. Advances in Psychiatric Treatment (in press).

Healy D, Nutt D (1998) Prescriptions, licenses and evidence. Psychiatric Bulletin 22: 680–684.

Healy D, Savage M, Michael P et al (2001) Psychiatric bed utilisation: 1896 and 1996 compared. Psychological Medicine 31: 779–790.

Huston D, Locher M (1996) Redundancy, disaggregation and the integrity of medical research. Lancet 347: 1024–1026.

Johnstone F, Rickard I, Healy D (1995) The costs of psychotropic medication. British Journal of Psychiatry 167: 112–113.

Klein DF (1996) Reaction patterns to psychotropic drugs and the discovery of panic disorder. In: Healy D, ed. The psychopharmacologists, vol 1, pp 329–352. London: Arnold.

Liebenau J (1987) Medical Science and Medical Industry. Basingstoke, UK: Macmillan.

McGhee RA, Wolfe DA (1991) Psychological maltreatment: toward an operational definition. Developmental Psychopathology 3: 3–18.

McKeown T (1979) The role of medicine. Oxford: Basil Blackwell.

Marsh P (1989) Prescribing all the way to the bank. New Scientist 18 November: 50–55.

Melville A, Johnson C (1982) Cured to death. Sevenoaks, UK: New English Library.

O'Donnell M (1991) Battle of the clotbusters. British Medical Journal 302: 1259–1261.

Pellegrino E (1979) The sociocultural impact of twentieth century therapeutics. In: Vogel MJ, Rosenberg CE, eds. The therapeutic revolution, pp 245–266. Philadelphia, PA: University of Pennsylvania Press.

Rawlins MD (1990) Development of a rational practice of therapeutics. British Medical Journal 301: 729–733.

Rennie D (1999) Fair conduct and fair reporting of clinical trials. Journal of the American Medical Association 282: 1766–1768.

Sheehan D (2000) Angles on panic. In: Healy D, ed. The psychopharmacologists, vol 3, pp 479–504. London: Arnold.

Sneader W (1990) The prehistory of psychotherapeutic agents. Journal of Psychopharmacology 4: 115–119.

Valenstein ES (1986) Great and desperate cures. New York: Basic Books.

Vogel MJ, Rosenberg CE, eds (1979) The therapeutic revolution. Philadelphia, PA: University of Pennsylvania Press.

Further reading

Ayd FJ (1995) Lexicon of psychiatry, neurology and the neurosciences. Baltimore, MD: Williams & Wilkins.

Baldessarini RJ, Cohen BM, Teicher MH (1988) Significance of antipsychotic doses and plasma levels in the pharmacological management of the psychoses. Archives of General Psychiatry 45: 79–91.

Cunningham-Owens DG (1999) A guide to the extrapyramidal side-effects of antipsychotic drugs. Cambridge: Cambridge University Press.

Dukes MNG, Swartz B (1988) Responsibility for drug-induced injury. Amsterdam: Elsevier.

Espie C (1991) The psychological treatment of insomnia. Chichester, UK: John Wiley.

Fink M (2000) Electroshock: restoring the brain. New York: Oxford University Press.

Gilbert PL, Harris J, McAdams LA, Jeste DV (1995) Antipsychotic withdrawal in schizophrenic patients: a review of the literature. Archives of General Psychiatry 52: 173–188.

Glenmullen J (2000) Prozac backlash. New York: Simon & Schuster.

Haikan E (1998) Venus envy. A history of cosmetic surgery. Baltimore, MD: Johns Hopkins University Press.

Healy D (1996, 1998, 2000) The psychopharmacologists, vols 1–3. London: Arnold.

Healy D (1997) The antidepressant era. Cambridge, MA: Harvard University Press.

Healy D (2001) The creation of psychopharmacology. Cambridge, MA: Harvard University Press.

Healy D, Nutt D (1997) British Association for Psychopharmacology consensus on childhood and learning disabilities psychopharmacology. Journal of Psychopharmacology 11: 291–294.

Healy D, Tranter R (1999) Pharmacopsychiatric stress syndromes. With commentaries by Ashton H, Baldessarini R, Haddad P and by Anderson I, Hollister L, Tyrer P. Journal of Psychopharmacology 13: 287–290.

Klerman GL (1990) The psychiatric patient's right to effective treatment: implications of Osheroff vs Chestnut Lodge. American Journal of Psychiatry 147: 409–418.

May PR, Van Putten T, Yale C et al (1976) Predicting individual responses to drug treatment in schizophrenia. Journal of Nervous and Mental Diseases 162: 177–183.

Melville A, Johnson C (1982) Cured to death. Sevenoaks, UK: New English Library.

Stone AA (1990) Law, science and psychiatric malpractice: a response to Klerman's indictment of psychoanalytic psychiatry. American Journal of Psychiatry 147: 419–427.

Tranter R, Healy D (1998) Neuroleptic discontinuation syndromes. Journal of Psychopharmacology 12: 306–311.

Waterhouse JM, Minors DS, Waterhouse ME (1990) Your body clock: how to live with it, not against it. Oxford: Oxford University Press.

Appendix:
Mental health websites

www.depression.org

National Foundation for Depressive Illness, Inc.
PO Box 2257
New York
NY 10116
Tel: 1800 239 1265

www.nsf.org.uk

National Schizophrenia Foundation
30 Tabernacle Street
London EC2A 4DD
Tel: 020 7330 9100/01
National Advice Service: 020 8974 6814; advice@nsf.org.uk

www.mind.org.uk

MIND – The Mental Health Charity
15–19 Broadway
London E15 4BQ
Tel: 020 8522 1728

www.mindinfo.co.uk

Mental Health Information & Links

hounslowcmht@88lampton.freeserve.co.uk

Hounslow Community Mental Health Team
88 Lampton Road
Hounslow
Middlesex TW3 4DW
Tel: 020 8583 3496

www.ndmda.org

National Depressive and Manic Depressive Associations
730 N.Franklin #501
Chicago
IL 60610
USA
Tel: 001 312 642 0049

www.mentalhelp.net
Mental Help Net
570 Metro Place North
Dublin
OH 43017
USA
Tel: 001 614 764 0143

www.thewindsofchange.org
The Winds of Change
7301 Alma Drive
Plano
TX 75025
USA
Tel: 001 972 528 2811

www.depressionalliance.org
Depression Alliance
35 Westminster Bridge Road
London SE1 7JB
Tel: 020 7633 0557

www.phobics-society.org.uk
National Phobics Society
Zion Community Resource Centre
339 Stretford Road
Hulme
Manchester M15 4ZY
Tel: 08707 700 456

www.social-anxiety.org
No contact details available

www.mdf.org.uk
Manic Depression Fellowship
Castle Works
21 St George's Road
London SE1 6ES
Tel: 020 7793 2600

www.sane.org.uk
SANE
1st Floor
Cityside House
40 Adler Street
London E1 1EE
Tel: 020 7375 1002

www.aware.ie

Aware
72 Lower Leeson Street
Dublin 2
Ireland
Tel: 01 661 7211

www.mentalhealth-jami.org.uk

The Jewish Association for the Mentally Ill
16A North End Road
London NW11 7PH
Tel: 020 8458 2223

www.healingwell.com

Location: Waltham, MA, USA
Fax: 801 912 1553

Index